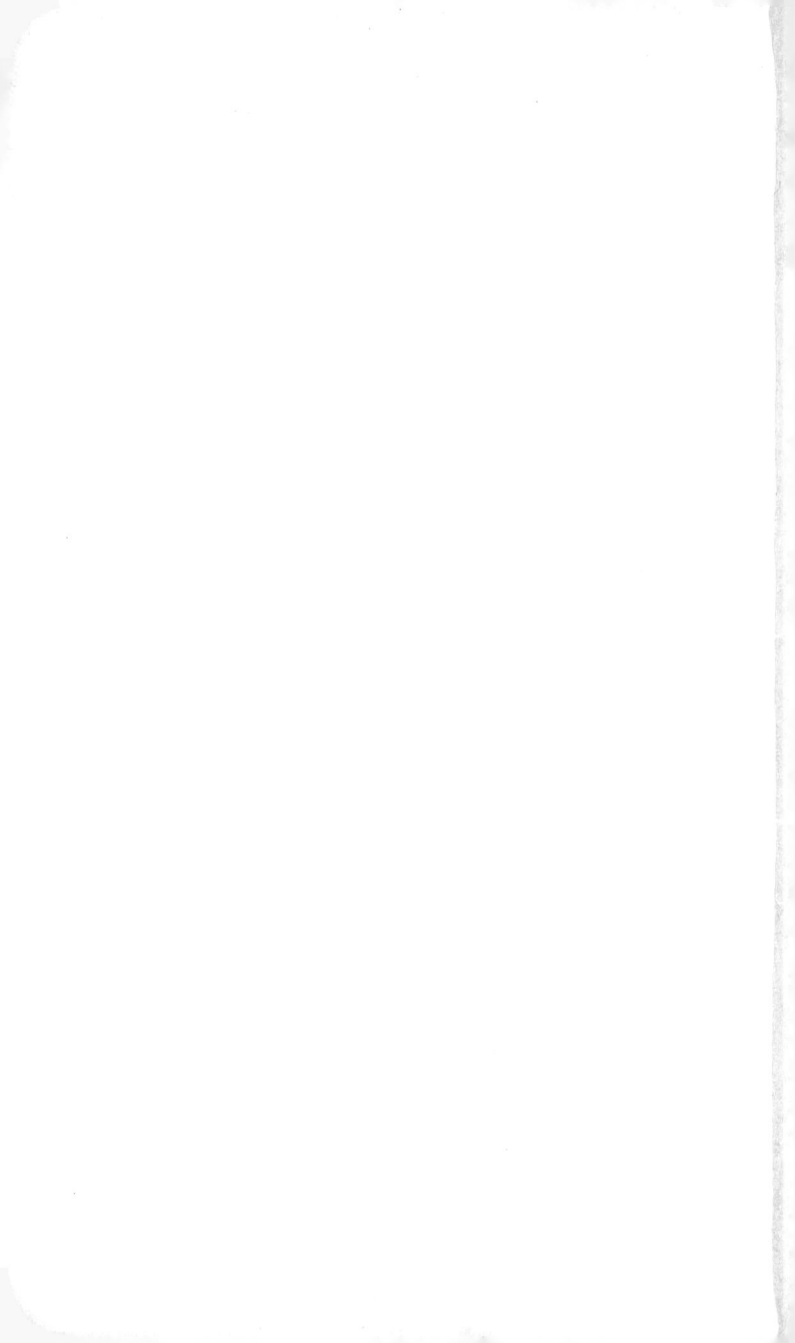

Gastroenterology and Hepatology Manual

Professor Segal

*To my wife Arlene for her unstinting devotion and
to my dear children Rosh, Perry, Hadass and their families
for their continuing understanding and support.*

Professor Pitchumoni

To my wife Prema Pitchumoni and to all my students

Professor Sung

To members of the GI team at Prince of Wales Hospital

Gastroenterology and Hepatology Manual

A Clinician's Guide to a Global Phenomenon

Isidor Segal
C.S. Pitchumoni
Joseph Sung

The McGraw·Hill Companies

Sydney New York San Francisco Auckland
Bangkok Bogotá Caracas Hong Kong
Kuala Lumpur Lisbon London Madrid
Mexico City Milan New Delhi San Juan
Seoul Singapore Taipei Toronto

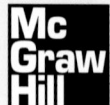

Notice

Medicine is an ever-changing science. As new research and clinical experience broaden our knowledge, changes in treatment and drug therapy are required. The editors and the publisher of this work have checked with sources believed to be reliable in their efforts to provide information that is complete and generally in accord with the standards accepted at the time of publication. However, in view of the possibility of human error or changes in medical sciences, neither the editors, nor the publisher, nor any other party who has been involved in the preparation or publication of this work warrants that the information contained herein is in every respect accurate or complete. Readers are encouraged to confirm the information contained herein with other sources. For example, and in particular, readers are advised to check the product information sheet included in the package of each drug they plan to administer to be certain that the information contained in this book is accurate and that changes have not been made in the recommended dose or in the contraindications for administration. This recommendation is of particular importance in connection with new or infrequently used drugs.

First published 2011

Text © 2011 McGraw-Hill Australia Pty Ltd
Illustrations and design © 2011 McGraw-Hill Australia Pty Ltd
Additional owners of copyright are acknowledged in on-page credits.

Every effort has been made to trace and acknowledge copyrighted material. The authors and publishers tender their apologies should any infringement have occurred.

National Library of Australia Cataloguing-in-Publication Data

Author: Segal, Isidor.
Title: Gastroenterology and hepatology manual : a clinician's
        guide to a global phenomenon / Isidor Segal, C.S. Pitchumoni, Joseph Sung.
ISBN: 9780070285576 (pbk.)
Notes: Includes index.
Subjects: Gastroenterology--Handbooks, manuals, etc.
Other Authors/Contributors: Pitchumoni, C.S., Sung, Joseph.
Dewey Number: 616.33

Published in Australia by
McGraw-Hill Australia Pty Ltd
Level 2, 82 Waterloo Road, North Ryde NSW 2113

Acquisitions editor: Elizabeth Walton
Associate editor: Fiona Richardson
Art direction and cover design: Astred Hicks
Internal design: Peta Nugent
Senior production editor: Yani Silvana
Permissions editor: Haidi Bernhardt
Copy editor: Ross Blackwood
Proofreader: Anne Savage
Indexer: Russell Brooks
Typeset in Zapf Humanist 601 BT, 8/10.5 by Mukesh Technologies, India
Printed in China on 80gsm matt art by iBook Printing Ltd

Foreword

Rapid globalisation is affecting all aspects of life, and the practice of medicine is no exception. *Gastroenterology and Hepatology: a Clinician's Guide to a Global Phenomenon* is a thoughtful attempt to address the issues related to the teaching and clinical practice of gastroenterology and hepatology in the current climate. The book is creatively organised and the chapters have been written by a team of international experts in the field.

Gastroenterology and Hepatology contains carefully selected topics that are of particular importance to the practice of gastroenterology and hepatology throughout the world. Chapter 1, for example, provides a scholarly, coherent discussion of the underlying factors that are propelling the development of diseases that are similar worldwide, and of the evolution from regional to global medicine, particularly in the field of gastroenterology and hepatology.

The popularity of international travel has resulted in travellers being exposed to new gastrointestinal and liver disorders that are not present in their homelands. The chapters devoted to international travel medicine provide useful information on the diagnosis and management of gastrointestinal and liver disorders both for travellers from different parts of the world to a common destination and for travellers from one region to varied regions.

The editors have cleverly divided clinical gastrointestinal and liver disorders into groups, such as diseases that are common in West but seem to spreading to the East, diseases that are common in emerging countries and spreading globally, and diseases that represent the melting pot. Other chapters discuss diseases—including gastrointestinal and liver cancers—that have different epidemiology, pathophysiology and clinical behaviour in different parts of the world.

Chapters discussing gastrointestinal and hepatic disorders of global importance include: one on the differences in the diagnostic tools that are used by practitioners for diagnosis and management of the same disorders in different parts of the globe; chapters dealing with important liver disorders of international interest because of the diversity of their epidemiology and clinical presentation; and chapters on biliary and pancreatic disorders that discuss global diversity in epidemiology, aetiology, clinical manifestations and management of these disorders.

Finally, the book includes a chapter on Chinese traditional medicine and another on Indian traditional medicine, both focused on gastrointestinal and liver diseases. Throughout the world, the vast majority of these diseases are being treated with alternatives to conventional medicine practised in the West. Moreover, many of the practitioners of alternative forms of medicine are now also formally trained in Western medicine. This understanding of different types of therapies will no doubt be beneficial for patients.

This unique compilation, written by talented, scholarly contributors with expertise in international medicine, is a pioneering work in global gastroenterology and hepatology. Students and practitioners who care for patients in the global environment will find this book very useful.

Raj K. Goyal, MD
Mallinckrodt Professor of Medicine
Harvard Medical School
VA Boston Health Care
Boston, Massachusetts 02132

Contents

About the editors

Isidor Segal FRACP, FRCP (UK), AGAF, Master World Gastroenterology Organisation (WGO)

Professor Segal established the African Institute of Digestive Diseases in 1999. The model of this institute has been used by the WGO to establish 13 training centres in countries such as Morocco, Pakistan, Bangkok, Egypt, Chile, Bolivia and Argentina.

Professor Segal has held many positions in the WGO, including: member of the Education and Training Committee and Vice Chairman African and Middle East Zone. He has published more than 200 papers and has recently co-edited two books and is a visiting lecturer at universities around the world. He is currently working in the Gastroenterology Division at Prince of Wales Hospital, Sydney.

C.S. Pitchumoni MD, MACP, MACG, AGAF, MPH

Professor Pitchumoni is the Adjunct Professor of Medicine at New York Medical College, Clinical Professor of Medicine at both Robert Wood Johnson School of Medicine at New Brunswick, New Jersey, and at Drexel University in Philadelphia, USA. Currently he is also Chief of Gastroenterology, Hepatology and Clinical Nutrition at Saint Peter's University Hospital in New Brunswick.

Professor Pitchumoni has more than 40 years of teaching and research experience as a clinical gastroenterologist.

Joseph Sung MD, PhD

Professor Sung is the President of the Chinese University of Hong Kong (CUHK) and Mok Hing Yiu Professor of Medicine. Before this appointment, he was Director of the Institute of Digestive Disease, Chairman of the Department of Medicine and Therapeutics, and Associate Dean of Medicine at CUHK. He is a gastroenterologist with special interest in gastrointestinal bleeding, digestive cancer and hepatitis infection. He has published more than 650 full papers in scientific journals and edited or co-edited seven books.

About the contributors

M. Abdullah, Indonesia
Division of Gastroenterology, Department of Internal Medicine, Faculty of Medicine, University of Indonesia, Jakarta.

R.M. Agrawal, USA
Associate Professor of Medicine, Drexel University College of Medicine, Philadelphia.

Associate Clinical Chief, Research and Education, Division of Gastroenterology, Hepatology and Nutrition, Department of Medicine, Allegheny General Hospital, Pittsburgh.

D.V. Alcid, USA
Professor of Medicine and Pathology, University of Medicine and Dentistry, Robert Wood Johnson Medical School, New Brunswick, New Jersey.

Director, Microbiology Laboratory, St. Peter's University Hospital, New Brunswick, New Jersey.

D. Amarapurkar, India
Bombay Hospital and Medical Research Centre; Mumbai and Jagjivanram Western Railway Hospital, Mumbai.

T.L. Ang, Singapore
Department of Gastroenterology, Changi General Hospital.

R. Banerjee, India
Consultant Gastroenterologist, Asian Institute of Gastroenterology, Hyderabad, Andhra Pradesh.

Z. Bian, Hong Kong, China
School of Chinese Medicine, Hong Kong Baptist University.

M. Bilal, USA
University of Tennessee Health Science Center, Memphis.

P. Chang, Australia
Gastroenterology Division, Prince of Wales Hospital, Sydney.

J. Chaganti, Australia
Senior Lecturer in Radiology, University of New South Wales, Sydney.

Senior Consultant, Radiology, St Vincent's Hospital, Sydney.

G.M. Dusheiko, England
Professor of Medicine, Centre for Hepatology, Royal Free Hospital and University College London Medical School.

S.S. Fedail, Sudan
Consultant Physician and Gastroenterologist, Chairman, Fedail Hospital, Khartown.

K.M. Fock, Singapore
Department of Gastroenterology, Changi General Hospital.

A.Y. Garcia, Cuba
Department of Gastroenterology, National Institute of Gastroenterology, Havana.

K.L. Goh, Malaysia
Professor of Medicine, Head of Gastroenterology and Hepatology, University of Malaya, Kuala Lumpur.

E.V. Gomez, Cuba
Director of Research, National Institute of Gastroenterology, Havana.

R. Jackson, Australia
Paediatric Gastroenterologist, Prince Of Wales Private Hospital, Sydney.

S.S. Jhangiani, USA
Attending, Departments of Internal Medicine, Gastroenterology and Clinical Nutrition, Montefiore Medical Center, New York.

Assistant Professor of Medicine, New York Medical College, Valhalla, New York.

Founder and Chairman, www.NutritionVista.com.

Founder and Chairman, Doctors for a Healthier Bronx.

J.C. Joshi, India
Consulting Gastroenterologist and Hepatologist, Samvedana Clinic, Jolly Centre, Mumbai.

A. Karstaedt, South Africa
Division of Infectious Diseases, Department of Medicine, Chris Hani Baragwanath Hospital and the University of the Witwatersrand, Johannesburg.

S.R. Lin, China
Peking University Third Hospital, Peking.

S. Nair, USA
Professor of Medicine, Medical Director of Liver Transplantation, University of Tennessee Health Science Center, Memphis.

C.J. Ooi, Singapore
Head and Senior Consultant, Department of Gastroenterology and Hepatology, Director, Inflammatory Bowel Disease Centre, Singapore General Hospital.

Associate Professor, Duke-NUS Graduate Medical School.

Clinical Associate Professor, Yong Loo Lin School of Medicine, NUS.

H. Paradwala, India
Consulting Physician, Saifee Hospital and Prince Aly Khan Hospital, Mumbai.

N.Y. Pathak, India
Senior Research Fellow, Medical Research Centre, Kasturba Health Society, Mumbai.

C.S. Pitchumoni, USA
Clinical Professor of Medicine, Robert Wood Johnson School of Medicine, New Brunswick, New Jersey.

Chief of Gastroenterology, Hepatology and Clinical Nutrition, Saint Peter's University Hospital, New Brunswick, New Jersey.

A.A. Rani, Indonesia
Head, Division of Gastroenterology, Department of Internal Medicine, Faculty of Medicine, University of Indonesia, Jakarta.

D.N. Reddy, India
Chairman, Chief Gastroenterologist, Asian Institute of Gastroenterology, Hyderabad, Andhra Pradesh.

S. Riordan, Australia
Professor of Medicine, Head of Department of Gastroenterology and Hepatology, Prince of Wales Hospital and the University of New South Wales, Sydney.

S.K. Sarin, India
Professor and Head of Department of Hepatology, Institute of Liver and Biliary Sciences, New Delhi.

I. Segal, Australia
Gastroenterology Division, Prince of Wales Hospital, Sydney.

S. Shah, India
Previous Head of Department of Gastroenterology, Sir J.J. Hospital, and Grant Medical College Honorary Gastroenterologist at Jaslok, Saifee and Breach Candy Hospital, Mumbai.

P. Sharma, India
Assistant Professor, Department of Hepatology, Institute of Liver and Biliary Sciences, New Delhi.

O. Shrivsatav, India
Consultant, Infectious Diseases and HIV Medicine, Sir H.N. Hospital, Jaslok Hospital, Saifee Hospital, Specialty Clinics, Breach Candy Hospital, Unit Head, Kasturba Hospital for Communicable Diseases, Mumbai.

D. Singhal, India
Department of Gastroenterology and Gastrointestinal Surgery, Pushpawati Singhania Research Unit for Liver, Renal and Digestive Diseases, New Delhi.

E.A. Soler, Cuba
General Director, National Institute of Gastroenterology, Havana.

J.D. Sollano, Philippines
Professor of Medicine, University of Santo Tomas, Manilla.

J. Sung, Hong Kong, China
President of the Chinese University of Hong Kong (CUHK) and Mok Hing Yiu Professor of Medicine.

R.K. Tandon, India
Department of Gastroenterology and Gastrointestinal Surgery, Pushpawati Singhania Research Unit for Liver, Renal and Digestive Diseases, New Delhi.

S. Tejavanija, Thailand
Medical Staff, Department of Endocrinology and Clinical Nutrition, Phramongkutklao Hospital, Bangkok.

K.T. Thia, Singapore
Consultant, Gastroenterology and Hepatology, Inflammatory Bowel Disease Centre, Singapore General Hospital.

R. Toney, USA
Senior Gastroenterology Fellow, Allegheny General Hospital, Drexel University College, Division of Gastroenterology, Hepatology and Nutrition, Department of Medicine, Pittsburgh.

J. Tu, Australia
Clinical Research Fellow, Gastrointestinal and Liver unit, Prince of Wales Hospital, Sydney.

A.D.B. Vaidya, India
Research Director, ICMR Advanced Centre of Reverse Pharmacology in Traditional Medicine, Medical Research Centre, Kasturba Health Society, Mumbai.

S.W. Wong, Australia
Senior Lecturer, Colorectal Surgeon, Prince of Wales Hospital, University of New South Wales, Sydney.

J.C.Y. Wu, Hong Kong, China
Professor, Institute of Digestive Disease, Chinese University of Hong Kong.

S.D. Xiao, China
Shanghai Renji Hospital, Shanghai Jiaotong, University School of Medicine, Shanghai Institute of Digestive Diseases, Shanghai.

Acknowledgments

Gastroenterology and hepatology continue to progress at an accelerating pace. Exciting new advances in techniques, treatments, diagnostic strategies and positive research outcomes have resulted in a new world for medical practitioners.

A silent ripple has spread like a global tsunami that has made a term like 'Western diseases' obsolete. Obesity, inflammatory bowel disease, gastro-oesophageal-reflux disease, colorectal cancer and other Western diseases are now common in the burgeoning emerging populations of India, China and other Asian and Pacific rim countries.

We have been fortunate to have the commitment of internationally renowned experts from around the world to address the global presentation of these diseases in their various geographic regions. These invited contributors are at the cutting edge of both research and clinical aspects of gastroenterology and hepatology and are able to provide an unprecedented insight into the global phenomena of the diseases.

The editors are honoured by the excellence of the work of these international authors, who have been partners in a sometimes difficult process. They have generously continued to give their time and energy in order to ensure the success of the book.

We believe the book may serve to bridge current knowledge for students, trainees, medical practitioners and researchers in digestive diseases.

The format of the publication facilitates ease of access to the specific information required by users. In addition to the core text, chapters also include key points, tables, summaries and recommended reading.

The editors are enormously indebted to the dedicated team at McGraw-Hill for their guidance, patience and zest in getting the book to press. In particular we are very grateful to Fiona Richardson, who was the driving force behind the scenes and who encouraged the enthusiastic participation of the other team members. We are most grateful to Lizzy Walton, Ross Blackwood and Yani Silvana for being part of this creative team and for their professional interest in the provision of a distinctive book.

Isidor Segal, C.S. Pitchumoni and Joseph Sung

Section 1

An overview

Chapter 1: Introduction

I. Segal, C.S. Pitchumoni, J. Sung

In this century, new economic forces arising from the emergence of China and India—the two most populous countries in the world—have impacted on the epidemiology of disease and modified the way we think about diseases. The winds of change have altered geographical pathology and have globalised patterns of disease. Internecine strife, regional wars and famine have caused a flood of refugees seeking relief in safe havens from dire living conditions; ironically, many carry diseases to their new environments.

There has also been a rapid change from rural to urban environments, and intra- and intercontinental migration has exacerbated the situation. Changes in diet, alcohol consumption, physical exercise and quality of life have promoted an epidemic of obesity and diabetes, the latter condition becoming a worldwide phenomenon.

The increase in international travel and the speed with which large populations move has accelerated the transfer of pathogens, seen for example in the recent SARS and Swine Flu epidemics. Multiculturalism is now an established fact in most countries.

Many diseases previously found only in regional areas have thus been internationalised, becoming a part of the disease spectrum in other domiciles. These include viral hepatitis B and C, hepatocellular cancer and traveller's diarrhoea.

Disturbances in immunity due to the spread of AIDS and the use of new, powerful drugs have lowered immunological function and facilitated the reappearance of diseases that had been regarded as exotic, along with the reoccurrence of previously uncommon diseases such as tuberculosis in developed countries.

The major developments in technology, particularly internet access, have condensed distance and made disease information swiftly and readily available, broadening our knowledge in the identification of unusual pathogens occurring in various countries.

This book delineates the tidal effect of all these changes on gastroenterology and hepatology. We have gathered together an international array of authors who each contributes unique expertise in their field.

The book is aimed at students, interns, fellows and health care providers. It encompasses the changes outlined above, and also contains chapters devoted to clinical examination and an outline of how to approach common problems encountered at the bedside. The format and style of the book allows common clinical problems to be identified and recognised within the framework of a global perspective.

QUICK FLICK 1

Chapter 2: A global phenomenon: medicine without frontiers

I. Segal (Australia)

Key points
▶ Climate change.
▶ Urbanisation.
▶ Xenobiotics: smoking, alcohol, volatile hydrocarbons, occupational disease, exposure to low-dose ionising radiation and air pollution.
▶ Dietary changes: obesity and junk food.
▶ Exercise trends.

○ Introduction

This is perhaps the most beautiful time in human history; it is really pregnant with all kinds of creative possibilities made possible by science and technology which now constitute the slave of man—if man is not enslaved by it.
Dr Jonas Salk (1914–1995), developer of the polio vaccine.

Globalisation has shifted the course of medicine. There are no longer any sharp divisions between geographical regions in terms of the prevalence and types of disease to be found in them: it is becoming more difficult to label diseases in terms of their geographic location. Environmental, economic, technological and social changes are evolving so rapidly in the twenty-first century that a paradigm shift is needed in order to categorise diseases that previously were restricted by geographical location.

The following discussion focuses on factors contributing to these changes: climate change, urbanisation, xenobiotics, dietary changes and exercise trends.

Climate change
The dynamics of disease patterns are changing due to climate change. In many places the Earth's temperature is rising; some have predicted that the average global temperature will rise by 3 to 7 degrees by 2100.

Warming is escalating, and significant rises have occurred in recent decades. Human activities enhance the natural greenhouse effect by generating greenhouse gases that trap heat in the atmosphere. If this continues at or above the current rate, average global temperatures are predicted to continue to rise, bringing significant long-term effects for people, the environment and disease patterns.

Burning fossil fuels such as coal, natural gas and oil for powering factories, industrial plants, home environments and cars, along with continued tree-clearing for extended building development as populations increase, all exacerbate greenhouse gas problems.[1]

Health conditions are most susceptible to changes in climate, particularly in the very young, the very old or those with heart and respiratory problems. Change also affects microbial contamination pathways and transmission mechanisms such that water-borne, food-borne, rodent-borne and vector-borne diseases increase, especially malaria and diarrhoeal diseases.

If temperatures rise 2 to 3 degrees Celsius by 2030, as some predictions maintain, the risk of malaria would increase by between 3 and 5 per cent and diarrhoeal diseases would increase by 10 per cent. The latter would particularly affect children, among whom mortality and morbidity from diarrhoea is already high in some developing countries. An example of this is seen in the spread of malaria to the previously malaria-free region of the Eastern Highlands of Kenya, where warmer, wetter weather has resulted in high rates of illness and death.[2]

McMichael et al. cite the known and probable health hazards of climate variability and health change. They include temperature extremes, more daily death events and disease events due mainly to very hot days and the effects of floods, with more injuries, deaths and resultant infectious diseases, mental health disorders, increased allergic disorders and greater risk of diarrhoeal diseases, especially salmonellosis (poisoning by contaminated food).[3]

The risk of water-borne infections such as cholera may increase, and the incidence of mosquito-borne infections tends to increase with warming and changes in rainfall; similarly, tick-borne infections may increase.

Recent climate change has already contributed to altered food yields in some regions, causing changes in temperature, rainfall, soil moisture, pest activity and plant disease that have reduced food production and increased the risk of malnutrition. It is evident that swift and aggressive international action is required to deal with the situation.

Urbanisation

Asia is the most rapidly urbanising continent. Between 1970 and 1990 the world's urban population rose by 1038 million, of which Asian cities accounted for 589 million (56%). At the current rate, in China 870 million people—more than half the projected population—will be living in cities within less than a decade.[4]

In 2008 the proportion of the world's population living in urban areas crossed the 50 per cent mark. Most observers believe that essentially all population growth from now on will be in cities. The transition is happening chaotically, resulting in unorganised urban landscapes in which many of the poorest people are rapidly absorbed into urban slums. Urbanisation is a health hazard for certain vulnerable populations, and this demographic shift threatens to create a humanitarian disaster. The threat comes both in the form of rising rates of endemic disease and a greater potential for epidemics and even pandemics.

Most people who relocate to cities are in search of employment. Many find that their only option is to live in dense, unplanned, illegal settlements lacking basic public infrastructure. These slums make up an increasing proportion of some growing cities. Increased population density in urban areas that lack proper water supply and sanitation magnifies the risk of communicable diseases being transmitted. Poor urban areas readily become breeding grounds for emerging infections and potential pandemics. Although slum residents may live close to health care providers, they generally have little access to high-quality care. Fundamental public health-related services, such as a safe water supply, sanitation and oral rehydration therapy, remain important. As the world becomes increasingly urban, the health of the urban poor may suffer and the stage could be set for devastating pandemics of infectious disease.[5]

In addition to these growing problems, rapid and unplanned urbanisation has important ramifications with regard to urban pollution and health due to inadequate drainage and solid waste services, poor urban and industrial waste management, air pollution (especially from particulates) and overcrowding, as well as such factors as depletion of water and forest resources.

Asia's economic growth is expected to continue. In order to achieve sustainable development there will be an enormous need for waste disposal facilities, roads, ports, power plants, water mains, airports and communication systems. The issue of access is important and the cost of infrastructure will be trillions of dollars.

The quality of education among the marginalised poor is variable and generally of a low standard. Access to health care is also low in poorer areas with overcrowded poor-quality housing, lacking potable water and with substandard sanitation.

In sub-Saharan Africa the traditional rural population is rapidly moving to cities; more than half of the population of approximately 700 million already live in urban areas.

UN-Habitat, the United Nations Human Settlements Program, has stated that Africa's chaotic urbanisation, together with the HIV/AIDS pandemic, was the biggest threat to the world's poorest continent. It was estimated that, by 2000, 51 per cent of Africans would be living in cities and towns, and

Africa would cease to be a rural continent. In the more developed countries, 84 per cent of the inhabitants will be urban dwellers by 2030.[6]

In agreement with this, according to a new report issued by the United Nations Population Division, virtually all population growth expected in the next 30 years will be concentrated in urban areas. By 2030 the worldwide population living in urban areas is projected to reach 60 per cent.[7]

Xenobiotics

Xenobiotics are substances foreign to living systems. The term includes drugs, pesticides, pollutants, carcinogens, volatile petrochemicals, food additives and polluted working environments. The following discussion focuses on some of the important xenobiotics.

Smoking

Smoking is a risk factor for many diseases. Lung cancer is the most serious, but other lung conditions such as chronic airways disease and emphysema are also related to smoking, which has been identified as the second most important risk factor for death from any cause worldwide. China, with a population of 1.3 billion, is the world's largest producer and consumer of tobacco and a large proportion of deaths in China are attributable to smoking.

It had also been predicted that smoking would cause approximately 930 000 adult deaths in India by 2010, mainly from tuberculosis and respiratory disease in both men and women, and from heart disease and cancer in men.

The three leading causes of death attributable to smoking in the United States are cancer, cardiovascular disease and respiratory disease in men and respiratory disease in women.[8]

Alcohol

Alcohol abuse causes 3.5 per cent of all deaths and disability in the world, and its impact is more than five times as significant as illegal drugs on human health globally.[9]

Alcohol consumption in South-East Asia is rising, particularly among youths and young adults in both rural and urban areas. This may be due to economic growth, increasing trade liberalisation and globalisation. Many countries in Asia, including India, Sri Lanka, Malaysia and Thailand, cannot provide accurate consumption figures since local cheap illicit brews are consumed in unknown quantities.[10]

It is common knowledge that alcohol leads to health-related and social problems. In the digestive system alcohol is a leading cause of cirrhosis and pancreatitis and is also related to cancers of the mouth, oropharyngeal, esophageal, liver and colorectal cancer. Diabetes is also implicated in the disease pattern.

Volatile hydrocarbons

A 1998 study carried out in Soweto, South Africa, suggested that exposure to volatile hydrocarbons, particularly petrochemicals, increases susceptibility to pancreatitis.[11] Braganza et al. had also earlier suggested that occupational exposure to volatile hydrocarbons may be related to idiopathic and alcohol-related pancreatitis.[12]

Chronic exposure to xenobiotics such as smoke from coal fires and kerosene fumes from Primus stoves, along with long-term alcohol abuse and smoking, were cited as major contributing causes of pancreatitis. Both acute and chronic pancreatitis appear to be endemic among the Soweto population. Case control studies all identified the same three environmental factors in each disease: heavy alcohol consumption, marked exposure to industrial chemicals and a low intake of fruit, which is a major source of vitamin C.

Occupational health

People in various occupations may be exposed to xenobiotic substances that have serious deleterious effects on health. It has been suggested that there is an association between breast cancer and workshop exposure. The authors believe that it is worth exploring exposure to chemicals metabolised into reactive chemicals such as organic solvents and rubber and plastic chemicals.[13]

Occupations cited as having possible links with chronic pancreatitis and pancreatic cancer include employment in automobile engine and parts manufacture, service and maintenance, as well as dry cleaning, catering, cooking and serving, gasoline production, glue manufacture, oil refining, petrochemical industries and steel manufacture.[14]

Exposure to low-dose ionising radiation

Imaging procedures are an important source of exposure to ionising radiation and can result in high cumulative effective doses of radiation, which have been linked to the development of solid cancers and leukaemia. Thus the growing use of medical imaging procedures has resulted in the risks of radiation exposure becoming relevant.[15]

It has been reported that the per capita dose of radiation from medical imaging in the United States has increased by a factor of nearly six since the early 1980s, the largest contributors to total effective doses being X-ray computed tomography (CT) scans and nuclear imaging, most of which occurred in outpatient settings. The United States has the world's highest per capita imaging rate; as many as two per cent of cancers may be attributable to radiation exposure during CT scanning.

Radiation-induced cancer might not appear for years. While the danger from individual scans may seem to be small, the effect is cumulative, so that exposure to even moderate degrees of medical radiation is an important yet potentially avoidable public health threat—one should be aware of the potential for radiation-induced carcinogenesis.[16]

Air pollution

Air pollution is an important cause of increased morbidity and mortality worldwide. It has been suggested that sustained reduction of fine-particulate air pollution exposure would result in improved life expectancy.[17]

Dietary changes

Western influences and modernisation of lifestyle in Asian populations has resulted in an alarming increase in the prevalence of obesity, both in children and adults.

Obesity

The health risks associated with increased prevalence of obesity, particularly type 2 diabetes, have also shown a similar increase. Other diseases associated with the obesity metabolic syndrome that have also indicated this pattern include cardiovascular disease, hypertension, gallstones and certain cancers.

The health risks associated with obesity in Asian countries occur at a lower body mass index (BMI) than that observed in Western populations. This suggests that the current World Health Organization (WHO) criteria for defining 'overweight' and 'obese' using BMI may not be appropriate for some populations in the Western Pacific region. In addition, the pattern of metabolic disease differs in Asians, who tend to preferentially increase abdominal fat. Pacific Islanders tend to be prone to diabetes at greater BMIs.

It is notable that obesity and under-nutrition occur side by side within the same population in some developing countries. Specific populations affected by the obesity epidemic include China, India, Japan, Korea, Malaysia, Singapore, Taiwan, Thailand and the Philippines.[18]

Junk food

There has been a marked increase in childhood obesity both in developed and developing countries. Parallelling this has been a great increase of food advertising in the media, particularly on television programs targeting children. Television has been singled out as the most easily modifiable influential factor on diet. A survey carried out in six Asian nations—India, Indonesia, Malaysia, Pakistan, South Korea and the Philippines—showed, for example, that 30 per cent of Malaysian children watch over eight hours of television daily during holidays, exposing them to more than two and a half hours of advertisements a day. A similar trend, although not as marked, was observed in the other countries surveyed; of these, only South Korea and the Philippines have legislation regulating the advertising of fast food and confectionery.

Child obesity has reached epidemic proportions in some countries and is on the increase in others. Approximately 17.6 million children five years and under are estimated to be overweight worldwide.

This trend has spread from the developed to the developing nations. The long-term prognosis of this obesity epidemic is poor health with an increased risk in adulthood of premature death from heart disease, and early onset of diabetes and certain cancers. These can no longer be regarded as Western diseases. A WHO report has emphasised that the incidence of cardiovascular diseases has rapidly increased in India and China. The incidence of diabetes is expected to rise 20 per cent worldwide over the next two decades. This trend is partly due to obesity, unhealthy diets and sedentary life styles. South-East Asia is witnessing the fastest spread of the epidemic. In India and China the incidence is projected to rise by 50 per cent within the next two decades, affecting younger people than in the developed countries.[18]

This trend is known as 'the nutrition transition'. Interestingly, nutrition problems in Asia cover the entire spectrum from diseases due to deficiency to those due to excess. Global availability of cheap vegetable oils and fats has resulted in greatly increased fat consumption among low-income nations. As the nutrition transition has progressed, diets containing traditional root vegetables and coarse grains are being replaced by refined rice and wheat along with other food products containing a greater proportion of dietary fats and sweeteners.[19]

Television is the most powerful variable influencing child obesity, contributing to it by two mechanisms: it reduces energy expenditure through lowered physical activity at the same time as it increases dietary energy intake, either during viewing or as a result of advertising. It has been observed that the greater a child's advertising exposure the more frequently snacking occurs and the lower the child's nutrient efficiency. Most food advertising aimed at children is for foods and beverages high in sugars, fat and/or salt.

Exercise

Many countries throughout the world are facing an increased incidence of chronic diseases involving the cardiovascular, pulmonary and skeletal systems, and cancer. Obesity and Type 2 diabetes are reaching epidemic proportions. Regular exercise has been shown to reduce the risk for all of these diseases. It has been emphasised that regular physical activity has numerous health benefits and is an essential component of a healthy lifestyle. Aerobic activity in particular brings about health benefits.[19]

The above is in the context of surveys that show that about 30 per cent of Americans are inactive (sedentary) in their leisure time, approximately 45 per cent are insufficiently active and only about 25 per cent are active at recommended levels. Trends in leisure activity over time have been flat—although there has been a gradual decline in the percentage of individuals who are inactive and a greater decline in older age groups.[20]

The recommended levels of exercise are at least 30 minutes of moderate-intensity physical activity on five or more days each week. This should be integrated into a 'lifestyle intervention' program that integrates physical activity into daily life.[21]

A study by Lorig et al. (1999) has suggested that intervention is feasible and beneficial beyond usual care in terms of improved health status, and can decrease hospitalisation with a substantial savings in health care cost.[22]

QUICK FLICK

2

Summary

In conclusion, the breakdown of barriers to the spread of disease has ramifications that impact on global health and may signal what one may expect in the future. Awareness, adjustment and adaptability will be the key to the practice of medicine worldwide.

References

1. United States Environmental Protection Agency. Climate change [internet]. Available from: www.epa.gov/climatechange.

2. Schuman EK. Global climate change and infectious diseases. *N Engl J Med.* 2010; 362(12):1061–3.

3. McMichael AJ, Woodruff RE, Hales S. Climate change and human health: present and future risks. *Lancet.* 2006; 367(9513):859–69.

4. Forbes D, Lindfield M. Urbanisation in Asia: lessons learned and innovative responses. Australian Agency for International Development; 1997.

5. Patel BR. Urbanisation: an emerging humanitarian disaster. *N Engl J Med.* 2009; 361(8):741–3.

6. UN warns of urbanisation in Africa. *IOL* [internet] 2005 June 17. Available from: www.iol.co.za.

7. UN Department of Economics and Social Affairs: Population Division [internet]. Available from: www.un.org/esa/population/unpop.htm.

8. Dongfeng G, Tanika NK, Wu X, Chen J, Samet JM, Huang J, Zhu M, Chen J, Chen C-S, Duan X, Klag MJ, He J. Mortality attributable to smoking in China. *N Engl J Med.* 2009; 360(2):150–9.

9. Assunta M. Impact of alcohol consumption on Asia. *The Globe* 2001; issues 3 & 4.

10. World Health Organization South-East Asia Office. Alcohol consumption control—policy options in the South-East Asia region. Regional Committee 59th Session, Agenda Item 10, SEA/RC59/15 (Rev.2). 2006 22–25 August.

11. Segal I. Pancreatitis in Soweto, South Africa. *Digestion*. 1998; suppl. 4:25–35.

12. Braganza J, Jolly JE, Lee WR. Occupational chemicals and pancreatitis: a link?. *Int J Pancreatol*. 1986; 1:9–19.

13. Labreche F. Occupations and breast cancer. Ontario Occupational Disease Panel [internet] 1997; Available from: www.canoshweb.org/odp/htm/breastca.htm.

14. Jeppe CV, Smith MD. Transversal descriptive study of xenobiotic exposures in patients with chronic pancreatitis and pancreatic cancer. *Int J Pancreatol*. 2008; 9:235–9.

15. Fazel R, Krumholz HM, Wang Y et al. Exposure to low-dose ionising radiation from medical imaging procedures. *N Engl J Med*. 2009; 361(9):849–57.

16. Lauer MS. Elements of danger: the case for medical imaging. *N Engl J Med*. 2009; 361(9):841–3.

17. Pope CA III, Ezzati M, Dockery DW. Fine-particulate air pollution and life expectancy in the United States. *N Engl J Med*. 2009; 360(4):376–86.

18. Inoue S, Zimmet P, Caterson I, Chunming C, Ikeda Y, Khalid AK, Kim YS, Bassett, J. The Asia–Pacific perspective: redefining obesity and its treatment. Regional Office for the WPRO, WHO, International Association for the Study of Obesity and the International Obesity Task Force. 2000.

19. Escalante de Cruz A, Phillips S, Visch M, Bulan Saunders D. The junk food generation: a multi-country survey of the influence of television advertisements on children. Consumers International, Asia Pacific Office, Kuala Lumpur [internet] 2004; Available from: www.consumersinternational.org/news-and-media/publications.

20. Powers SK. Research in exercise science: a road map for the future. *Arch Exerc Health Dis*. 2010; 1(1):1–2.

21. Buchner DM. Physical activity. Chapter 14. In: Goldman L, Ausiello D, editors. Cecil medicine. 23rd ed. Philadelphia: Saunders Elsevier; 2008, p.64–70.

22. Lorig KL, Sobel DS, Stewart AL, Brown Jr BW, Ritter PL, Gonzalez VM, Laurent DD, Holman HR. Evidence suggesting that a chronic disease self-management program can improve health status while reducing utilization and costs: a randomized trial. *Med Care*. 1999; 37(1):5–14.

Section 2

Gastrointestinal diseases

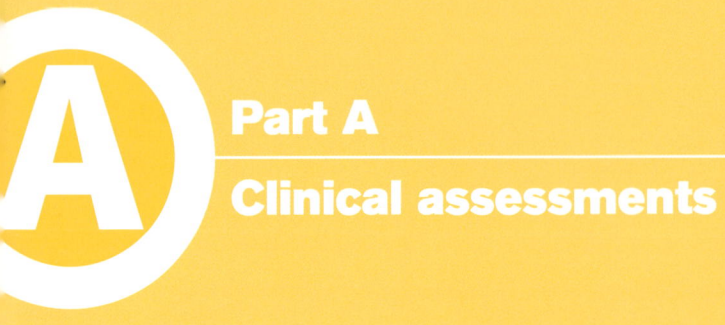

Part A

Clinical assessments

Chapter 3: Acute and chronic abdominal pain

S. Wong (Australia)

Key points

- ▶ Visceral pain results from distension, is localised to the midline, and is usually dull or colicky in nature and not worse on movement.
- ▶ Parietal pain is accurately localised to the site of inflammation, is constant, exacerbated by movement, and associated with signs of peritonism.
- ▶ Referred pain is felt in an area of the body other than the site of origin and is usually sharp and persistent.
- ▶ Management of acute abdominal pain depends on the disease but the trend is towards more conservative and minimally invasive treatments.
- ▶ Patients with generalised peritonitis present with sudden onset of severe generalised constant abdominal pain which is worse with movement.
- ▶ Sources of primary peritonitis include spontaneous bacterial peritonitis in cirrhosis, haematogenous, respiratory, tuberculosis, peritoneal dialysis, female genital tract and nephrotic syndrome.
- ▶ Secondary peritonitis results from perforated viscus (e.g. peptic ulcer disease, diverticulitis and appendicitis) or from blood due to a ruptured ectopic pregnancy.
- ▶ Urgent laparotomy is usually required in patients with secondary peritonitis.
- ▶ There are four main pathological processes in the gastrointestinal tract: infection, obstruction, haemorrhage and ischaemia.

▶ It is important to exclude acute urinary retention and medical causes for acute abdominal pain and be aware of attenuated signs in the elderly and immunosuppressed patients.

○ Introduction

History, clinical examination and focused investigations are the mainstay of an accurate diagnosis in the assessment of acute abdominal pain. With chronic abdominal pain, it is important to differentiate functional pain, abdominal wall pain and bloating.

○ Diagnosis

An accuracy of 80 per cent is achievable by experienced surgeons and this can be improved with laboratory tests and imaging. Analysis of a comprehensive history and physical examination is the mainstay of clinical diagnosis. Algorithms involving a combination of history, physical findings and laboratory results can be used to improve diagnostic accuracy—for example, use of the Alvarado score (see below) for acute appendicitis.

Alvarado score

The maximum Alvarado score is 10, based on eight items:

- symptoms are migration of pain (1), anorexia (1) and nausea/vomiting (1)
- signs are right iliac fossa tenderness (2), rebound pain (1) and temperature >37.5 (1)
- laboratory results are leukocytosis (2) and shift to the left (1).

Important components of the history include the nature of the pain, associated symptoms, and a relevant systems review. The aims of the physical examination include assessment of haemodynamic stability and hydration status, identifying the cause of the abdominal pain and detecting signs of peritoneal irritation. Inspection, auscultation, percussion and palpation are important components of a thorough examination. Vaginal and rectal examinations can sometimes be valuable.

The clinical findings should help direct subsequent focused investigations. Blood tests can assist with the diagnosis and subsequent management. Leukocytosis points to an infective cause, abnormal liver function tests indicate hepatic or biliary pathology, and a high lipase level indicates a diagnosis of pancreatitis. A serum pregnancy test should be performed in all women of childbearing age who present with abdominal pain. Metabolic acidosis indicated by arterial blood gas analysis supports a diagnosis of mesenteric ischaemia or severe intraperitoneal sepsis.

QUICK FLICK
3

Urinalysis and urine culture is important in the diagnosis of urinary tract infection and renal colic.

Simple radiological investigations in the form of chest and abdominal X-rays (CXR and AXR) can assist with diagnoses such as pneumonia, perforated viscus, bowel obstruction and ureteric calculus. An upper abdominal ultrasound is warranted if hepatobiliary or pancreatic pathologies are suspected. A pelvic ultrasound can help distinguish acute gynaecological conditions from appendicitis. A contrast abdominal–pelvic computed tomography (CT) scan can be useful in conditions such as appendicitis, diverticulitis, pancreatitis, ruptured abdominal aneurysm, mesenteric ischaemia, retroperitoneal pathology, and perforated viscus. CT scanning can help clarify the diagnosis, indicate the need for surgery (e.g. ruptured aneurysm), direct non-surgical management (e.g. retroperitoneal haematoma), assist with further interventional treatments (e.g. drainage of diverticular abscess), and indicate the severity of the surgical condition (e.g. necrosis in pancreatitis).

Visceral pain is mediated by the autonomic nervous system and results from distension, stretch or pressure. It is often caused by obstruction of the gastrointestinal tract. Visceral pain is localised to the midline: epigastric region for foregut pain, periumbilical region for midgut pain, and suprapubic region for hindgut pain. Anatomically, the transition between the foregut and the midgut is the second part of the duodenum and the transition between the midgut and the hindgut is the distal two-thirds of the transverse colon. This also corresponds to the blood supply: coeliac, superior mesenteric and inferior mesenteric arteries. The pain is usually dull or colicky in nature and not worse on movement. Consider the embryology when patients present with visceral pain.

Parietal pain is accurately localised to the site of inflammation because the parietal peritoneum is innervated by somatic nerves. The pain is caused by irritation of the parietal peritoneum by the inflamed organ or fluid. The pain is sharp, constant in nature and worse with movement. Patients present with signs of peritonitis, which include rebound tenderness and involuntary guarding. Consider the anatomy when patients present with parietal pain (see Table 3.1).

Referred pain is felt in an area of the body other than the site of origin (see Table 3.2). The pain is usually sharp and persistent. The region of the referred pain and the organ of origin usually share a common central sensory pathway.

○ Management

Initial management of patients with acute abdominal pain includes resuscitation and stabilisation, rehydration, analgesia, and appropriate treatment depending on the initial diagnosis. Subsequent treatments include immediate surgery, delayed surgery, and conservative treatment with regular reassessment.

Table 3.1 Abdominal pain location and diagnoses

Right upper quadrant	Left upper quadrant
Cholecystitis	Pancreatitis
Cholangitis	Splenic infarct
Hepatitis	Splenic haemorrhage
Fitz-Hugh-Curtis syndrome	
Right iliac fossa	**Left iliac fossa**
Appendicitis	Diverticulitis
Acute gynaecological conditions	Acute gynaecological conditions
Meckel's diverticulitis	Ureteric colic
Bacterial ileitis	Pyelonephritis
Crohn's disease	
Mesenteric adenitis	
Right colonic diverticulitis	
Ureteric colic	
Pyelonephritis	
Perforated peptic ulcer	

Table 3.2 Referred pain and origin

Shoulder tip pain	Subphrenic abscess
	Ruptured spleen
Shoulder blade pain	Biliary pathology
Back pain	Pancreatitis or pancreatic cancer
	Aorta
Leg pain	Irreducible obturator hernia
Lower abdominal pain	Testicular torsion
Back and groin pain	Ureteric colic

Acute appendicitis

Acute appendicitis is the most common emergency abdominal condition. It is probably a disease of progressive pathology. Studies have shown that perforation usually occurs prior to hospital presentation, not due to in-hospital delays. Perforation significantly increases the morbidity of the condition. Early surgical removal is recommended but delayed surgery in patients without perforation for 12–24 hours has not been shown to compromise patient outcome.

QUICK FLICK

3

Regular reassessment in hospital can reduce the negative appendicectomy rate in cases where the diagnosis is in doubt. There is an inverse relationship between overall perforation and negative appendicectomy rates. Imaging such as CT and ultrasound scans has been shown to have high predictive accuracy in the diagnosis of appendicitis. Laparoscopy, especially in female patients, can be used for diagnostic and therapeutic purposes.

An appendiceal phlegmon, without signs of generalised peritonitis, can be treated conservatively with antibiotics and close observation. A colonoscopy to exclude caecal (cancer) or terminal ileal (Crohn's disease) pathology is advisable after resolution of the acute attack. Interval appendicectomy after conservative treatment may not be warranted because the risk of a recurrent attack is slight.

Acute cholecystitis and acute cholangitis

Early laparoscopic cholecystectomy is recommended for patients with acute cholecystitis. A meta-analysis has shown early versus delayed (after six weeks) laparoscopic cholecystectomy to be associated with a longer operative time, shorter total length of hospital stay, and no increase in the open conversion and complication rates. The therapeutic procedure of choice for patients with cholangitis is endoscopic retrograde cholangiopancreatography (ERCP) and stone extraction or placement of a biliary stent. Patients should undergo cholecystectomy once the infection resolves if gallstones are responsible for the cholangitis.

Acute diverticulitis

Management of acute diverticulitis depends on whether it is uncomplicated or complicated. Difficulty may occur in deciding the timing and place of surgery. Most patients with uncomplicated diverticulitis can be managed non-operatively. Decisions should be based on individual circumstances.

In managing complicated diverticulitis, Hartmann procedure remains a safe and quick operation for patients with faecal peritonitis or those who would not cope well physically from an anastomotic leak. With better experience, utilisation of single-stage or laparoscopic procedures in managing complicated diverticulitis is gaining favour as a safe alternative to more radical and multi-stage procedures in selected patients. A single-stage procedure in experienced hands can be equally successful in an emergent setting. Where possible, operations should be converted from an emergency to a semi-elective one by utilising techniques such as radiological or laparoscopic-guided drainage of collections.

Acute pancreatitis (see Chapter 29)

The treatment of mild acute pancreatitis is conservative and supportive. Severe attacks characterised by infected necrosis of the pancreatic tissue may require surgical intervention.

Patients with gallstone pancreatitis have been traditionally treated by early ERCP removal of common bile duct stones followed by cholecystectomy prior to discharge from hospital. A better outcome may be achieved by laparoscopic cholecystectomy, intra-operative cholangiogram and antegrade sphincterotomy.

There is conflicting data about the use of antibiotic prophylaxis in severe acute pancreatitis. The use of either enteral or parenteral nutrition is associated with a lower risk of death in acute pancreatitis compared with no supplementary nutrition. Early initiation of enteral feeding rather than parenteral nutrition is both feasible and beneficial. Enteral nutrition has been shown to be associated with a lower risk of infectious complications. The detection of necrosis alone is not an indication for surgery. Even in the presence of infected necrosis, appropriate antibiotic usage, critical care support and radiological drainage can improve outcome. If surgery is indicated, delayed surgery after four weeks and minimally invasive procedures (e.g. retroperitoneal approach) may result in better outcomes.

Generalised abdominal pain

Patients with generalised peritonitis present with sudden onset of severe, generalised, constant abdominal pain that is worse with movement. Physical examination reveals generalised abdominal tenderness, rebound tenderness, involuntary guarding and a high temperature. The patient is usually dehydrated and unwell. Other signs include hyperventilation and reduced mental alertness. Investigations may demonstrate leukocytosis, metabolic acidosis, and pneumo-peritoneum on erect CXR or CT scan.

The causes include primary peritonitis (such as spontaneous bacterial peritonitis in patients with cirrhosis) or secondary peritonitis (from perforated viscus or blood). Other sources of primary peritonitis include haematogenous, respiratory, tuberculosis, peritoneal dialysis, female genital tract and nephrotic syndrome. Familial Mediterranean fever is a congenital cause of recurrent peritonitis and fever. The more common perforated viscus causes of peritonitis are peptic ulcer disease, colonic diverticular disease, and appendicitis. Women with a ruptured ectopic pregnancy can present with generalised peritonitis and hypotension. Generalised tenderness and rebound tenderness is common but involuntary guarding may be absent. Abdominal wall rigidity is more common with chemical peritonitis. Diffuse peritonitis should be distinguished from the severe pain of acute pancreatitis. Urgent laparotomy is usually required in patients with secondary peritonitis.

▷ Classifications

There are four main pathological processes in the gastrointestinal tract: infection, obstruction, haemorrhage and ischaemia. Most abdominal pathologies involve one or a combination of these processes. Acute abdominal pain can be classified into one of four general categories to guide assessment: peritonitis, bowel obstruction, vascular catastrophe, and non-specific abdominal pain.

Peritonitis

Peritonitis can be localised or generalised. Surgical assessment and management is usually indicated in patients with symptoms and signs of peritonitis.

Bowel obstruction

Symptoms

The four main symptoms of bowel obstruction are abdominal pain, vomiting, abdominal distension, and constipation/obstipation. The nature of the four symptoms may help differentiate between a small bowel and large bowel aetiology. Small bowel obstruction is associated with periumbilical abdominal pain, non-bile-stained or feculent vomiting, abdominal distension depending on the proximity of the obstruction, and constipation as a late symptom. Lack of abdominal distension in proximal small bowel obstruction can mislead inexperienced doctors into a misdiagnosis of gastroenteritis. Large bowel obstruction pain may be situated in the periumbilical or suprapubic regions depending on the site of obstruction. An incompetent ileocaecal valve results in more feculent vomiting and abdominal distension, and is associated with a delayed presentation.

Causes

Common causes of small bowel obstruction are adhesions and external hernias. Other causes can be classified to origins outside the bowel wall, in the bowel wall, and in the bowel lumen. Volvulus and internal hernias are other external causes. Strictures in the bowel wall can be benign or malignant. Benign strictures can be caused by Crohn's disease, radiation enteritis, ischaemia of a small bowel anastomosis, and medications (such as potassium or non-steroid anti-inflammatory drugs). Malignant strictures are most commonly due to carcinoid tumours and adenocarcinomas. Lymphoma, gastrointestinal stromal tumours (GISTs), and metastatic tumours such as melanoma are other small bowel tumours. Intra-luminal causes of small bowel obstruction include gallstone ileus and bezoars. Common causes of large bowel obstruction are cancer, diverticular stricture, and volvulus.

Treatment

The initial treatment includes bowel rest, rehydration with intravenous fluids, analgesia, and drainage with a nasogastric tube. An erect and supine AXR may show dilated bowel loops with air–fluid levels. Small bowel is usually in a central position with a ladder appearance (valvulae conniventes or plicae circulares) and large bowel is usually in a peripheral position with lines that do not go right across the lumen (haustra). Adhesive small bowel obstruction can be managed conservatively at first, but will require operative intervention if there are signs of ischaemia (constant severe pain, signs of peritonitis, fever, and high white cell count). A gastrograffin small bowel series at 48 hours may assist in selecting out the cases which require surgical intervention. Small bowel obstruction due to a hernia or unknown cause usually requires an operation for resolution.

An abdominal CT scan or gastrograffin enema study can be used to differentiate mechanical large bowel obstruction from pseudo-obstruction. A caecal diameter greater than 10 cm usually warrants urgent treatment. Pseudo-obstruction can be treated conservatively, with neostigmine, or by colonoscopic decompression. Mechanical large bowel obstruction can be treated by decompression of a sigmoid colon volvulus, resection and anastomosis, resection and stoma, diverting proximal stoma, or colonic stent.

Vascular catastrophe

Patients presenting with an abdominal vascular catastrophe usually present with severe pain but relatively benign signs. Symptoms of a ruptured abdominal aortic or iliac artery aneurysm include severe abdominal, flank or back pain and hypotension. A pulsatile abdominal mass may be palpable. The symptoms can be mistaken for ureteric colic. In haemodynamically stable patients, an abdominal CT scan can confirm the diagnosis before surgery. In haemodynamically unstable patients, urgent surgery is required to prevent death. Repair can be performed via a laparotomy or via an endovascular approach.

Acute mesenteric ischaemia can be due to thrombosis, embolus, or non-occlusive low flow states. The patient usually presents with severe abdominal pain. The abdominal findings are disproportionally mild. Findings of lactic acidosis and leukocytosis are supportive of the diagnosis. The mortality is high but urgent laparotomy, small bowel resection, and mesenteric artery thrombectomy or embolectomy may save the patient's life. However, short bowel syndrome and requirement of total parenteral nutrition may be a long-term problem. In acute mesenteric ischaemia secondary to low flow states, conservative treatment with anticoagulation can be therapeutic.

Non-specific abdominal pain

After excluding peritonitis, bowel obstruction and abdominal vascular catastrophe, a diagnosis of non-specific abdominal pain can be considered. The aetiology may represent minor versions of mesenteric adenitis, ovulation pain, or torsion of appendix epiploicae. Other diagnoses such as peptic ulcer disease, gastritis and gastro-oesophageal reflux can be confirmed on upper gastrointestinal endoscopy.

○ Pitfalls

Elderly and immunosuppressed patients may have attenuated signs.

Patients with acute urinary retention may present with signs of an acute abdomen. Patients are typically male and may not be able to provide a good history (e.g. dementia, stroke, or language barriers).

A diagnosis of rectus sheath or retroperitoneal haematoma should be considered in a patient with new onset abdominal pain if they are on heparin or warfarin treatment.

Medical causes of acute abdominal pain should be excluded (see Table 3.3).

Table 3.3 Medical causes of abdominal pain

Endocrine	Diabetic ketoacidosis
	Adrenal insufficiency
	Hypothyroidism or hyperthyroidism
Metabolic	Hypercalcaemia
	Porphyria
	Lead toxicity
	Uraemia
Haematological	Acute leukaemia
	Sickle cell anaemia
	Henoch-Schönlein purpura
Cardio-respiratory	Inferior acute myocardial infarction
	Right heart failure
	Pneumonia
	Pulmonary infarction
Gastrointestinal	Inflammatory bowel disease
	Hepatitis
	Disaccharidases deficiency
Infective	Herpes zoster
Renal	Pyelonephritis
Psychiatric	Münchausen's syndrome

○ Abdominal pain in the tropics

Tropical diseases can mimic common Western conditions and should be considered in overseas travellers and immigrants (see Table 3.4). Travel from one country to another has become more common and rare diseases from a

Table 3.4 Tropical infection, organism and abdominal pain

Malaria (protozoa)	*Plasmodia falciparum* or *P. vivax*	Severe abdominal pain Splenomegaly
Leishmaniasis (protozoa)	*Leishmania donovani*	Splenomegaly
Amoebiasis (protozoa)	*Entamoeba histolytica*	Amoebic colitis Amoebomas of rectum and caecum Hepatic abscess
Giardiasis (protozoa)	*Giardia lamblia*	Abdominal cramps
Cryptosporidiosis (protozoa)	*Cryptosporidium hominis* and *C. parvum*	Abdominal cramps Biliary disease including sclerosing cholangitis
Round worm (nematode)	*Ancylostoma* (hookworm) *Ascaris lumbricodes* *Strongyloides stercoralis*	Epigastric pain Small bowel obstruction, intussusception and perforation Hepatobiliary and pancreatic diseases Hyperinfection syndrome—generalised abdominal pain
Tapeworm (cestode)	*Taenia saginata* and *T. solium*	Subcutaneous nodules
Liver fluke (trematode)	*Clonorchis sinensis* *Opisthorchis* spp. *Metorchis conjunctus*	Cholangitis, cholangiohepatitis, and cholangiocarcinoma Pancreatitis
Schistosomiasis (trematode)	*Schistosoma mansoni* and *S. japonicum*	Colorectal mass Bladder involvement and ureteric obstruction Hepatomegaly, splenomegaly and portal hypertension
Tuberculosis	*Mycobacterium tuberculosis*	Peritonitis Small intestinal obstruction and perforation Ileocaecal tuberculosis
Hydatid disease	*Echinococcus granulosus*	Ruptured hydatid cyst Hepatic and splenic cyst
Trypanosomiasis	*Trypanosoma cruzi*	Chagas disease—megacolon
Actinomycosis	*Actinomyces israelii*	Inflammation of the appendix and ileocaecal region

QUICK FLICK

3

remote part of the world can be encountered in another part of the world. Knowledge of the clinical presentations of tropical diseases may assist doctors with the correct diagnosis and appropriate treatment. Full blood count for eosinophilia, stool cultures, serological tests, and imaging studies may assist with the diagnosis.

▷ Chronic abdominal pain

Chronic abdominal pain is common and impacts significantly on patient well-being. Chronic abdominal pain may be functional, abdominal wall pain or functional bloating. Organic diseases should be excluded before commencement of treatment.

Aetiology

Functional gastrointestinal disorders such as functional abdominal pain syndrome (FAPS) or irritable bowel syndrome (IBS) are common. Symptoms of IBS may predominantly be associated with constipation, diarrhoea, or abdominal pain. There may be psychosocial precipitants for the presentation. FAPS differs from IBS in that symptoms are largely unrelated to food intake or defaecation.

Chronic abdominal wall pain is often misinterpreted as visceral or functional abdominal pain. It is somatic pain caused by cutaneous nerve entrapment. Carnett's test is diagnostic and is positive if there is an increase in pain at one site when the patient tenses the abdominal muscle by sitting up while the doctor applies pressure on the patient's forehead. Injection of local anaesthesia at the trigger point usually relieves the pain. Fasciotomy of the anterior rectus sheath over the affected anterior intercostal nerve can potentially relieve the pain.

Abdominal bloating is a common symptom and can be difficult to treat. The symptoms are usually worse during the day. Treatment options include laxatives, probiotics, antibiotics to treat bacterial overgrowth, and activated charcoal.

Exclusion of organic disease

Features that suggest an organic aetiology include weight loss, rectal bleeding, and change in bowel habits. Chronic pain features that suggest organic disease include recent onset, precise anatomical positions, and direct relationship to bowel function. Initial tests should include blood tests such as erythrocyte sedimentation rate, AXR, ultrasound or CT scan. Other tests to consider include gastroscopy, colonoscopy, small bowel imaging or capsule endoscopy, imaging of pancreas, gastrointestinal transit studies, and laparoscopy.

Treatment of chronic functional abdominal pain

Management of these patients includes establishing an effective trusting doctor–patient relationship and multimodal treatment. This includes centrally acting medications (such as antidepressants and anticonvulsants), pain management, behavioural modification and psychosocial support. There is some evidence of benefit for antispasmodic drugs for abdominal pain but no clear evidence of benefit for antidepressants or bulking agents.

Summary

Relevant in the diagnosis of acute abdominal pain are a thorough history, clinical examination and focused investigations. Initial management of patients with acute abdominal pain includes resuscitation, stabilisation, rehydration, analgesia and appropriate treatment depending on the initial diagnosis. The most common surgical emergencies are acute appendicitis, cholecystitis, diverticulitis and pancreatitis.

There are four main pathological processes: infection, obstruction, haemorrhage and ischaemia. Most abdominal pathologies involve one or a combination of these processes. Medical causes of abdominal pain should be excluded.

Recommended reading

Camilleri M. Management of patients with chronic abdominal pain in clinical practice. *Neurogastroenterol Motil*. 2006 Jul; 18(7):499–506.

Clouse RE, Mayer EA, Aziz Q, Drossman DA, Dumitrascu DL, Monnikes H, Naliboff BD. Functional abdominal pain syndrome. *Gastroenterology*. 2006 Apr; 130(5):1492–7.

Cooke R. Diseases caused by parasites. In: Selected topics in basic surgical sciences. Royal Australasian College of Surgeons. 1988; pp 1–47.

Dang C, Aguilera P, Dang A, Salem L. Acute abdominal pain. Four classifications can guide assessment and management. *Geriatrics*. 2002 Mar; 57(3):30–42, 35–6, 41–2.

Green JM. When is faster better? Operative timing in acute care surgery. *Curr Opin Crit Care*. 2008; 14:423–7.

Newton E, Mandavia S. Surgical complications of selected gastrointestinal emergencies: pitfalls in management of the acute abdomen. *Emerg Med Clin North Am*. 2003 Nov; 21(4):873–907, viii.

Schafer TW, Skopic A. Parasites of the small intestine. *Curr Infect Dis Rep*. 2007 Jan; 9(1):60–8.

sphincter (LES) (<10 mm Hg) as well as the transient LES relaxations (TLESRs) just prior to the episode of reflux in patients who have normal LES pressure (>10 mm Hg), are the most frequent mechanism for reflux.

Typical reflux symptoms are heartburn and acid regurgitation after meals, either with or without mucosal breaks of the oesophagus, and are caused by reflux of gastric content into the lumen of the oesophagus (see Figure 4.1). Bile acid and digestive enzymes also can cause oesophageal mucosal damage.

Atypical reflux symptoms include epigastric pain or epigastric discomfort, bloating, dysphagia, chest pain, nausea and early satiety. Extraoesophageal GERD-related symptoms—chronic cough, pharyngitis, hoarseness, wheezing and non-cardiac chest pain, among others—may also be present with heartburn and regurgitation.

Clinical manifestations of complications caused by erosive oesophagitis, including oesophageal stricture, ulcer and bleeding, are characterised by, for example, dysphagia, retrosternal pain, upper gastrointestinal bleeding and anaemia (see Figure 4.1).

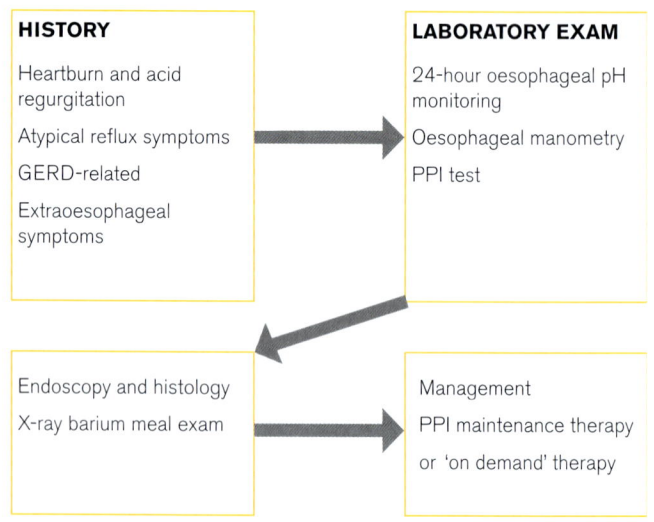

Figure 4.1 Algorithm for diagnosis and management of GERD

When Barrett's oesophagus is complicated by adenocarcinoma, the clinical manifestations may be the alarm symptoms, such as dysphagia, anaemia, weight loss, haematemesis and melaena (see Tables 4.1–4.3).

Table 4.1 Typical reflux symptoms

• Heartburn	• Acid regurgitation
Atypical GERD symptoms	
• Epigastric pain • Eructation • Bloating • Dysphagia	• Epigastric discomfort • Chest pain • Nausea • Early satiety

Table 4.2 GERD-related extraoesophageal symptoms

• Chronic cough • Hoarseness • Non-cardiac chest pain	• Pharyngitis • Wheezing

Table 4.3 Symptoms of complications in erosive oesophagitis (stricture, ulcer) and Barrett's oesophagus (oesophageal adenocarcinoma)

• Dysphagia • Upper gastrointestinal bleeding • Weight loss	• Retrosternal pain • Anaemia • Haematemesis and melaena

◑ Diagnosis of GERD

GERD should be considered if the patient has typical reflux symptoms: heartburn and acid regurgitation, without pyloric or upper gastrointestinal tract obstruction.

Diagnosis based on reflux symptoms

Upper gastrointestinal endoscopic examination is useful for the diagnosis of GERD, and it may determine whether it is erosive oesophagitis, NERD or Barrett's oesophagus. When the patient is suspected to have GERD, endoscopic examination is generally performed first, especially for patients with frequent and severe reflux symptoms or alarm symptoms, or with a family history of gastrointestinal cancer.

Erosive oesophagitis

Endoscopic examination can detect hiatus hernia, oesophageal mucosal breaks, oesophageal stricture or ulcer, and upper gastrointestinal ulcer or cancer.

Endoscopic examination

The endoscopic lesions of erosive oesophagitis may be divided into four grades according to the Los Angeles Classification. If no oesophageal mucosal break is found at endoscopy despite the presence of reflux symptoms,

NERD can be diagnosed. Diagnosis of Barrett's oesophagus is made mainly by endoscopic examination and biopsy of the distal oesophagus. The typical sign of Barrett's oesophagus under endoscopy is the appearance of orange-red columnar epithelium proximal to the oesophageal gastric junction (EGJ).

X-ray barium meal examination

X-ray barium meal examination of the oesophagus can show whether there are mucosal lesions, strictures or hiatus hernia and whether there is a reflux of the barium meal from the stomach to the oesophagus.

24-hour oesophageal pH monitoring

Oesophageal pH monitoring over 24 hours confirms reflux of gastric contents and gastric acid into the oesophagus, the relation between the symptoms and acid reflux episode, and the response to therapy.

Oesophageal manometry

Oesophageal manometry reflects the barrier function of the EGJ, and can help to locate the position of the oesophageal pH electrode.

Impedance measurement combined with pH monitoring

Impedance measurement combined with pH monitoring is used to determine the relationship between acid reflux and its symptoms (see Figure 4.2).

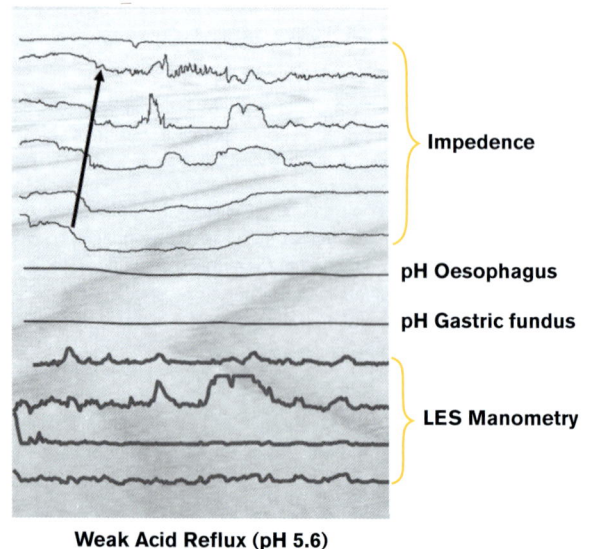

Impedence

pH Oesophagus

pH Gastric fundus

LES Manometry

Weak Acid Reflux (pH 5.6)

Figure 4.2 Relationship between impedance, pH and LES manometry

Impedance measurement monitors the presence of non-acidic or weakly acidic reflux, or gas reflux. Non-acidic/weakly acidic reflux events occur regularly during acid inhibition therapy.

Determination of the oesophageal reflux of bile acid

The presence and degree of bile acid reflux can be reflected by the determination of bilirubin in gastric juice. However, the reflux of the duodenal contents coexists with the reflux of gastric contents, and symptoms may be improved after acid inhibition (see Tables 4.4 and 4.5).

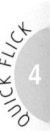

Table 4.4 Diagnosis of GERD

- GERD is diagnosed if typical reflux symptoms are present
- Endoscopy is useful for differentiating the three types of GERD: erosive oesophagitis, NERD and Barrett's oesophagus
- Los Angeles endoscopic grading scheme for oesophagital severity
- Histopathology: when columnar epithelial metaplasia or intestinal metaplasia is found in distal oesophageal mucosa, Barrett's oesophagus can be diagnosed
- X-ray barium meal examination: oesophageal stricture, hiatus hernia and reflux of barium meal into the oesophagus
- 24-hour oesophageal pH monitoring: reflux of gastric acid and gastric contents into the oesophagus, and the relationship between symptoms and acid reflux
- Oesophageal manometry: reflects the barrier function of the EGJ and helps to locate the position of the oesophageal pH electrode
- Gastric juice bilirubin: presence or degree of bilirubin reflux from duodenum into the stomach
- Proton-pump inhibitor (PPI) test: in NERD the reflux symptoms disappear after taking the PPI, but not in functional heartburn.

Table 4.5 Los Angeles endoscopic grading scheme for erosive oesophagitis

- Grade A: One (or more) mucosal breaks no longer than 5 mm that do not extend between the tops of two mucosal folds
- Grade B: One (or more) mucosal breaks more than 5 mm long that do not extend between the tops of two mucosal folds
- Grade C: One (or more) mucosal breaks that are continuous between the tops of two or more mucosal folds but involve <75 per cent of the circumference
- Grade D: One (or more) mucosal breaks that involve at least 75 per cent of the oesophageal circumference.

Source: Lundell LR, Dent J, Bennett JR et al. Endoscopic assessment of oesophagitis: clinical and functional correlates and further validation of the Los Angeles classification. *Gut*. 1999; 45:172

⟁ Diagnosis of NERD

The natural course of NERD is not yet well known; however, most NERD patients do not develop erosive oesophagitis. The diagnosis of NERD is made if the reflux symptoms are present without oesophageal mucosal breaks at endoscopy. However, the squamous epithelium of the lower oesophagus may show the mean intercellular space diameter to be greater than those in the controls under transmission electron microscope or light microscope. The PPI test is one of the most practical methods for the diagnosis of NERD. The marked improvement of reflux symptoms after PPI treatment denotes the association between the reflux symptoms and acid reflux. When heartburn is the chief complaint without oesophageal mucosal breaks, NERD can be differentiated from functional heartburn in which there is no evidence of acid reflux, giving a negative PPI test result (see Tables 4.6 and 4.7).

Table 4.6 Ultrastructure change in NERD

In NERD, where the distal oesophagus is normal at endoscopy but the mean intercellular space diameter is greater than normal controls under transmission electron microscope and light microscopy.

Table 4.7 Diagnosis of NERD

- The patient has reflux symptoms
- No mucosal breaks in distal oesophagus at endoscopy
- A positive PPI test
- Functional heartburn should be considered if PPI test is negative
- No evidence of the pathological acid reflux or no relationship between GER symptom and reflux episode in functional heartburn.

⟁ Diagnosis of Barrett's oesophagus

Barrett's oesophagus itself does not induce symptoms; the clinical manifestations of Barrett's oesophagus are mainly reflux symptoms, such as heartburn, acid regurgitation, retrosternal pain and dysphagia. However, sometimes no reflux symptoms are present.

Diagnosis of Barrett's oesophagus is made on the basis of endoscopic examination and biopsy of oesophageal mucosa. When columnar epithelial metaplasia is found in the distal oesophagus and confirmed by histopathology, Barrett's oesophagus can be diagnosed.

Endoscopic examination indicates that the squamous-columnar epithelial junction (SCJ) and the oesophageal gastric junction (EGJ) are two important markers for the recognition of Barrett's oesophagus. The endoscopic marker of the SCJ is the dentate Z line formed by the junction of oesophageal squamous-columnar epithelium. The endoscopic marker of the EGJ is the junction between the tubular oesophagus and the saccular region of the stomach. Its location under endoscopy is the proximal border of gastric mucosal rugae and/or the longitudinal lattice-like blood vessel terminal of the distal oesophagus. The typical appearance of Barrett's oesophagus at endoscopy is the orange-red columnar epithelium proximal to the EGJ—that is, the dissociation of SCJ and EGJ. The length of Barrett's oesophagus is the distance from the EGJ to the SCJ. Four-quadrant biopsy sampling is recommended. Routinely, starting from the EGJ, biopsy specimens are taken from four quadrants at 2 cm intervals. There are three histological types: (1) gastric cardiac glandular type; (2) gastric fundic glandular type; and (3) specialised intestinal metaplasia type. There are two grades of dysplasia in Barrett's oesophagus: low-grade dysplasia and high-grade dysplasia.

Depending on the length of the columnar metaplastic epithelium, Barrett's oesophagus can be typed as:

1. long-segment Barrett's oesophagus (LSBE): columnar metaplastic epithelium involving the whole circumference of oesophagus and having a length ≥3 cm; or
2. short-segment Barrett's oesophagus (SSBE): columnar metaplastic epithelium not involving the whole circumference of oesophagus or, alternatively, involving the whole circumference but having a length <3 cm.

According to the morphology at endoscopy, three types may be defined: (1) whole circumference type (dentate form); (2) tongue type; or (3) island type. The Prague C and M classification assesses the circumference (C) and maximal (M) extent of the endoscopically viewed Barrett's segment: that is, circumference metaplasia (C) when the length of mucosa involves the whole circumference, and maximal proximal extension of metaplastic segment (M) represents the maximal length of the metaplastic mucosa. As examples, C3–M5 represents a 3 cm long oesophageal circumferential columnar epithelium and a non-circumferential or tongue-like extension that is 5 cm above the EGJ; C0–M3 represents no whole circumference metaplasia and a tongue-like extension that is 3 cm above the EGJ.

Barrett's oesophagus carries with it the risk of developing oesophageal adenocarcinoma, so that patients with Barrett's oesophagus should be followed up regularly for early detection of dysplasia and early adenocarcinoma (see Table 4.8 overleaf).

Table 4.8 Diagnosis of Barrett's oesophagus

- The typical appearance of Barrett's oesophagus is the orange-red columnar epithelium proximal to the EGJ

- When columnar epithelial metaplasia is found in the distal oesophagus and confirmed by histopathology, Barrett's oesophagus can be diagnosed

- The length of Barrett's oesophagus is the distance from EGJ to SCJ. There are three forms according to morphology at endoscopy: dentate form, tongue form and island form. There are three histological types of Barrett's oesophagus: gastric cardiac glandular type, gastric fundic glandular type, and specialised intestinal metaplasia type. There are two grades of dysplasia in Barrett's oesophagus: low-grade dysplasia and high-grade dysplasia

- According to the length of columnar metaplastic epithelium, Barrett's oesophagus can be typed as long-segment Barrett's oesophagus (LSBE) (length ≥3 cm) and short-segment Barrett's oesophagus (SSBE) (length <3 cm)

- Prague C and M classification: circumferential metaplasia (C) represents the length of metaplastic mucosa involving the whole circumference; maximal proximal extension of metaplastic segment (M) represents the maximal length of the metaplastic mucosa.

⊙ **Management**

The aims of treatment of GERD are healing oesophagitis; alleviating symptoms; improving the quality of life and preventing complications (see Table 4.9).

Table 4.9 Aims of management

- Healing oesophagitis
- Alleviating symptoms
- Improving quality of life
- Preventing complications.

It is important to change the patient's lifestyle: elevating the head of the bed, no food three hours before sleep, avoiding a high-fat diet, abstaining from alcohol and smoking, and reducing body weight.

Acid inhibition therapy: PPI and H_2-receptor antagonist (H_2RA) are common acid inhibition drugs in the treatment of GERD. PPI is the most effective drug for GERD and its related diseases. Short-term clinical trials in erosive oesophagitis patients with PPI have demonstrated that healing of erosive lesions of oesophagus and improvement of reflux symptoms is more rapid than with H_2RA. PPI treatment may also improve the reflux symptoms in NERD and extraoesophageal symptoms of GERD patients. As GERD is a chronic disease, maintenance therapy of acid inhibition is needed for controlling reflux symptoms and preventing complications. Treatment on demand is sometimes advocated—that is, the drug is used only when the symptoms appear and until symptoms are alleviated.

Prokinetic therapy

Prokinetics can be used as an adjuvant of acid inhibitory drug therapy in treatment (see Table 4.10).

Table 4.10 Acid inhibition therapy

- PPI and H_2RA are common acid inhibition drugs for GERD
- PPI is the most effective therapy for GERD and its related diseases
- PPI ordinary dose (one tablet) twice a day for eight weeks
- PPI treatment may improve the reflux symptoms in erosive oesophagitis NERD- and GERD-related extraoesophageal symptoms
- PPI treatment 'on demand' is a form of intermittent treatment, particularly for NERD
- Prokinetic therapy: Domperidone, Mosapride and Itopride are used as an adjuvant of acid inhibitory treatment.

Surgical therapy

Complications and mortality rate of anti-reflux surgery are closely related to the experience and technique of surgeons performing the operation.

Endoscopic therapy

Endoscopic anti-reflux therapy should only be performed by experienced endoscopists in some patients with GERD. Endoscopic ablation therapy or endoscopic oesophageal mucosal resection may be considered in Barrett's oesophagus patients with dysplasia or early adenocarcinoma (see Tables 4.11 and 4.12).

Table 4.11 Indications for endoscopic therapy

- Anti-reflux treatment may produce good results when performed by expert endoscopists
- Complications such as oesophageal stricture, dysplasia and early oesophageal adenocarcinoma are the indications for endoscopic treatment.

Table 4.12 Indications for surgical therapy

- Anti-reflux surgery may produce good results when performed by expert surgeons
- Complications such as oesophageal stricture and adenocarcinoma are the indications for surgical operation.

Summary

Gastro-oesophageal reflux disease (GERD) is a chronic disease, in which gastric contents reflux recurrently into the lower part of the oesophagus. GERD may be divided into three types: erosive oesophagitis, non-erosive reflux disease (NERD) and Barrett's oesophagus.

GERD is a common disease in Western countries and is becoming increasingly common in Asian countries. NERD is more common than erosive oesophagitis: about 70 per cent of GERD is NERD, the other 30 per cent being erosive oesophagitis. Barrett's oesophagus is the premalignant disease of oesophageal adenocarcinoma.

Typical reflux symptoms are heartburn and acid regurgitation after meals.

The clinical manifestations of complications caused by erosive oesophagitis include oesophageal stricture, ulcer and bleeding. Upper gastrointestinal endoscopic examination is useful for the diagnosis of GERD, and it may determine whether it is erosive oesophagitis, NERD or Barrett's oesophagus. Endoscopic examination is generally performed first. The endoscopic lesions of erosive oesophagitis may be divided into four grades according to the Los Angeles Classification. If no oesophageal mucosal break is found at endoscopy despite the presence of reflux symptoms, NERD can be diagnosed. Diagnosis of Barrett's oesophagus is made mainly by endoscopic examination and biopsy of the distal oesophagus.

Twenty-four hour oesophageal pH monitoring, oesophageal manometry and impedance measurement combined with pH monitoring are further tests that can be carried out in assessing GERD. The PPI test is a practical method for the diagnosis of NERD.

Diagnosis of Barrett's oesophagus is made on the basis of endoscopic examination and biopsy of oesophageal mucosa showing columnar epithelial metaplasia. Patients with Barrett's oesophagus should be followed up regularly for the early detection of dysplasia and early oesophageal adenocarcinoma.

The aims of treatment of GERD are to heal oesophagitis, alleviate symptoms, improve the quality of life and prevent complications. Change in patient's lifestyle, acid inhibition therapy such as PPI and H_2-receptor antagonist (H_2RA) and prokinetics are important management methods for GERD. Endoscopic therapy and anti-reflux surgery are sometimes used in particular circumstances.

Information for patients

What is GERD?

GERD is a chronic and common disease worldwide, especially in Western countries, but it is rare in African countries. The prevalence of GERD has been increasing in Asian countries in recent years. There are three types of GERD: erosive oesophagitis, NERD and Barrett's oesophagus. Typical reflux symptoms are heartburn and acid regurgitation. PPI is the drug of choice in the treatment of GERD.

What happens in GERD?

Excessive reflux of acid fluid is the main mechanism responsible for reflux symptoms, heartburn and acid regurgitation. Lowering the lower oesophageal sphincter (LES) pressure and acid-clearing capacity of the oesophagus, and the transient LES relaxations (TLESRs) just prior to the episode of reflux in patients who have normal LES pressure are important mechanisms for GERD.

In Asian countries, erosive oesophagitis is usually mild or moderate. Patients with NERD have normal lower oesophagus mucosa despite the presence of the reflux symptoms heartburn and acid regurgitation. However, in patients with Barrett's oesophagus the clinical manifestations are mainly reflux symptoms; Barrett's oesophagus itself does not have symptoms. When columnar epithelial metaplasia is found in the distal oesophagus and confirmed by histopathology, Barrett's oesophagus can be diagnosed.

How are patients managed who have erosive oesophagitis and NERD?

The aims of treatment of GERD are to heal oesophagitis, alleviate the symptoms, improve quality of life and prevent complications, and we use PPI to achieve these aims. The oesophageal breaks will heal if the gastric $pH>4$ persistently, and the reflux symptoms will be alleviated by using PPI. The reflux symptoms normally disappear in patients with NERD after treatment with PPI, so 'on demand' treatment is usually effective.

How are patients with Barrett's oesophagus managed?

We would follow-up the patients diagnosed with Barrett's oesophagus. If the histopathology shows high-grade dysplasia or early adenocarcinoma, it would be ablated or resected endoscopically or surgically.

Recommended reading

Fock KM, Talley NJ, Fass R, Goh KL, Katelaris P, Hunt R, Hongo M, Ang TL, Holtmann G, Nandurkar S. Asia–Pacific consensus on the management of gastroesophageal reflux disease: update. *J Gastroenterol Hepatol*. 2008; 23:8–22.

Gaddam S, Sharma P. Advances in endoscopic diagnosis and treatment of Barrett's esophagus. *J Dig Dis*. 2010; 11:323–33.

Lin SR, Xu GM, Hu PJ, Zhou LY, Chen MH, Ke MY, Yuan YZ, Fang DC, Xiao SD. Chinese consensus on gastroesophageal reflux disease (GERD). *J Dig Dis*. 2007; 8:162–9.

Moayyedi P, Talley NJ. Gastro-oesophageal reflux disease. *Lancet*. 2006; 367:2086–100.

Talley NJ, Lauritsen K, Tunturi-Hihnala N, Lind T, Moum B, Bang C, Schulz T, Omland TM, Delle M, Junghard O. Esomeprazole 20 mg maintains symptom control in endoscopy-negative gastro-oesophageal reflux disease: a controlled trial of 'on demand' therapy for 6 months. *Aliment Pharmacol Ther*. 2001; 15:347–54.

Chapter 5: Irritable bowel syndrome

J. Wu (Hong Kong, China)

Key points

▶ Irritable bowel syndrome (IBS) is one of the most common human digestive disorders, affecting between 5 and 20 per cent of the adult population worldwide.

▶ IBS is associated with significant morbidity, quality of life impairment, absenteeism and burden on health care resources.

▶ The aetiology of IBS is poorly understood. The mechanism probably involves a combination of biological, psychological and social factors.

▶ IBS is a symptom-based clinical diagnosis based on the fulfilment of a set of diagnostic criteria. There is no reliable diagnostic biological marker that is readily available in clinical practice.

▶ The diagnostic yield of investigations such as colonoscopy, blood and stool tests are very low in patients with typical IBS symptoms. Selected investigation is indicated only in patients with alarm symptoms or atypical clinical features.

▶ There is no effective conventional medical treatment for IBS. The management of IBS should involve reassurance, education, early detection of concomitant psychological disorders and symptom-targeted medical therapy.

◒ Introduction

IBS is one of the most common digestive disorders, affecting between 5 and 20 per cent of the adult population worldwide. It is a chronic functional bowel disorder characterised by recurring abdominal pain and disturbed bowel movements for which no organic bowel pathology is identifiable. Although IBS is not associated with increased mortality, it is associated with significant morbidity, quality of life impairment and absenteeism, and it creates a substantial burden on the health care system.

◒ Epidemiology

IBS used to be considered a disease of affluence. Early studies from Asia suggested that the prevalence of IBS was below 5 per cent. More recent studies, however, have suggested a trend of higher prevalence in more affluent Asian countries. Owing to the variation in diagnostic criteria, the reported prevalence of IBS in the community varies substantially, ranging between 3 and 12 per cent, comparable with observations in the West. There is no significant ethnic and gender difference in the prevalence of IBS in Asia, but it is more prevalent in populations with higher educational and socioeconomic levels.

Pathophysiology

The underlying pathophysiological mechanism of IBS is poorly understood. There is mounting evidence that IBS is caused by the interaction of various biological and psychosocial factors. This 'biopsychosocial' pathophysiological model constitutes a variety of dysfunctions of the 'brain–gut axis'—a lowered pain threshold due to increased sensitivity to stimuli in the gastrointestinal tract or abnormal processing of the visceral pain signals in the central nervous system (visceral hypersensitivity), abnormal bowel motility, strong association with psychological disorder (e.g. generalised anxiety disorder) and childhood adversity (including child abuse), abnormal neurohormonal responses to physiological stress or stimuli such as excessive serotonin (5-HT) response after meals, or hypothalamic–pituitary–adrenal response to psychological stress. Recent evidence also suggests that previous gastrointestinal infection, activated gut immunity, altered gut microbiota and genetic factors may also play a role in the pathogenesis of IBS.

Clinical features

IBS is characterised by recurrent episodes of abdominal pain or discomfort associated with changes in bowel frequency (diarrhoea or constipation) or stool consistency (watery or hard stool) during the pain attacks. The character of the abdominal symptoms is highly variable, ranging from bloating, to distension sensation, to colicky cramps of variable severity. It can be generalised or localised anywhere in the abdomen. Typically, the pain is provoked by psychological stress and meals, and is relieved or significantly alleviated after bowel movements. It seldom lasts overnight and it tends to subside during sleep. Other common bowel symptoms include a transient sense of incomplete evacuation after bowel opening, and mucus in stool. Physical examination is generally unremarkable but mild abdominal distension and exaggerated bowel sounds may be detected.

Patients with IBS often have some co-morbid conditions. Upper gastrointestinal symptoms such as dyspepsia and reflux are more prevalent in these patients, and overlapping functional gastrointestinal disorders such as functional dyspepsia and gastro-oesophageal reflux disease are common.

Many IBS patients also suffer from various psychological co-morbidities such as generalised anxiety disorder and depression, observed in specialist or primary care as well as population setting. Another feature seen in IBS patients is somatisation—the tendency to experience psychological distress in the form of somatic symptoms and to seek medical help for these symptoms. Symptoms of somatisation, which include chronic pelvic pain, fibromyalgia, chronic low back pain and tension headache, are common in IBS patients.

Although most patients with this symptom complex are suffering from IBS, similar symptoms can be present in other organic diseases. Important differential diagnoses that may mimic IBS include thyrotoxicosis, inflammatory bowel disease, chronic enteric infections and colon cancer, especially in patients with symptom onset after the age of 50, or with a positive family history. Gynaecological pathology should always be considered in female patients with predominant lower abdominal pain and relatively mild disturbance of bowel movements. Lactose intolerance shares marked similarity to IBS except that the symptoms are specifically associated with the consumption of dairy product. In Western populations, coeliac disease may present with IBS-like symptoms but it is exceedingly rare in Asian populations.

○ Diagnosis

IBS is a clinical diagnosis based on the classical symptom complex of intermittent abdominal pain associated with altered bowel movements. Several sets of diagnostic symptom criteria have been established for IBS. The Manning criteria were the earliest and are the time-honoured symptom criteria for daily clinical use, but their sensitivity is reduced in IBS patients with constipation as a predominant symptom (see Table 5.1). Furthermore, the Manning criteria are less accurate in male patients.

Table 5.1 Manning criteria for irritable bowel syndrome

Chronic or recurrent abdominal pain for at least six months, associated with:

- abdominal pain relieved with defecation
- abdominal pain associated with more frequent stools
- abdominal pain associated with looser stools
- abdominal distension
- feeling of incomplete evacuation after defecation
- mucus in the stools.

The Rome criteria were established after 1991 and have been revised regularly. Despite their higher specificity, the Rome criteria may be too stringent for many patients with milder disease and therefore they are more suitable for use in clinical trials rather than in daily clinical practice (see Table 5.2).

Table 5.2 Rome III criteria for irritable bowel syndrome

Recurrent abdominal pain or discomfort* at least three days per month during the last three months, associated with *two or more* of the following:

1. Improvement with defecation
2. Onset associated with a change in frequency of stool
3. Onset associated with a change in form (appearance) of stool.

*   *Remarks*
- *Criteria fulfilled for the previous three months with symptom onset at least six months prior to diagnosis*
- *Discomfort means an uncomfortable sensation not described as pain.*

IBS can be further classified into several subtypes based on the predominant disturbance of bowel movement (see Table 5.3).

Table 5.3 Subtypes of irritable bowel syndrome

1. IBS with constipation (IBS-C): hard or lumpy stools ≥25% and loose (mushy) or watery stools <25% of bowel movements

2. IBS with diarrhoea (IBS-D): loose (mushy) or watery stools ≥25% and hard or lumpy stool <25% of bowel movements

3. Mixed IBS (IBS-M): hard or lumpy stools ≥25% and loose (mushy) or watery stools ≥25% of bowel movements

4. Unsubtyped IBS: insufficient abnormality of stool consistency to meet criteria for IBS-C, D or M.

Visceral hypersensitivity, as demonstrated by increased rectal sensitivity to mechanical distension in barostat studies, has been considered a common biological feature of IBS; however, the role of visceral hypersensitivity as a diagnostic marker has not been clearly defined.

Some investigations may be useful in patients with IBS-like symptoms, especially if alarm symptoms or atypical features are present. The diagnostic yield of these investigations in non-selected patients is very low, however, if the IBS diagnostic criteria are fulfilled. Common blood tests for IBS include haemoglobin level, erythrocyte sedimentation rate (ESR) and thyroid function test. Serology testing for coeliac disease has been advocated as a routine test for IBS patients in the West but this is unlikely to be useful for

Asian populations. Stool occult blood testing may be used as a screening tool for colonoscopy; stool microbiological tests are indicated in selected patients with features suggesting enteric infections. Colonoscopy should be considered in patients older than 50 or those with features suspected of being associated with colon cancer or inflammatory bowel disease (see Tables 5.4 and 5.5).

Table 5.4 Differential diagnoses of irritable bowel syndrome

- Thyrotoxicosis
- Chronic enteric infections (e.g. giardiasis, salmonellosis)
- Inflammatory bowel disease
- Lactose intolerance
- Coeliac disease
- Colon cancer
- Drugs (e.g. metformin, artificial sweetener).

Table 5.5 Features that justify investigation

- Rectal bleeding
- Progressive weight loss
- Family history of colon cancer
- Recurring fever
- Persistent and severe diarrhoea
- Frequent nocturnal attacks of abdominal pain and diarrhoea
- Anaemia
- Malabsorption
- Onset of symptom after age 50.

QUICK FLICK

5

◌ **Management**

The management of IBS should always begin with the establishment of a therapeutic doctor–patient rapport, patient reassurance and supportive counselling (see Table 5.6 overleaf). The bothersome symptoms and quality of life impairment should be acknowledged with empathy even though there is neither organic pathology nor risk of complication and mortality. Introducing the concept of 'brain–gut axis' dysfunction may help the patient to understand the cause of their bowel symptoms in the absence of bowel pathology.

The clinician should also help identify the stressors that trigger the symptoms. Common dietary factors include high fat content and gas-forming food such as indigestible carbohydrates, artificial sweetener and added sugar. Early detection of concomitant psychological disorders such as anxiety and depression should be an essential part of the initial evaluation and management

Table 5.6 Management of irritable bowel syndrome

Non-pharmacological

- Patient reassurance and counselling
- Dietary and lifestyle modification
- Early detection and intervention of psychological disorder
- Cognitive behavioural therapy.

Pharmacological

Abdominal pain
- Anticholinergics: hyoscine
- Smooth muscle relaxants: mebeverine
- Tricyclic antidepressants (TCAs): nortriptyline, imipramine, amitriptyline
- Serotonin reuptake inhibitors (SSRIs): paroxetine, sertraline, fluoxetine

Diarrhoea
- Antidiarrhoeals: loperamide, diphenoxylate
- 5-HT$_3$ receptor antagonists: alosetron, cilansetron

Constipation
- Bulk-forming agents: ispaghula, psyllium, dietary fibre
- Laxatives: polyethylene glycol
- 5-HT$_4$ receptor agonists: tegaserod, prucalopride
- Chloride channel activator: lubiprostone.

of all IBS patients. Sleep disturbance, psychological stress as triggering factors of most symptom attacks, marked avoidance behaviour to prevent triggering symptoms, and somatisation, are features suggesting a high likelihood of psychological disorders whose successful treatment may contribute to significant improvement of bowel symptoms. Psychotherapy, notably cognitive behavioural therapy, has been shown to be effective in refractory IBS patients.

There is no cure for IBS. No single conventional pharmacological therapy for IBS can provide all-round effective control of its whole symptom complex. Because of the complexity of the mechanism, there is no unique target receptor that mediates all IBS symptoms. Current medical therapies are primarily used for symptomatic treatment. Anticholinergics and smooth muscle relaxants are the two most commonly used drugs for treating abdominal pain. Aggravation of abdominal bloating, constipation and anticholinergism are the major side effects. Antidiarrhoeal drugs such as loperamide provide effective control of diarrhoea but may also precipitate disturbing constipation, especially in patients with mixed-type IBS. Dietary fibre and osmotic laxative such as lactulose are the recommended first-line therapies for constipation; however, these agents induce significant fermentation and poorly tolerated bloating symptoms in many patients. There is increasing evidence supporting the efficacy and tolerability of polyethylene glycol (PEG) as the first-line treatment for constipation. The new agent lubiprostone, a chloride channel activator, has been approved for the treatment of IBS with constipation. Generally, these symptom-targeted first-line therapies have been limited by marginal therapeutic benefit, introduction of side effects or even exacerbation of IBS symptoms. Combining these drugs invariably results in more side effects, poor adherence and further quality of life impairment. Antidepressants have been shown to be effective in improving symptoms and psychological well-being but their use is limited by intolerance of side effects and poor acceptance by patients. Modulators of serotonin (5-HT) receptors, which include 5-HT_3 antagonist and 5-HT_4 agonist, have been developed with initially promising therapeutic effects in recent years. Unfortunately, their use is limited by the risk of severe adverse effects. Severe complications of constipation and fatal ischaemic colitis have been associated with the use of alosetron (5-HT_3 antagonist) and increased cardiovascular events have been observed in users of tegaserod (5-HT_4 agonist).

Complementary and alternative medicines (CAM) remain popular for treating IBS owing to the lack of effective conventional treatment. Peppermint oil, probiotics, traditional Chinese medicine, exclusion diets based on immunological testing, and gut-directed hypnotherapy have all been reported to be promising treatment for IBS.

QUICK FLICK 5

Summary

Irritable bowel syndrome is one of the most common digestive disorders associated with significant morbidity. Owing to a poor understanding of the mechanism and the lack of a biological marker, the diagnosis is still based on symptom criteria; selected investigation is indicated only in patients with alarm symptoms or atypical clinical features. There is no effective conventional medical treatment for IBS and the use of available drugs is limited by side effects and poor tolerance.

The management of IBS should involve reassurance, education, early detection of concomitant psychological disorders and symptom-targeted medical therapy.

Information for patients

What is IBS?

Irritable bowel syndrome (IBS) is a common functional bowel disorder whose symptoms are intermittent attacks of abdominal pain, distension and bloating. These are often accompanied by changes in bowel movement such as constipation or diarrhoea. Despite these troubling symptoms, IBS is not related to any serious condition such as infection, cancer or other bowel inflammation.

What is the cause of IBS?

The cause is still not exactly understood. A number of physical, psychological and social factors contribute to it: psychological stress, previous serious infection of the bowel, adverse life events and dietary habits have been implicated. These factors lead to abnormal functioning of the bowel and the nervous system. The bowel becomes more sensitive to pain or other stimuli and it contracts in a more erratic way.

How is IBS diagnosed?

There is no single investigation that can confirm the diagnosis of IBS. The diagnosis of IBS can be confirmed with a high degree of certainty in most cases, however, based on a combination of typical symptoms.

Is investigation necessary?

Investigation is generally unnecessary and additional tests add little value in the diagnosis. However, some investigations such as blood tests or colonoscopy may be necessary if there are symptoms that are not compatible with a diagnosis of IBS. Colonoscopy is also necessary if the symptoms occur after the age of 50.

What is the treatment of IBS?

Unfortunately, there is no effective cure for IBS. Current drugs are used mainly for controlling the symptoms. Commonly used drugs include anti-spasmodics, laxatives and anti-diarrhoeal drugs. These can be used 'on demand' to prevent the symptom attacks if triggering factors are anticipated. Psychological disorders such as anxiety and depression may be present in some patients with IBS and treatment of these conditions may help to relieve the symptoms.

Recommended reading

Brandt LJ, Chey WD, Foxx-Orenstein AE, Schiller LR, Schoenfeld PS, Spiegel BM et al. An evidence-based position statement on the management of irritable bowel syndrome. *Am J Gastroenterol*. 2009 Jan; 104: suppl 1:S1–35.

Gwee K-A, Bak Y-T, Ghoshal UC, Gonlachanvit S, Lee OY, Fock KM, Chua ASB et al. Asian consensus on irritable bowel syndrome. *J Gastroenterol Hepatol*. 2010 July; 25(7):1189–205.

Longstreth GF, Thompson WG, Chey WD, Houghton LA, Mearin F, Spiller RC. Functional bowel disorders. *Gastroenterology*. 2006 Apr; 130(5): 1480–91.

Mayer EA. Clinical practice. Irritable bowel syndrome. *N Engl J Med*. 2008 Apr 17; 358(16):1692–9.

Spiller R, Aziz Q, Creed F, Emmanuel A, Houghton L, Hungin P, Jones R, Kumar D, Rubin G, Trudgill N, Whorwell P. Guidelines on the irritable bowel syndrome: mechanisms and practical management. *Gut*. 2007 Dec; 56(12):1770–98. Erratum in: *Gut*. 2008 Dec; 57(12):1743.

Chapter 6: Changing patterns of inflammatory bowel disease in a global context (ulcerative colitis)

K. Thia, C. Ooi (Singapore)

Key points

▶ A rising incidence and prevalence of ulcerative colitis (UC) is reported in Asia—industrialisation appears to play an important role.

▶ There are significant differences in genetic susceptibility between Caucasian and Asian inflammatory bowel disease (IBD) patients.

▶ In developing countries, a careful exclusion of infectious enterocolitis is pertinent before UC diagnosis.

▶ Treatment strategies for UC are based on clinical activity, extent of disease, patient preferences, and mainly follow evidence from Western studies.

▶ IBD patients on immunosuppressive therapies should be actively screened for opportunistic infection.

▶ Surveillance colonoscopy should be recommended for all IBD patients who meet established criteria; image enhanced endoscopy can improve the detection of dysplasia.

○ Introduction

Inflammatory bowel disease (IBD) comprises the two main subtypes Crohn's disease (CD) and ulcerative colitis (UC), which are idiopathic, chronic relapsing inflammations affecting the gastrointestinal tract. Up to 10–15 per cent of IBD cases may be categorised as indeterminate colitis when CD or UC cannot be clearly assigned from established criteria. Furthermore a change in diagnosis between CD and UC can occur in a small proportion of cases over time as the disease evolves.

As far as possible, UC and CD will be discussed separately here. Due to the overlapping nature of these IBD subtypes, however, certain topics—aetiology and risk factors, general diagnostic approach, general management, pregnancy and cancer surveillance issues—will be discussed together. Most of the information on IBD has been derived from studies performed among Western patients, but similar or unique features among non-Caucasian IBD populations will be presented where evidence is available.

⟡ Definition and classification of UC

UC is a lifelong disease characterised by diffuse inflammation, usually affecting only the mucosa and confined to the colon. It is traditionally classified as proctitis (rectal involvement only), left-sided (involving the sigmoid colon with or without involvement of the descending colon) or extensive colitis (involvement which extends beyond the splenic flexure) based on endoscopy findings. The extent of disease involvement is important as it influences the form of treatment as well as the frequency of colorectal cancer surveillance.

⟡ Epidemiology of UC

UC frequently affects young people between the ages of 30 and 40 years, although it can affect individuals of any age. There appears to be a slightly predominant male prevalence in some high-incidence Western countries, but gender distribution in Asia appears to be equal. Since World War II, UC incidence in European and North American countries has begun to plateau, whereas rising incidence rates have been noted in traditionally low-prevalence regions such as eastern Europe, South America and Asia. Overall, the incidence rate of UC varies widely, between 0.5–24.5 per 100 000 inhabitants worldwide. Southern Asian migrants settled in Western countries have a greater risk of developing UC than people of European descent.

The highest incidence rate for UC that has been reported in Asia was observed among Punjabi Indians, at 6 per 100 000 person-years. The emergence of IBD in Asia, particularly in Japan, Korea and China, cannot be explained by better disease awareness or better diagnosis. Urbanisation, along with Western diet and other unidentified environmental factors, could be potential risk factors for IBD. A temporal trend in Asia of increasing UC incidence that precedes CD by 10–20 years has been reported, similar to observations from Western population studies. In Asia, as in the rest of the world, there is convincing evidence of a rising prevalence of IBD, probably due to increased incidence as well as the more or less normal life expectancy of IBD patients.

⟡ Aetiology and risk factors of IBD

To date, the aetiologies of UC and CD remain elusive, although evidence suggests that mucosal injury in the bowel results from an inappropriate inflammatory response to intestinal microbes in a genetically susceptible host. The genetic component is larger in CD than in UC. A family history of IBD is more common among Caucasian patients than Asian patients—in the West, first-degree relatives of patients with UC have a ten- to fifteen-fold risk of developing the disease. The differences in genetic susceptibility and the low prevalence of IBD in Asia possibly accounts for the differential rates of familial aggregation.

The nucleotide-binding oligomerisation domain protein 2/caspase recruitment domain protein 15 (NOD2/CARD15) mutations—present in two per cent of Caucasian and Jewish CD populations—do not appear in CD populations from East Asia and Turkey. Furthermore, il-23 receptor (il-23), autophagy-related 16-like 1 (*ATG16L1* gene), IBD5 locus and the gene desert on chromosome 5p12.1, all important susceptibility loci among Caucasian CD patients, are not found in Japanese CD patients. In recent studies the tumour necrosis factor superfamily, member 15 (TNFSF15) genetic polymorphism was found to be significantly represented in Japanese and Korean CD patients.

Smoking has been established as a risk factor, increasing the risk and worsening the clinical course of CD, but is protective in UC. While no significant association between smoking and CD has been observed in small studies in East Asia, the protective effect on UC has been reported among Japanese and Chinese patients.

Non-selective anti-inflammatory drugs (NSAIDs) appear to exacerbate the clinical activity of IBD.

Studies on the role of appendectomy, diet (including refined sugars), drugs, seasonal variation, water supply, social circumstances, hygiene factors and vaccination have been largely controversial and inconclusive.

⟡ Clinical features and disease course in UC

The cardinal symptom of UC is bloody diarrhoea; associated symptoms include abdominal cramps, urgency and tenesmus. Most guidelines use a cut-off point of 'more than six weeks' of diarrhoea to differentiate IBD from infectious diarrhoea. Paradoxically, patients with proctitis may complain of constipation. About 15 per cent of UC patients may present with severe colitis at first. There may be accompanying symptoms of weight loss, fever and tachycardia. Extraintestinal manifestations such as arthritis, episcleritis and erythema nodosum may complicate presentation in 10 per cent of cases and may precede bowel symptoms in rare cases (see Table 6.1).

Table 6.1 Extraintestinal manifestation of IBD

Site	Specific conditions
Bone	Arthritis, arthralgia, spondyloarthropathy including ankylosing spondylitis
Eyes	Episcleritis, uveitis, iritis
Skin	Erythema nodosum, pyoderma gangrenosum
Liver	Primary sclerosing cholangitis, non-alcoholic fatty liver disease
Haematological	Venous thromboembolism (associated with active disease)
Other	Nephrolithiasis, gallstones (CD)

At presentation, about 40 per cent of adult UC cases have proctitis, 40 per cent have left-sided colitis and up to 20 per cent suffer from extensive colitis. Progression of disease extent over time is observed in both Western and Asian UC patients. In the first 3–7 years after diagnosis, 25 per cent of UC patients are in remission, 18 per cent experience persistent activity every year and 57 per cent suffer from intermittent relapses. The disease extent and clinical course in terms of disease relapse rates are generally similar among Asian UC patients. One in four UC patients requires colectomy after 10 years of disease. Studies from Japan and Korea suggest lower colectomy rates, although it is unclear if this is related to a milder course of disease or lower acceptance of colectomy among Asians.

▷ Diagnosis of IBD

There is no 'gold standard' test for IBD. In clinical practice, the diagnosis of IBD is based on clinical evaluation, supported by a constellation of biochemical, endoscopic, radiological and histological evidence (Figure 6.1 overleaf). Considering the socioeconomic background and risk factors of the patient is important in the diagnostic work-up. It is imperative to exclude common mimickers of IBD such as infectious colitis, medication-related symptoms (particular non-steroidal anti-inflammatory agents), ischaemia, vasculitis and functional disorders such as irritable bowel syndrome (Table 6.2 overleaf).

QUICK FLICK

6

Table 6.3 Investigations relevant in inflammatory bowel disease (IBD) diagnosis

Evaluations	Findings	Comments
Laboratory tests		
Full blood count and iron indices	Anaemia, thrombocytosis, iron deficiency	Reflect disease activity and blood loss; risk of thromboembolism in marked thrombocytosis
C-reactive protein (CRP) erythrocyte sedimentation rate (ESR)	Usually elevated	May be normal in small bowel CD
Liver function tests	Elevated alkaline phosphatase, bilirubin and gamma glutamyl-transferase (GGT) may suggest primary sclerosing cholangitis (PSC)	PSC is rare among Asian IBD patients
Microbiological stool tests		
Bacterial cultures	Examples: *Salmonella, Shigella, Campylobacter* spp.	Consider specific testing, e.g. for *Yersinia*
Clostridium difficile toxin	May present together with IBD or a flare-up of symptoms	Pseudomembranes seen during endoscopy is pathognomonic
Ova, cysts and parasites		Multiple fresh samples needed
Mycobacterium tuberculosis (TB)	Useful in TB-endemic areas	Not a sensitive test; consider chest X-ray, tuberculin skin test, intestinal tissue TB polymerase chain reaction (PCR), interferon gamma release assays (e.g. TB gold quantiferon, T-spot)
Imaging studies		
Plain abdominal radiography	Useful to exclude toxic megacolon and intestinal obstruction	Order based on clinical suspicion

Evaluations	Findings	Comments
Small bowel series, small bowel follow-through	More widely available, useful to exclude small bowel disease	Requires experienced radiologist to interpret well
CT abdomen and pelvis/ CT enterography (CTE)	Useful to exclude complications such as strictures, fistulas and abscesses in CD; CTE can distinguish active inflammation from fibrosis	Avoid unnecessary testing due to radiation exposure
Magnetic resonance enterography (MRE)	Useful to exclude complications such as strictures, fistulas and abscesses in CD; MRE can distinguish active inflammation from fibrosis	Requires high-resolution scanners, useful to avoid radiation exposure
Endoscopy		
Ileocolonoscopy	Look for ulcers and inflammation; attempts should always be made to intubate ileum if IBD is suspected. Obtain systematic biopsies from entire colon	Perform with care or avoid if IBD activity is severe/ fulminant
Upper endoscopy	Look for ulcers and inflammation	Useful if upper GI symptoms present
Capsule endoscopy	Usually performed for obscure GI bleeding; non-invasive but does not allow for biopsies	Risk of capsule retention if small bowel stricture present
Balloon-assisted enteroscopy	Useful to obtain biopsies of isolated small bowel ulcers or inflammation detected on capsule endoscopy or imaging	Usually performed to diagnose IBD, or for therapy of bleeding small bowel ulcers

QUICK FLICK

6

○ Management

The broad aims of treatment are induction and maintenance of remission of symptoms to provide an improved quality of life, reducing the need for long-term corticosteroids and minimising cancer risk.

The management of IBD should be based on the subtype (whether UC or CD), disease location, disease severity, presence of extraintestinal manifestations, complications, prior response, tolerance to medication and patient access to diagnostic and treatment options. It is important to engage patients in active participation during the therapeutic decision-making process, and concerns relating to quality of life issues should be addressed. The treatment options are decided on the basis of the balance between drug efficacy and medication side effects. In general, it is always prudent to exclude other disease conditions which may produce symptoms such as diarrhoea or abdominal pain similar to those of an IBD flare-up before escalating or switching therapy (see Table 6.4). It is recommended that, where possible, objective evidence of disease activity—inflammatory markers, radiology and/or endoscopy—should be obtained before starting or changing therapy.

Table 6.4 Differential causes of inflammatory bowel disease (IBD) exacerbation

Types of conditions	At risk groups
Diarrhoea and/or haematochezia	
Lactose intolerance	Dietary changes
Bacterial overgrowth	Particularly in CD with previous surgery and strictures
Bile salt malabsorption	Previous ileal resection in CD
Medication-induced	Intolerance to antibiotics, e.g. aminosalicylates
Functional diarrhoea	Concomitant functional bowel disorder
Infectious complications	Consider cytomegalovirus and tuberculosis infection, especially if receiving immunosuppression (steroids/biological therapy), or *Clostridium difficile* if exposed to antibiotics
Cancer	Particularly for longstanding colitis in UC and CD
Anorectal sphincter dysfunction	For CD patients with multiple perianal surgery, and older patients with IBD
Pain	
Gallstone disease	CD patients at risk for gallstone disease
Diverticular disease	Diverticulitis may occur in older patients with concomitant IBD
Functional bowel disease	Concomitant irritable bowel syndrome
Peptic ulcer disease	Non-steroidal anti-inflammatory agents and steroids

There is no known specific diet that either exacerbates IBD or helps to resolve inflammation; for patients with cramping and diarrhoea, however, restriction of fresh fruits, vegetables, caffeine and/or sorbitol-containing products may improve symptoms. It is also useful to consider general preventative health measures in managing IBD patients, including a review of immunisation status, before introducing immunosuppressive therapies (Table 6.5). Vaccination against influenza and pneumococcal infection is recommended for patients already on immunosuppressant drugs, and patients should be screened for hepatitis B, HIV and tuberculosis before they are started on immunosuppressives or anti-tumour necrosis factor (TNF) agents.

Table 6.5 General preventative health measures

Health measure	Comment
Compliance	Adherence should be checked at each visit with patients
Smoking	Encourage cessation, especially in CD patients
Regular exercise	For all IBD patients, unless active flare; emphasis on management of anxiety and illness related stressors
Vaccines	Avoid live vaccines if receiving immunosuppressive medication. Routine vaccination should be completed preferably before treatment of IBD
	Patients on immunosuppressives should be vaccinated against influenza and pneumococcal infection, and for tetanus and meningococcus (in appropriate setting)
	Patients started on infliximab and steroids should be routinely screened for hepatitis B, HIV and TB
Cervical cancer screening for women	Emphasise compliance with Pap smear testing, as IBD patients on steroids/immunosuppressants are at increased risk. Consider human papillomavirus (HPV) vaccination in women receiving immunosuppressives
Colon cancer surveillance	IBD patients should be appropriately offered surveillance for colorectal cancer and dysplasia

QUICK FLICK

6

With current appropriate and effective medical therapies, clinical improvement of symptoms should occur within two to four weeks, with maximal improvement being observed at 12 to 16 weeks. Patients who achieve remission should be considered for maintenance therapy. Patients who do not respond should be offered alternative therapies. Special attention should be given to common and/or significant side effects associated with IBD medications (Table 6.6 overleaf).

Table 6.6 Commonly used inflammatory bowel disease (IBD) medications: dosages and side effects

Type	Dose	Important side effects
Aminosalicylates (includes sulphasalazine, olsalazine, balsalazide, asacol, salofalk, pentasa)	Sulphasalazine 4–6 g per day in 4 divided doses; mesalazine 2–4.8 g per day in 3 divided doses; balsalazide 6.75 g per day in 3 divided doses	Side effects more frequent for sulphasalazine: nausea, vomiting, headaches, dyspepsia and anorexia. Rare: pancreatitis, allergic reaction, bone marrow suppression, interstitial nephritis, haemolytic anaemia, acute intolerance (bloody diarrhoea)
Corticosteroids (prednisone, prednisolone)	Induction dose 40–60 mg per day, or up to 1 mg/kg per day with slow taper	Gastroduodenal mucosa injury, impaired wound healing, glaucoma, Cushingoid features, mood disturbances, metabolic bone disease, metabolic disturbances (hyperglycaemia, hyperlipidaemia, accelerated atherogenesis), opportunistic infection, adrenal insufficiency
Budesonide	Induction dose 9 mg per day for 8–12 weeks	Small risk of bone loss and adrenal insufficiency
Metronidazole	For perianal CD, up to 1.5 g in 3 divided doses	Nausea, peripheral neuropathy, disulfiram-like reaction
Ciprofloxacin	For perianal CD, up to 1g in 2 divided doses	Tendonitis, tendon rupture, *Clostridium difficile*
Azathioprine/6-mercaptopurine (6-MP)	Azathioprine: 2–3 mg/kg per day; 6-MP: 1–1.5 mg/kg per day	Flu-like symptoms, leucopaenia/bone marrow suppression, hepatotoxicity, pancreatitis, lymphoma
Methotrexate	Induction of CD, parenteral 25 mg per week	Nausea, vomiting, diarrhoea, stomatitis, hepatoxicity, pneumonitis

Type	Dose	Important side effects
Anti-tumour necrosis factor agents (infliximab, adalimumab and certolizumab pegol)	Infliximab (intravenous) at 5 mg/kg at weeks 0, 2 and 6 (induction) and 5 mg/kg every 8 weeks (maintenance). Adalimumab (subcutaneous) 160 mg at week 0, 80 mg at week 2 (induction) and 40 mg every other week (maintenance) Certolizumab pegol (subcutaneous) 400 mg at weeks 0, 2 and 4, then every 4 weeks (maintenance)	Infusion reaction with acute and delayed hypersensitivity reactions (infliximab only), injection site reactions, autoimmunity, increased risks of opportunistic infections (especially *Mycobacterium tuberculosis* and fungal infections), lymphoma

UC management: induction of response and remission

For UC, therapeutic decisions depend on the endoscopic extent of the disease (proctitis, left-sided or extensive) and the severity of the IBD activity (see Figure 6.2 overleaf).

Assessment of UC disease activity

For simple practical use, UC activity can be categorised as:

- mild (up to four bloody stools daily, with no systemic toxicity)
- moderate (four to six bloody stools daily, with minimal toxicity)
- severe (more than six bloody stools daily and signs of toxicities such as fever, tachycardia, anaemia and raised erythrocyte sedimentation rate)
- fulminant (more than 10 bloody stools, continuous bleeding, frequent need for transfusion, abdominal tenderness and colonic dilatation on abdominal radiology).

Mild to moderate disease

In general, first-line therapy for mild to moderate UC consists of aminosalicylates (sulphasalazine, olsalazine, mesalamine or balsalazide) which are effective for induction and maintenance of remission. A newer mesalamine in a multimatrix formulation allows for once-daily dosing. Patients with proctitis or left-sided colitis may also be treated with topical mesalamine (mesalamine suppository for proctitis and mesalamine enema for distal colitis) or in combination with oral mesalamine.

Topical corticosteroids are also effective in the acute therapy of distal colitis but less effective in maintaining remission. Some patients achieve

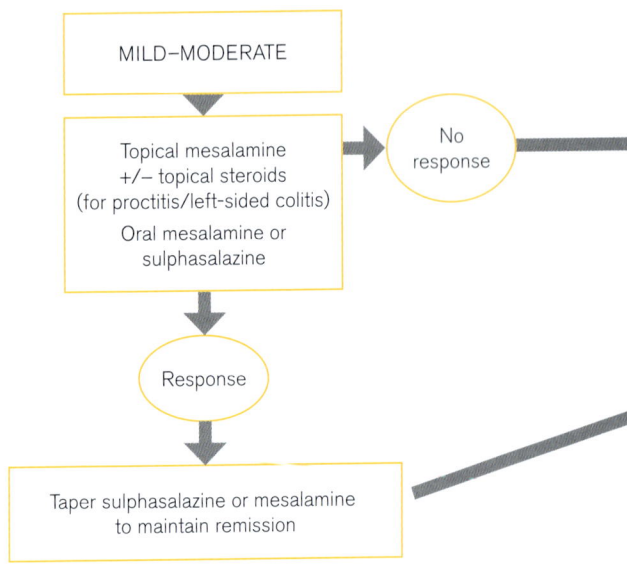

Figure 6.2 Medical therapy of ulcerative colitis (UC)

maximal benefit from a combination of oral and topical mesalamine therapy. Aminosalicylates are generally tolerated well, and toxicities are rare and mostly idiosyncratic in nature. Mesalamine therapy has similar efficacy and is better tolerated than sulphasalazine, but because sulphasalazine is substantially cheaper it is the preferred first-line therapy for UC in many Asian countries.

Moderate to severe disease
Patients who have moderate to severe disease, or whose disease resists optimal aminosalicylate doses, should be treated with oral prednisolone for quicker control of disease activity. Once patients respond to corticosteroids, they should be gradually tapered off: corticosteroids are not effective in the long term as they fail to maintain remission and often result in significant side effects. The thiopurines 6-mercaptopurine (6-MP) or azathioprine are the next line of treatment for patients who do not respond to, or cannot be weaned off, corticosteroids. Their efficacy is limited by the slow onset of action to achieve maximal effect, but in the long term they are effective as a steroid-sparing agent.

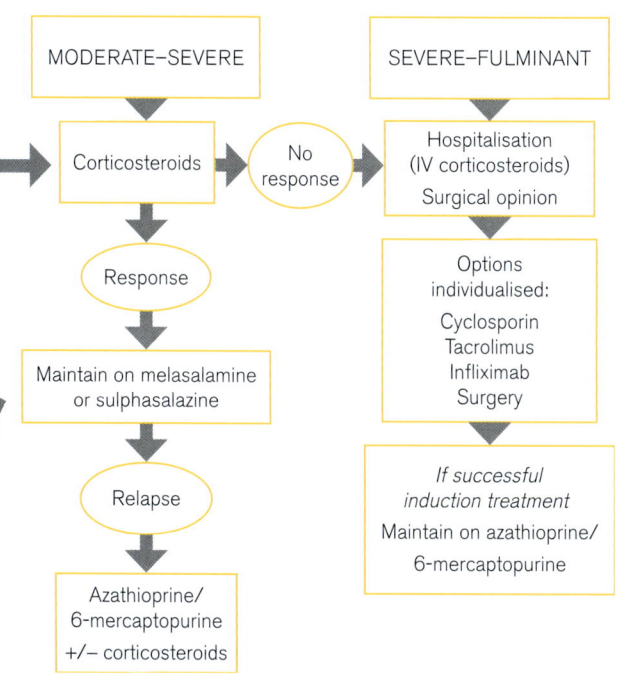

Methotrexate has not been proven to be effective in UC when administered as weekly oral doses of 12.5 mg per day; neither higher doses nor parenteral route administration have yet been evaluated in controlled trials.

Severe to fulminant disease

Patients with severe or fulminant UC, or those who do not respond to oral corticosteroids, should be admitted to hospital for intravenous corticosteroids. Prompt and careful evaluation to exclude concomitant infection such as cytomegalovirus or *Clostridium difficile* is necessary. General supportive measures are also appropriate in this setting (Table 6.7 overleaf). A withdrawal trial of aminosalicylates should be considered if the disease flare-up coincided with a recent increase in dose or addition of aminosalicylates. Cyclosporin, tacrolimus and infliximab are all effective in patients with severe UC who are refractory to intravenous corticosteroids. Early co-management with a colorectal surgeon should occur in the care of severely active UC, so that timely colectomy can be performed to prevent complications.

Table 6.7 General supportive measures for severe colitis

Measure	Comment
Intravenous fluids and electrolyte replacement	Avoid hypokalaemia and hypomagnesaemia
Sigmoidoscopy and biopsy	Careful examination, to rule out cytomegalovirus (CMV) infection
Stool culture and assay	In particular to rule out *Clostridium difficile* infection
Subcutaneous heparin	To reduce risk of thromboembolism
Nutritional support for malnourished	Enteral feed has fewer complications than parenteral nutrition
Withdrawal of drug	Stop anticholinergics, antidiarrhoeals, opioids and NSAIDS. Stop aminosalicylates if hypersensitivity reaction suspected.
Antibiotics	Consider if infection is suspected
Blood transfusion	To keep Hb>10 g/dL

UC management: maintenance of remission

First-line therapy for maintenance of remission is oral aminosalicylates. Rectal mesalamine can be used as maintenance therapy as an alternative to oral dosing in patients with left-sided colitis or proctitis.

For patients who relapse while on optimal doses of aminosalicylates, those who are steroid-dependent and those with severe UC flare requiring induction therapy with cyclosporine or tacrolimus, maintenance therapy with 6-MP or azathioprine should be considered. Infliximab is effective for remission maintenance, and is also effective as a steroid-sparing agent. Adalimumab administered subcutaneously is an alternative to infliximab therapy.

Surgical management in UC

Emergency surgery is indicated for patients with life-threatening complications such as perforation, refractory rectal bleeding or toxic megacolon, and those not responding to medical therapies. Early and close interaction between gastroenterologists and surgeons is necessary to ensure colectomy is undertaken at the best time for such patients.

Elective surgery may be indicated in patients with dysplasia or cancer, or among those with medically refractory disease or showing intolerance to long-term immunosuppressive therapies. The most widely performed surgery for UC is the ileal J-pouch anal anastomosis. Post-operatively, patients may develop complications such as pouchitis, high stool frequency, faecal incontinence or sub-fertility, and repeat surgery may be required.

Cancer surveillance in IBD

There is greater risk of developing colorectal cancer (CRC) in both UC and CD patients than in the average population. More CRC and dysplasia data exists for UC than for CD. The CRC risk is significantly associated with longer disease duration, extensive colitis, poorly controlled disease and primary sclerosing cholangitis. Early meta-analysis studies suggested a risk of CRC of 18 per cent after 30 years of UC disease but more recent data suggests a lower risk rate (2–8%); small studies of relatively shorter disease duration suggest that the risk of CRC among Asian UC patients appears to be lower than for Western patients.

Current international guidelines recommend annual or biannual surveillance colonoscopy, with protocol biopsies for left-sided or extensive UC patients who have had the disease for at least eight to ten years. For CD patients with eight to ten years of disease and with more than one-third of the colon involved, surveillance colonoscopy should be performed at similar intervals.

Compared to common CRC, colitis-associated CRC is often multiple and infiltrative, arising from flat mucosa rather than from the usual adenoma-cancer polyp sequence. These flat dysplastic lesions are more clearly seen using image-enhanced endoscopy (dye-spray chromoendoscopy, narrow-band imaging and autofluorescence imaging) rather than standard white light. Evidence is also accumulating that supports the use of other enhanced imaging techniques such as confocal microscopy for IBD CRC surveillance.

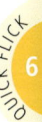

Pregnancy and fertility issues in IBD

In general, IBD patients do not have decreased fertility compared to the general population, but active disease, as well as surgery that involves tubal function, can affect fertility. Sulphasalazine (but not mesalamine) can cause oligospermia, but this is reversible upon stopping the drug.

In pregnancy, the clinical course of IBD is determined by the level of disease activity at the point of conception. Patients in remission at the time of pregnancy are likely to remain in remission during pregnancy; patients are advised to be in clinical remission before attempting pregnancy.

The mode of delivery should be influenced predominantly by obstetric necessity and indication, in conjunction with the gastroenterologist and/or colorectal surgeon. Caesarean section should be preferred among those with perianal or rectal disease. The incidences of low birth weight and prematurity are not increased in UC but appear to be increased in CD, and active disease is a risk factor.

There is no conclusive evidence that the risk of stillbirth or congenital abnormalities is increased in IBD patients. In general, medical therapy for IBD (except methotrexate) should be continued during pregnancy because the benefits of medications outweigh the risks.

Summary

There are two main subtypes of inflammatory bowel disease (IBD—Crohn's disease (CD) and ulcerative colitis (UC)—which comprise idiopathic, chronic relapsing inflammation affecting the gastrointestinal tract.

UC is classified as proctitis (rectal involvement only), left-sided (involving the sigmoid colon with or without also involving the descending colon) or extensive colitis (involvement which extends beyond the splenic flexure). It frequently affects young people between the ages of 30 and 40 years. There appears to be a slight male predominance in some high-incidence Western countries but gender distribution appears equal for UC in Asia. Since World War II, rising UC incidence has been noted in traditionally low-prevalence regions such as eastern Europe, South America and Asia. Regarding aetiology, a negative association between smoking and UC has been noted.

The cardinal symptom of UC is bloody diarrhoea; associated symptoms include abdominal cramps, urgency and tenesmus. Extraintestinal manifestations such as arthritis, episcleritis and erythema nodosum may complicate presentation in 10 per cent of cases, and rarely it may precede bowel symptoms. It is imperative to exclude common mimickers of IBD such as infectious colitis, medication-related (particularly non-steroidal anti-inflammatory agents), ischaemia, vasculitis and functional disorders such as irritable bowel syndrome. The broad aims of treatment are to induce and maintain symptom remission to provide an improved quality of life for the patient, to reduce the need for long-term corticosteroids, and to minimise the risk of cancer.

For practical purposes, disease activity can be categorised as *mild* (up to 4 bloody stools daily, and no systemic toxicity), *moderate* (4–6 bloody stools daily and minimal toxicity), *severe* (more than 6 bloody stools daily and signs of toxicities) and *fulminant* (more than 10 bloody stools, with continuous bleeding, frequent need for transfusion, abdominal tenderness and colonic dilatation on abdominal radiology).

The drugs used for maintenance of remission are oral aminosalicylates and rectal mesalamine. For patients who relapse while on optimal doses of aminosalicylates, for those who are steroid-dependent, and for those with severe UC flare requiring induction therapy with cyclosporine or tacrolimus, maintenance therapy with 6-MP and azathioprine should be considered. Infliximab or adalimumab is effective for maintaining remission and as a steroid-sparing agent.

Emergency surgery is indicated for patients with life-threatening complications such as perforation, refractory rectal bleeding or toxic megacolon, and for patients not responding to medical therapies. The risk of developing colorectal cancer (CRC) is greater for both UC and CD patients than for the average population.

The clinical course of IBD during pregnancy is correlated with the level of disease activity at the time of conception.

Recommended reading

Abraham C, Cho JH. Inflammatory bowel disease. *N Engl J Med*. 2009; 361(21):2066–78.

Kornbluth A, Sachar DB, American College of Gastroenterology, Practice Parameters Committee. Ulcerative colitis practice guidelines in adults. *Am J Gastroenterol*. 2010; 105:501–23. doi:10.1038/ajg.2009.727. Erratum: *Am J Gastroenterol*. 2010; 105:500. doi:10.1038/ajg.2010.52.

Lakatos PL. Recent trends in the epidemiology of inflammatory bowel diseases: up or down? *Am J Gastroenterol*. 2008 Dec; 103(12):3167–82.

Nikolaus S, Schreiber S. Diagnostics of inflammatory bowel disease. *Gastroenterology*. 2007; 133:1670–89.

Ooi CJ, Fock K, Makharia G, Goh K, Ling K, Hilmi I, Lim W, Kelvin T, Gibson P, Gearry R, Ouyang Q, Sollano J, Manatsathit S, Rerknimitr R, Wei S, Leung W, de Silva H, Leong R. The Asia–Pacific consensus on ulcerative colitis. Asia–Pacific Association of Inflammatory Bowel Disease. *J Gastroenterol Hepatol*. 2010 Mar; 25(3):453–68.

Stange EF, Travis SPL, Vermeire S, Reinisch W, Geboes K, Barakauskiene A, Feakins, Fléjou JF, Herfarth H, Hommes DW, Kupcinskas L, Lakatos PL, Mantzaris GJ, Schreiber S, Villanacci V, Warren BF, European Crohn's and Colitis Organisation (ECCO). European evidence-based consensus on the diagnosis and management of ulcerative colitis: definitions and diagnosis. *J Crohns Colitis*. 2008; 2:1–23.

Thia KT, Loftus EV Jr, Sandborn WJ, Yang SK. An update on the epidemiology of inflammatory bowel diseases in Asia. *Am J Gastroenterol*. 2008 Dec; 103(12):3167–82.

Travis SPL, Stange EF, Lémann M, Øresland T, Bemelman WA, Chowers Y, Colombel JF, D'Haens G, Ghosh S, Marteau P, Kruis W, Mortensen NJMcC, Penninckx F, Gassull M, European Crohn's and Colitis Organisation (ECCO). European evidence-based consensus on the management of ulcerative colitis: current management. *J Crohns Colitis*. 2008; 2:24–62.

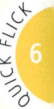
QUICK FLICK
6

Chapter 7: Changing patterns of inflammatory bowel disease in a global context (Crohn's disease)

K. Thia, C. Ooi (Singapore)

Key points

▶ The incidence of Crohn's disease (CD) is on an upward trend worldwide, even in Western countries where the incidence of ulcerative colitis (UC) is stable.

▶ Distinguishing CD from tuberculosis (TB) remains challenging. A high index of suspicion coupled with polymerase chain reaction (PCR) tissue testing for TB can expedite diagnosis and management.

▶ Wireless capsule endoscopy and small bowel enterosopic methods have improved the diagnosis of small bowel CD.

▶ Treatment strategies for CD are based on clinical activity, location, disease behaviour and patient preference, mainly in accordance with evidence from Western studies.

▶ The expense of anti-tumour necrosis factor (TNF) monoclonal antibodies limits their use in many developing countries.

○ Introduction

This chapter contains a concise overview of the epidemiology, clinical phenotypes and therapeutic options available for the treatment of Crohn's disease from a global perspective, with discussion of recent developments in small bowel imaging, enteroscopy and serological markers, and their specific roles in distinguishing it from ulcerative colitis.

The importance of differentiating between CD and gastrointestinal TB is covered in Chapter 10.

○ Definitions and classification

CD is characterised by patchy, transmural inflammation which may affect any part of the gastrointestinal tract. It is classified according to the disease location (terminal ileum, colonic, ileocolonic and upper gastrointestinal sites of involvement) and the pattern of disease (inflammatory, stricturing or penetrating).

Descriptive epidemiology

Evidence indicates that the incidence of CD is rising in many Western countries, unlike UC, which appears to be stable. Worldwide, the incidence rate of CD ranges between 0.1 and 16 per 100 000 inhabitants; however, the rate is increasing in some South American countries (Brazil, Chile and Puerto Rico), and also in Asian countries including Japan, Hong Kong, India and Korea. The prevalence of CD worldwide varies substantially from 2 to 350 per 100 000 persons. The Asian CD patient population is predominantly male, unlike Western CD populations which demonstrate equal gender distribution or a moderate female predominance. The peak age of CD diagnosis among both Asian and Caucasian patients lies between 20 and 30 years.

In many developing countries such as India, it has been suggested that improvements in sanitation and hygiene—with the disappearance of helminths coinciding with the emergence of IBD—have caused the increased numbers of diagnosed CD cases over the past decade.

Clinical features and disease course

The symptoms of CD vary considerably, often influenced by the site of disease but typically presenting with abdominal pain, diarrhoea and weight loss. More acute presentations may occur, and acute terminal ileitis secondary to CD may mimic the symptoms of acute appendicitis. Systemic symptoms such as fever, poor appetite and malaise are more frequently reported by CD compared to UC patients. Blood and/or mucus in stools are seen less frequently in CD colitis (40–50%) than in UC. About 5–10 per cent of CD patients have stomach and duodenal involvement. Perianal fistulas are present in 10 per cent of patients at the time of diagnosis and may be the only presenting complaint. Associated extraintestinal features include spondyloarthritis, peripheral arthritis, cutaneous manifestations and ocular inflammation (see Table 7.1 overleaf).

Based on the Vienna classification, CD at the time of diagnosis is confined to the terminal ileum in 47 per cent of cases, to the colon in 28 per cent, the ileum and colon in 21 per cent and the upper gastrointestinal tract in 3 per cent. There is considerable heterogeneity in the distribution of disease location reported worldwide. Among Asian CD patients, combined small bowel and colon involvement predominates at diagnosis. A more complicated course of CD may be predicted by baseline factors at diagnosis such as young age (<40 years), ileal involvement, perianal disease and early corticosteroid use. CD patients presenting with poor prognostic factors may be candidates for early immunosuppressive therapy.

After the first year of diagnosis, 10–30 per cent of cases will have an exacerbation, 15–25 per cent will have low activity, and 55–65 per cent will be in remission. In 70 per cent of CD patients at diagnosis, disease behaviour is purely inflammatory, stricturing in 17 per cent and penetrating

Table 7.1 Differentiation of ulcerative colitis and Crohn's disease

	Ulcerative colitis (CD)	Crohn's disease (CD)
Clinical features		
Haematochezia	Common	Occasional
Passage of mucus or pus	Common	Occasional (consider rectal/perianal disease)
Small bowel involvement	No (unless backwash ileitis)	Yes
Upper gastrointestinal tract	No	Yes
Abdominal mass	Uncommon (left lower quadrant if inflamed sigmoid)	Right lower quadrant
Fistula or abscess	No	Common
Perianal disease	Uncommon	Common
Smoking history	Non-smoker/recent cessation	Common
Laboratory features		
Anti-neutrophil cytoplasmic antibodies (ANCA)	Common	Uncommon (usually in isolated colonic CD)
Anti-saccharomyces cerevisiae antibodies (ASCA)	Uncommon	Common
Endoscopic features		
Rectal involvement	Always	30–50%
Morphology of ulcers	Usually shallow, extensive	Deep, longitudinal
Strictures	Rare, consider carcinoma	Occasional
Skipped inflammation	Uncommon (consider partially treated UC)	Common
Pathologic features		
Transmural mucosal inflammation	No	Yes
Creeping fat	No	Yes
Granulomas	No	Less common (up to 50%)
Fissures and skip lesions	Rare	Common

(fistula, abscess or both) in 13 per cent. Many studies point to an inexorable progression towards either a stricturing and/or penetrating phenotype with time. A similar evolution of CD behaviour has also been described among Chinese CD patients in Hong Kong. The lifetime risk of surgery for CD patients is 70–80 per cent, with a slightly decreased life expectancy. The surgical rates of CD patients in Asia vary considerably and further studies are needed to better understand the reasons for these differences.

Specific diagnostic issues in CD

UC diagnosis is supported by confluent inflammation seen on sigmoidoscopy and/or colonoscopy, whereas CD diagnosis is based on focal, asymmetric and often granulomatous inflammation. Granulomas are present in up to 50 per cent of patients. In about 10–15 per cent of patients with IBD (in the absence of distinctive features), it can be challenging in the setting of exclusive colonic involvement to confirm CD or UC. Such patients should be observed for diagnostic features that would distinguish the IBD subtypes over a period of time, and should be re-evaluated if clinically indicated by progressive symptoms or presence of complications (see Chapter 6, Table 6.1).

In 10 per cent of patients, CD affects the ileum beyond the reach of the endoscope, or affects only the proximal small bowel, and may present with stricturing and/or penetrating complications. Both computed tomography (CT) and magnetic resonance (MR) enterography are levels of radiological imaging for CD that can establish small bowel disease extent and activity based on wall thickness and contrast enhancement, and detect bowel strictures, abscesses and fistulas. CT is the more widely available technique, and is cheaper and less time-consuming than MRI—but considering the need for repeated abdominal imaging among young CD patients throughout the course of their disease, MRI would be preferred, if available, in order to minimise radiation exposure. Small bowel barium studies are still used in countries with limited resources.

Wireless capsule endoscopy (WCE) provides improved visualisation of the small bowel and is non-invasive; however, an appreciable capsule retention rate (up to 15 per cent) has been reported among known and suspected CD cases that have been evaluated with WCE. At present, WCE should be reserved for patients with high clinical suspicion for CD in spite of negative ileocolonoscopy and radiological examinations. WCE may be overly sensitive in cases of suspected CD, as 10 per cent of healthy subjects have clinically irrelevant mucosal breaks and erosions in the small intestine.

Small bowel enteroscopic techniques such as balloon-assisted enteroscopy allow deeper access into the small intestine for histological evaluation and may occasionally play interventional roles such as stricture dilatation; however, the risks involved with small bowel enteroscopy—prolonged sedation time, and perforation risks associated with adhesions in CD patients, for instance—need to be appreciated.

QUICK FLICK

7

Antibodies directed against certain microbial antigens have also been developed into serological tests that can be useful in distinguishing CD from UC, but they are not sufficiently sensitive nor specific enough to be used as screening tools (Table 7.2). Recent evidence suggests that the number and magnitude of CD-related immune markers may be associated with a greater severity of disease.

Table 7.2 Prevalence of serological markers of inflammatory bowel disease (IBD)

Serological marker	Crohn's disease	Ulcerative colitis	Healthy control	Sensitivity	Specificity
ASCA (anti-saccharomyces cerevisiae antibodies)	50–60%	5–15%	0–5%	50–60%	80–85%
ANCA (anti-neutrophil cytoplasmic antibodies)	6–20%	50–70%	0–2.5%	65–70%	80–85%
Anti-OmpC (*Escherichia coli* outer membrane porin C)	20–55%	10%	5%	20–55%	88.5%
Anti-I2 (*Pseudomonas fluorescens*-related sequences I2)	54%	10%	4%	42%	76%
Anti-CBir (flagellin)	50%	<5%	8%	–	–

Source: Adapted from Peyrin-Biroulet et al. IBD serological panels: facts and perspective. *Inflamm Bowel Dis.* 2007; 13:1561–6.

▷ Management of CD: induction of response and remission

The management plan for the CD patient should always take into account the clinical activity, site and behaviour of the disease.

Assessment of CD activity

Disease activity in CD patients can be defined using a practical assessment method:

- mild to moderate (ambulatory patients able to tolerate oral alimentation without dehydration, toxicity or abdominal tenderness, painful abdominal mass, obstruction, or more than 10 per cent weight loss)
- moderate to severe (failure to respond to mild disease therapy, more prominent symptoms of fever, weight loss, abdominal pain or tenderness, intermittent nausea and vomiting without obstruction, or significant anaemia)
- severe to fulminant (persisting symptoms on corticosteroids, high fevers, persistent vomiting, evidence of intestinal obstruction, rebound tenderness, cachexia or evidence of abscess).

Mild to moderate disease

Among CD patients with mild to moderate activity, ileal, ileocolonic and colonic involvement has traditionally been treated with oral mesalamine or sulfasalazine for ileocolonic or colonic disease in divided doses. Despite the widespread use of mesalamine, current evidence suggests that it is only minimally effective. Alternatively, antibiotics such as metronidazole or ciprofloxacin can be considered for patients with ileocolonic or colonic involvement, but who are not responding to sulphasalazine.

Controlled ileal release budesonide has better short-term efficacy than mesalamine, sulphasalazine or antibiotics in treating active disease confined to the ileum and/or right colon. Anti-tuberculous therapy has not been efficacious for either induction or maintenance of remission among CD patients (see Figure 7.1 overleaf).

Moderate to severe disease

For CD patients with moderate to severe disease, oral prednisolone is used to induce remission, then tapered off gradually when symptoms resolve. If intra-abdominal abscesses are present, appropriate antibiotic treatment is usually required together with percutaneous or surgical drainage. Elemental diet, which has poor palatability, is less effective than corticosteroids but can help avoid corticosteroid-related treatment toxicities.

Azathioprine and 6-MP (thiopurines) are effective in maintaining a steroid-induced remission, and parenteral methotrexate is effective for steroid-dependent and steroid-refractory CD. The anti-TNF monoclonal antibodies infliximab, adalimumab and certolizumab pegol are all effective for treating moderate to severely active CD when corticosteroids or immunosuppressive agents have failed. Infliximab monotherapy and infliximab combined with azathioprine are more effective than azathioprine alone for treating patients with moderate to severe CD for whom first-line therapy with mesalamine and/or corticosteroids has failed. The use of anti-TNF monoclonal antibodies is associated with TB reactivation and therefore all patients should be carefully screened for latent TB before starting anti-TNF therapy (history of exposure, chest radiology, tuberculin skin test, interferon (IFN) gamma release assays).

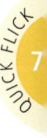

Extensive small bowel CD represents a more severe disease phenotype and should be treated with systemic corticosteroids and early immunosuppressive therapy such as thiopurines or methotrexate. Oesophageal and gastroduodenal CD can be treated with proton pump inhibitor (PPI) and, if necessary, systemic corticosteroids with thiopurines or methotrexate. In either situation, patients with moderate to severe disease who relapse have a lowered threshold for the use of anti-TNF monoclonal antibodies. Adjunctive nutritional support can be helpful, and surgical options such as bowel resection, strictureplasty and dilatation should be considered for obstructive symptoms.

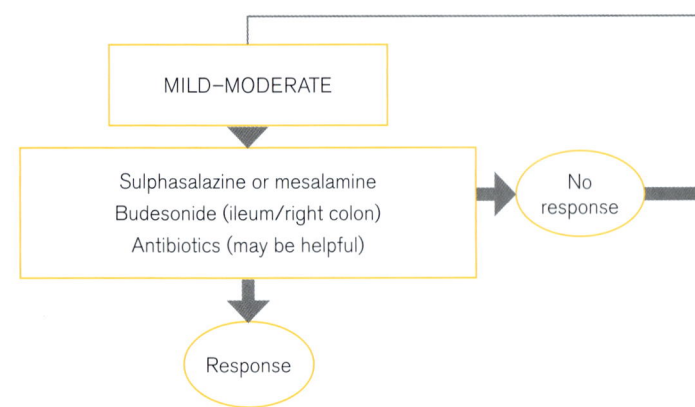

Figure 7.1 Medical therapy of Crohn's disease (CD)

The anti-alpha4 integrin antibody natalizumab is also effective in treating patients with moderate to severely active CD who are refractory to conventional CD therapies and anti-TNF monoclonal antibody therapy; however, natalizumab is associated with reactivation of JC polyomavirus and lethal progressive multifocal leukoencephalopathy (PML). As a result, natalizumab has very restricted use in CD, and enrolment in a drug safety monitoring program is mandatory for such patients.

Severe to fulminant disease
Patients should be hospitalised if their symptoms persist despite systemic corticosteroids or anti-TNF monoclonal antibody therapy, or if they present with high fever, frequent vomiting and evidence of intestinal obstruction or abscess. Surgical consult is necessary for patients with intestinal obstruction or with a tender abdominal mass. General supportive measures as for severe colitis should be instituted (see Chapter 6, Table 6.7).

The more severely ill patients with malnutrition and/or anticipated prolonged bowel rest should be supported with parenteral nutrition. Parenteral corticosteroids are indicated for severe to fulminant CD after

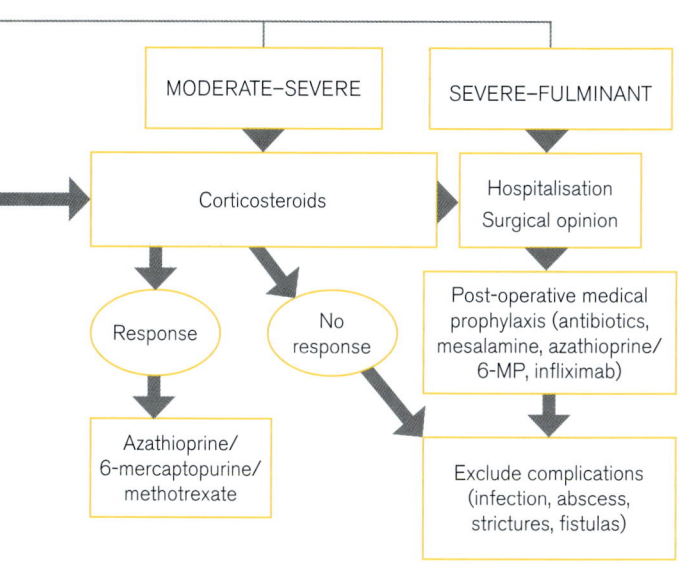

abscess has been excluded, and parenteral cyclosporine or tacrolimus may be effective in patients who do not respond to intravenous corticosteroids.

There is insufficient data to recommend the use of anti-TNF agents in the treatment of severe to fulminant CD. Failure to respond to medical therapies or worsening symptoms are reasons for surgical intervention.

Special considerations

In many developing countries, access to biological therapies such as anti-TNF monoclonal antibodies is limited and, due to cost, are infrequently used as first-line treatment or for regular maintenance therapy. Treatment options and recommendations for IBD patients should therefore take into consideration issues of local access and constraints on resources.

Patients on immunosuppressive therapies should be actively screened for opportunistic infection and, if necessary, advice sought from a specialist in infectious diseases.

The long-term use of combinational azathioprine/6-mercaptopurine and anti-TNF therapy is best avoided in young people because of the risk of hepatosplenic T-cell lymphoma.

QUICK FLICK

7

◐ Management of CD: maintenance of remission

Budesonide maintenance therapy appears to be effective for up to six months of usage in preventing relapses in ileal and/or right colon disease. Smoking should be discouraged in all CD patients. Sulphasalazine and mesalamine are not consistently effective in maintaining remission among CD patients after medical inductive treatment. Corticosteroids should not be used as long-term therapy to prevent relapses in view of toxicity in colonic CD. Azathioprine/6-MP and methotrexate are the most commonly used agents for maintenance therapy after control of acute disease with corticosteroids. The use of omega-3 fatty acids and probiotics remains controversial due to inconsistent efficacy data.

After achieving remission with an anti-TNF agent, maintenance with regular anti-TNF therapy is appropriate; however, in many resource-limited countries, maintenance anti-TNF therapy is not affordable for many patients. Infliximab monotherapy and infliximab combinational therapy with azathioprine are more effective than azathioprine for keeping moderate to severe CD patients in remission. Maintenance therapy with natalizumab is also effective. Following ileocolonic resection, metronidazole, mesalamine, azathioprine/6-MP or infliximab may prevent clinical and endoscopic relapses (post-operative prophylaxis).

Penetrating complications

Perianal abscesses and fistulas can occur in up to one-third of CD patients. Acute suppuration is an indication for surgical drainage with or without insertion of non-cutting setons. Fistulectomy and the use of advancement flaps in combination with medical therapy may be appropriate for persistent and complex fistulas. Non-suppurative, chronic fistulisation or perianal fissuring disease can be treated with antibiotics; long-term therapy of more than six months is often required. Such patients should be monitored for adverse drug effects. Other medical options include thiopurines, methotrexate or infliximab.

Surgcal management of CD

Surgical resection may be a reasonable option in moderate to severe ileocaecal disease failing to respond to initial immunosuppressive therapy. Where the expertise is available, a laparoscopic approach is preferred for ileocaecal resection because of early post-operative recovery and reduced morbidity. For intestinal complications or medical refractory disease, surgical resection, stricturoplasty or drainage of abscesses may be indicated.

Surgical intervention is also necessary for as many as two-thirds of CD patients to treat intractable haemorrhage, perforation, persisting or recurrent obstruction, abscesses not amenable to percutaneous drainage, dysplasia and cancer, and unresponsive fulminant disease. Patients who have active luminal disease and whose condition does not improve within seven to ten days of intensive inpatient medical therapy should be considered for surgery.

Summary

The incidence of CD appears to be on the increase in many Western countries, in South American countries such as Brazil, Chile, Puerto Rico, and in Asian countries such as Japan, Hong Kong, India and Korea. Unlike Western CD populations that demonstrate equal gender distribution or a moderate female predominance, there is a male predominance in Asian CD patients.

At the time of diagnosis CD is confined to the terminal ileum in 47 per cent of patients, the colon in 28 per cent, the ileum and colon in 21 per cent and the upper gastrointestinal tract in 3 per cent. There is considerable heterogeneity in the distribution of CD. Among Asian CD patients, combined small bowel and colon involvement predominates at diagnosis. Within the first year following diagnosis, the disease will have an exacerbated in 10–30 per cent of patients, 15–25 per cent will have low activity, and 55–65 per cent will be in remission.

Computed tomography (CT) and magnetic resonance (MR) enterography are standard radiological imaging techniques for CD, MRI being the preferred method for young CD patients in order to minimise radiation exposure. Small bowel barium studies are still used in resource-limited countries.

Non-invasive wireless capsule endoscopy (WCE) provides improved images of the small bowel. Small bowel enteroscopic techniques such as balloon-assisted enteroscopy allow deeper access into the small intestine for histological evaluation, and have occasional interventional roles such as stricture dilatation. Antibodies directed against certain microbial antigens have also been developed into serological tests which can be useful in distinguishing CD from UC, but they are not sufficiently sensitive or specific to be used as screening tools. The management plan for the CD patient should always take into account the clinical activity, site and behaviour of the disease.

Budesonide maintenance therapy appears to be effective for up to six months of use in preventing relapses in ileal and/or right colon disease. Smoking should be discouraged in all CD patients. Sulphasalazine and mesalamine are not consistently effective in maintaining remission among CD patients after medical inductive treatment. Corticosteroids should not be used as long-term therapy to prevent relapses in view of toxicity in colonic CD. Azathioprine/6-MP and methotrexate are the most commonly used agents for maintenance therapy after control of acute disease with corticosteroids. After achieving remission with an anti-TNF agent, maintenance with regular anti-TNF therapy is appropriate.

Surgical resection may be a reasonable option in moderate to severe ileocaecal disease when initial immunosuppressive therapy proves to be ineffective. A laparoscopic approach is preferred for ileocaecal resections.

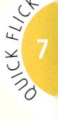

QUICK FLICK

7

For intestinal complications or medical refractory disease, surgical resection, stricturoplasty or abscess drainage may be indicated. Surgical intervention is also necessary in up to two-thirds of CD patients in order to treat intractable haemorrhage, perforation, persisting or recurrent obstruction, abscesses not amenable to percutaneous drainage, dysplasia and cancer and unresponsive fulminant disease.

Recommended reading

Abraham C, Cho JL. Inflammatory bowel disease. *N Engl J Med*. 2009; 361(21):2066–78.

Almadi MA, Ghosh S, Aljebreen AM. Differentiating intestinal tuberculosis from Crohn's disease: a diagnostic challenge. *Am J Gastroenterol*. 2009; 104:1003–12.

Amarapurkar DN, Patel ND, Rane PS. Diagnosis of Crohn's disease in India where tuberculosis is widely prevalent. *World J Gastroenterol*. 2008: 14(5):741–6.

Baumgart DC, Sandborn WJ. Inflammatory bowel disease: clinical aspects and established and evolving therapies. *Lancet*. 2007; 369(9573):1641–57.

Desai HG, Gupte PA. Increasing incidence of Crohn's disease in India: is it related to improved sanitation?. *Indian J Gastroenterol*. 2005: 24:23–4.

Lichtenstein, GR, Hanauer, SB, Sandborn, WJ, Practice Parameters Committee of American College of Gastroenterology. Management of Crohn's disease in adults. *Am J Gastroenterol*. 2009; 104:465.

Nikolaus S, Schreiber S. Diagnostics of inflammatory bowel disease. *Gastroenterology*. 2007; 133:1670–89.

Stange EF, Schreiber W, Schölmerich J, Reinisch W, Barakauskiene A, Villanacci V, Von Herbay A, Warren BF, Gasche C, Tilg H, Travis SSPL, Vermeire S, Beglinger C, Kupcinkas L, Geboes K, for the European Crohn's and Colitis Organisation (ECCO). European evidence-based consensus on the diagnosis and management of Crohn's disease: definitions and diagnosis. *Gut*. 2006; 55:1–15.

Travis SPL, Strange EF, Lémann M, Öresland T, Chowers Y, Forbes A, D'Haens G, Kitis G, Cortot A, Prantera C, Marteau P, Colombel J-F, Gionchetti P, Bouhnik Y, Tiret E, Kroesen J, Starlinger M, Mortensen NJ for the European Crohn's and Colitis Organisation (ECCO). European evidence based consensus on the diagnosis and management of Crohn's disease: current management. *Gut*. 2006; 55:16–35. doi:10.1136/gut.2005.081950b.

Chapter 8: Constipation

R. Agrawal, R. Toney (USA)

Key points

▶ Constipation is the most commonly occurring digestive problem in the general population.

▶ It is most prevalent in the United States, France, Brazil and South Korea, and least prevalent in Germany, the United Kingdom and Italy.

▶ In the West, it occurs most commonly in women and people of low income and poor education. In India, by contrast, constipation is more prevalent in men.

▶ Constipation can adversely affect quality of life and lead to increased health-related costs.

▶ It is diagnosed by obtaining a careful medical history and performing a detailed physical examination.

▶ Laboratory testing, imaging, and/or endoscopic evaluation are indicated only for patients with symptoms suggestive of a secondary cause.

▶ Treatment starts with a stepwise increase in dietary fibre and/or the introduction of osmotic laxatives.

▶ If initial therapies are unsuccessful, specialised testing may be necessary to rule out types of constipation that could be amenable to biofeedback. Surgical management may be indicated as a last resort.

▷ Introduction

Constipation is the most common digestive complaint in the general population. It is broadly defined as infrequent bowel movements—fewer than three per week—or movements that are painful or difficult to evacuate. Because constipation is generally a subjective interpretation, however, prevalence estimates vary between 12 and 19 per cent. One international survey found the prevalence to be 12.3 per cent in the general population, with the lowest reported incidence (5%–10%) for Germany, the United Kingdom and Italy, and the highest (10%–20%) reported in the United States, France, Brazil and South Korea. In general, the prevalence of constipation has not been well studied among the Asian population. Importantly, it may not be feasible to use the Western definition of constipation (<3 times per week) everywhere in the world: for example, an epidemiological study of patients with irritable bowel syndrome (IBS), conducted in India by the Indian Society of Gastroenterology Task Force, found that most subjects passed stools once or twice a day. In the Western population, by comparison, three or more bowel movements per week is considered normal.

While the prevalence of this disorder differs around the world, it is generally accepted, at least among the Western population, that constipation is more common in women than in men, in people older than 65, and in people with little daily physical activity, low income or poor education. Notably, constipation in India is more prevalent in men than in women.

The definition of constipation varies widely because patients have a tendency to focus on the symptoms associated with the disorder, while physicians focus more on stool frequency. Criteria have been developed in an effort to standardise the definition, with the most recent being the Rome III criteria described in Table 8.1 (see also Tables 5.2 and 5.3, Chapter 5). While these criteria are mainly used for research, they can also aid diagnosis in clinical practice. In brief: in order to meet the criteria for chronic constipation, a patient must have experienced at least two of the symptoms outlined in Table 8.1 for three months or more, with symptoms beginning not less than six months before the condition is diagnosed. In addition, patients should rarely have had loose stools unless the use of laxatives is documented. Furthermore, patients should not meet the criteria for IBS. The indicator of IBS-constipation predominant (IBS-C) is abdominal pain relieved by defecation.

Table 8.1 Rome III criteria for constipation and irritable bowel syndrome-constipation predominant (IBS-C)

Constipation	IBS-C
1. At least 2 of the following symptoms present for 3 months or more, with onset at least 6 months prior to diagnosis: • straining* • lumpy or hard stools* • sensation of incomplete evacuation* • sensation of anorectal obstruction/blockage* • manual manoeuvres to facilitate defecation (e.g. digital evacuation, support of the pelvic floor)* • fewer than 3 bowel movements per week 2. Loose stools rarely present without the use of laxatives 3. Insufficient criteria for IBS-C	Symptoms at least 3 days/month for the 3 months before diagnosis: 1. IBS-recurrent abdominal pain/discomfort associated with at least 2 of the following: • improvement with defecation • onset associated with change in stool frequency • onset associated with change in stool form 2. IBS-C: hard or lumpy stools ≥25% of defecations; loose or watery stools <25% of defecations without the use of laxatives

*   For at least 25 per cent of bowel movements.

In general, constipation is categorised as either 'primary' or 'secondary' (Table 8.2):

- if no cause can be identified, it is classified as primary or idiopathic constipation, which is subdivided into normal transit, slow transit or disorders of defecatory or rectal evacuation
- if the underlying reason can be found, it is termed secondary constipation.

Normal transit constipation is also referred to as functional constipation. In this subtype, patients believe they are constipated, but stool traverses at a normal rate through the colon, and stool frequency is normal. Patients may complain of hard stools, abdominal bloating or discomfort, and they may experience psychological distress regarding their symptoms. Many will respond to the addition of fibre to their diet or to an osmotic laxative.

Table 8.2 Causes of chronic constipation

Primary or idiopathic constipation	Secondary constipation		
	Neurogenic disorders	Non-neurogenic disorders	Drugs

Normal colonic transit
Slow transit
Dyssynergic defecation
	Peripheral
	Diabetes mellitus
	Autonomic neuropathy
	Hirschsprung disease
	Chagas disease
	Intestinal pseudo-obstruction
	Central
	Multiple sclerosis
	Spinal cord injury
	Parkinson's disease
		Hypothyroidism
		Hypokalaemia
		Anorexia nervosa
		Pregnancy
		Panhypopituitarism
		Systemic sclerosis
		Myotonic dystrophy
			Analgesics
			  NSAIDs
			Anticholinergics
			  antihistamines
			  antispasmodics
			  antidepressants
			  antipsychotics
			Cation-containing drugs
			  iron supplements
			  aluminium
			Neurally active drugs
			  opiates
			  antihypertensives
			  ganglionic blockers
			  vinca alkaloids
			  5-HT$_3$ antagonists

QUICK FLICK

8

Slow transit constipation refers to decreased colonic transit time leading to infrequent stools, often only once a week. Unlike normal transit constipation, it does not respond to fibre supplementation or laxatives because it is the result of decreased contractility of the colon. The pathophysiology is not well understood, but studies have shown decreased numbers of interstitial cells of Cajal that are thought to regulate gastrointestinal motility. Other studies have found abnormalities in the expression of excitatory and inhibitory neurotransmitters in myenteric plexus neurons. Hirschsprung's disease is considered to be a form of slow-transit constipation, as there are no ganglion cells in the distal bowel, causing bowel narrowing at the aganglionic segment. Patients may be asymptomatic until adulthood because only a short segment of bowel is involved.

Disorders of defecatory or rectal evacuation are also referred to as pelvic floor dyssynergia, obstructed defecation, outlet obstruction and anismus. These are usually due to dysfunction of the pelvic floor or anal sphincter. The defecatory mechanism is an intricately coordinated set of events that is best understood by appreciating the anatomy of the anorectum (Figure 8.1). Continence is maintained by contraction of the internal and external anal sphincters as well as the puborectalis muscle, which wraps around the anorectum causing the anorectal angle to be between 80° and 110°. During defecation, the puborectalis muscle relaxes, which allows the anorectal angle to straighten and descends the perineum 1.0–3.5 cm. This, combined with relaxation of the external anal sphincter, results in successful defecation. Any anatomical or neurological disorder can disrupt this process and lead to obstructed defecation which, if left untreated, could lead to megacolon or megarectum from chronic faecal retention.

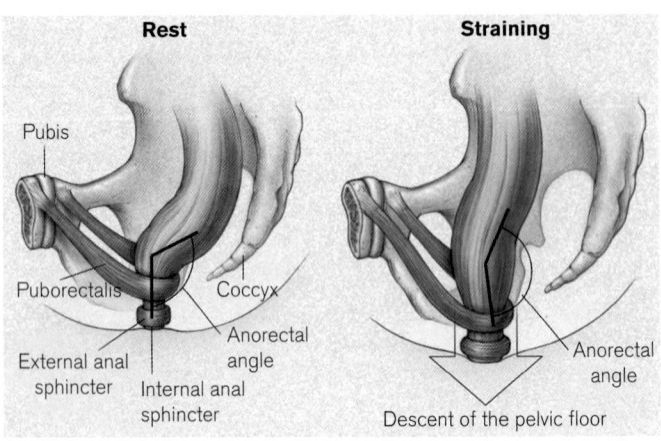

Figure 8.1 Pelvic floor anatomy during rest and straining

Source: Lembo A, Camilleri M. *N Engl J Med.* 2003;349:1360–1368.

These types of constipation can often be identified by performing a detailed history and physical examination. However, they can often overlap and will therefore require more than one treatment modality.

Diagnosis

The diagnosis of constipation requires a detailed history and physical examination. Questions regarding the duration of symptoms and any recent changes in bowel habits should be asked. Stool frequency, stool consistency, along with the presence or absence of pain or straining during defecation, should also be determined. Associated symptoms of abdominal bloating or discomfort, or the sensation of an abdominal mass, may also suggest the diagnosis. A comprehensive list of the patient's prescribed and over-the-counter medications should be obtained, and it should be confirmed whether their use preceded the symptoms of constipation. Obtaining a dietary history to assess the amount of fluid and fibre intake is informative, and it is important to know if the patient uses laxatives or manual manoeuvres in order to successfully defecate. Of note, if a patient reports several days without stools and then subsequently has loose stools, this may indicate constipation with overflow diarrhoea. An important question to ask patients is whether they have faecal incontinence, as some patients may not volunteer this information due to the embarrassing nature of this complaint. Incontinence may suggest faecal impaction. A gynaecological history should also be obtained, since weakened pelvic floor muscles from childbirth can be a contributing factor to constipation in some patients. Finally, it is important to note whether the patient is devoting enough time to bowel function, as some patients may ignore signals to defecate.

The physical examination should include a digital rectal examination, with the patient placed in the left lateral decubitus position. It should begin with an examination of the perineum to rule out anal fissures, external haemorrhoids, fistulas or scars. The anocutaneous reflex should be assessed by stroking the perineal skin with a cotton swab. An absence of reflex suggests neuropathy. The degree of perineal descent during simulated defecation should be observed. Reduced descent suggests inability to relax the pelvic floor, while excessive descent suggests laxity, both of which can lead to incomplete evacuation. On digital examination, the resting tone of the external anal sphincter should be assessed in addition to the degree of increased tone during a squeeze. If palpation of the puborectalis muscle, situated above the internal anal sphincter, elicits pain, spasm should be suspected. Finally, the patient should be asked to expel the examining finger with valsalva.

If there an underlying disorder is suspected, a complete blood count, basic metabolic panel with serum calcium, and thyroid function testing should be carried out. Alarm signs or symptoms (family history of inflammatory bowel disease or colon cancer, age over 50 years, sudden change in stool calibre, anaemia, weight loss or rectal bleeding) necessitate further investigation to rule out colon cancer as a structural cause for constipation. This can be performed with a referral either for colonoscopy or a barium enema.

Specialised testing to determine the type of primary constipation should be carried out only if first-line therapies prove ineffective, or if the history and physical examination suggest a disorder. Some tests are also useful for identifying good candidates for biofeedback or surgical management: these include balloon expulsion, defecography, anorectal manometry and colonic transit studies. Balloon expulsion is a simple screening test used to rule out pelvic floor dysfunction, by assessing if a patient can expel a balloon filled with 50 mL of warm water within three minutes. Defecography, for ruling out structural abnormalities, involves instilling 150 mL of thickened barium into the rectum and taking radiographs while the patient simulates defecation, allowing the anorectal angle and perineal descent to be measured.

Anorectal manometry and colonic transit study are described in Table 8.3. The results of these tests may be limited depending on the patient's level of cooperation, and no single test can adequately define pathophysiology.

Table 8.3 Specialised testing modalities for constipation

Testing modality	Description	Interpretation of results
Colonic transit study	24 radiopaque markers are ingested then a plain radiograph is taken on day 6 (120 hours later)	1. Normal transit: <5 markers remain in colon 2. Slow transit: >5 markers are scattered throughout the colon 3. Pelvic floor dyssynergia: >5 markers in rectosigmoid with near-normal transit in the remaining colon
Anorectal manometry	Measures: 1. Internal anal sphincter pressure at rest 2. External anal sphincter pressure at maximal voluntary contraction 3. The anorectal inhibitory reflex (relaxation of the internal anal sphincter during balloon distension) 4. Rectal sensation 5. Ability of the anal sphincters to relax during straining	1. Pelvic floor dyssynergia: inappropriate contraction of the anal sphincter at rest and while bearing down 2. Hirschsprung's disease: absent anorectal inhibitory reflex[*] 3. Anal fissure or anismus: high anal pressure at rest and rectal pain 4. Rectal hyposensitivity: suggested by an increased balloon volume distension required to induce urgency

[*] Most often seen in patients with enlargement of the rectum from retained stool and therefore insufficient distension of the rectal wall by the balloon.

○ Treatment

After secondary causes are excluded, successful treatment of constipation requires an algorithmic approach using patient response as an indication to increase pharmacologic therapy or to perform specialised testing (see Figure 8.2 overleaf). Initial management includes advising the patient to maintain adequate hydration and to engage in regular non-strenuous exercise. These measures assist with patients who are dehydrated, but there is little evidence that they successfully treat constipation in all patients. Patients should also be encouraged to establish a regular pattern of bowel movement that takes advantage of the times when the colon is most active—after waking, and also after a meal, the latter being due to the gastrocolonic reflex.

First-line therapy includes gradually increasing dietary fibre by 5 grams/day up to a total of 20–35 grams/day. A high-fibre diet increases stool weight and accelerates colonic transit. If a patient elects not to modify their diet, fibre supplementation can be used instead. They should be aware that bloating or flatulence can occur, but this will decrease over time. Results will not be immediate, so this regimen should be adhered to for several weeks. Note that patients with slow-transit constipation or dyssynergic defecation will not respond to fibre therapy.

If increasing dietary fibre is unsuccessful, medications should be initiated (see Table 8.4, pages 84–7). Available evidence supports using an osmotic laxative to begin with. These include polyethylene glycol (PEG), saline laxatives such as milk of magnesia, and non-absorbable sugars such as sorbitol or lactulose. The dose should be titrated until stools are soft, and the patient should be advised that it will take several days before the medication provides relief. PEG is slightly more effective than lactulose and has fewer bloating and flatulence side effects, since it is an inert substance and therefore not degraded by colonic bacteria. In addition, PEG is more cost-effective than lactulose despite being more expensive, according to a decision analysis model developed by the National Health Service of the United Kingdom. Studies carried out over a six-month period have indicated that PEG appears also to be safe for long-term use. Note that laxatives containing magnesium should be avoided in patients with cardiac dysfunction or renal insufficiency.

Stimulant laxatives such as senna and bisacodyl should be added only if patients do not respond to osmotic laxatives. Anthraquinone derivatives taken chronically can lead to pigmentation of the colon called melanosis coli. This condition does not lead to colon cancer and decreases over time once the laxative is discontinued. Concerns for cathartic colon using stimulant laxatives are not supported by the available data. All therapy should be titrated to the least expensive and most effective maintenance dose, with enemas, suppositories and stimulant laxatives used as needed for rescue

QUICK FLICK

8

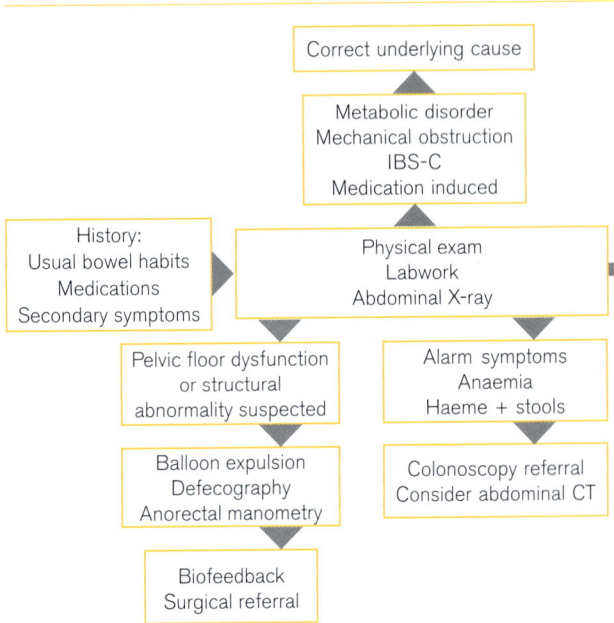

Figure 8.2 Overview for diagnosis and treatment of constipation

Table 8.4 Medications for constipation

Laxative	Adult dosing	Onset of action	Comments
Bulk forming: Increase retention of fluid in the stool leading to softer consistency, increased stool volume and increased GI motility			
Psyllium	Up to 20 g/day	12–72 h	Initial treatment option
Methylcellulose	Up to 20 g/day	12–72 h	Can be used daily
Calcium polycarbophil	2–4 tabs/day	24–48 h	Can cause bloating, flatulence and abdominal pain; take with water to avoid obstruction

```
                    ┌─────────────────┐   ┌─────────────────┐
┌──────────────────┐│ Stepwise addition of:│   │ Titrate down to │
│ Colon evacuation ││       MOM       │   │ simplest, most  │
│ then trial of fibre│   Lactulose    │→  │ effective dose  │
└──────────────────┘│ Polyethylene glycol │   │ PRN dulcolax as │
                    │  (continue fibre)│   │ rescue therapy  │
                    └─────────────────┘   └─────────────────┘
```

Colon evacuation then trial of fibre → Stepwise addition of: MOM, Lactulose, Polyethylene glycol (continue fibre) → Titrate down to simplest, most effective dose PRN dulcolax as rescue therapy

Consider specialised testing on medications (i.e. marker study)

Slow transit constipation

Normal transit constipation

- Prokinetics or lubiprostone
- Colectomy with ileorectal anastomosis (well selected patients)

- Continue other therapies
- Consider addition of lubiprostone

Laxative	Adult dosing	Onset of action	Comments
Osmotic agents: Retain water in the intestine by creating an osmotic gradient			
Saline laxatives			
Magnesium hydroxide (MOM)	15–30 mL once to twice daily	0.5–3 h	For occasional constipation.
Magnesium citrate	200 mL daily		Can be used to liquefy stools in outlet obstruction
Sodium phosphate	10–25 mL in 360 mL of water as needed		Electrolyte abnormalities (hypermagnesaemia, hyperphosphataemia, hyponatraemia, hypokalaemia); use with caution in patients with cardiac or renal insufficiency

QUICK FLICK

8

continued

Table 8.4 continued

Laxative	Adult dosing	Onset of action	Comments
Poorly absorbed sugars			
Lactulose	15–30 mL once to twice daily	24–48 h	Electrolyte abnormalities, bloating, flatulence, diarrhoea, abdominal cramping
Sorbitol	15–30 mL once to twice daily		
Glycerine suppositories	3 g per rectum/ day		
Polyethylene glycol (PEG)	17–36 g in 240 mL of liquid	24–48 h	Electrolyte abnormalities, bloating, flatulence, diarrhoea, abdominal cramping
			Do not use in patients with known or suspected bowel obstruction
Emollients: Act as detergents, enhancing interaction of water with stool, resulting in softer stool; stimulate peristalsis			
Docusate sodium	100 mg twice daily	24–72 h	Minimal role for outpatient treatment. Should not be used in patients with acute or suspected bowel obstruction.
			Abdominal cramping, electrolyte depletion
Mineral oil	5–15 mL orally at bedtime	6–8 h	Long-term use can cause fat-soluble vitamin depletion.
			Lipoid pneumonia in patients prone to aspiration of liquids
Stimulant laxatives: Decrease absorption of, and increase secretion of water and ions			
Bisacodyl	10–30 mg/day 10 mg PR daily	6–10 h	For rescue therapy.
Senna (anthraquinone)	2–4 tabs once daily	6–12 h	Potential for overuse/ abuse: hypokalaemia, metabolic alkalosis and fluid depletion are manifestations.
			Can cause electrolyte imbalances

Laxative	Adult dosing	Onset of action	Comments
Prokinetics: Increase gastrointestinal motility and intestinal secretion, reduce visceral hypersensitivity			
5-HT$_4$ receptor agonists			
Tegaserod	6 mg twice daily	18 h	Tegaserod withdrawn from the US market in 2007 and cisapride in 2000 due to increased risk of serious cardiovascular events.
Cisapride	10–20 mg 4 times daily		
			Newer agents being developed
Chloride channel activator: Stimulates small bowel epithelial cells to increase intestinal fluid			
Lubiprostone	24 µg twice daily	24 h	Does not cause serum electrolyte fluctuations
			Can cause nausea, headache, abdominal distension and diarrhoea
			Nausea can be reduced by taking with food

therapy. It should be noted that stool softeners such as docusate sodium and docusate calcium have only modest efficacy in relieving constipation if used in isolation, and are best used alongside stimulant laxatives.

Patients with faecal impaction require more immediate treatment. If left uncorrected, this condition can lead to bowel obstruction, ulceration or perforation. Initially, a digital disimpaction should be performed to fragment the faecal mass. Then either suppositories or enemas should be administered for bowel evacuation. Only after this is achieved should oral laxatives be initiated. Physically or mentally incapacitated patients and the institutionalised elderly are at highest risk of impaction. However it can be seen in patients of any age, or in those with chronic constipation. The best treatment is prevention, with a consistent bowel regimen for constipation.

For patients with constipation refractory to first-line medical management, further testing should be obtained to rule out slow-transit constipation or pelvic floor dyssynergia. In patients with documented slow-transit constipation, there are few prokinetics widely available to stimulate colonic motility. The 5-HT$_4$ receptor agonist tegaserod was found to be efficacious in placebo-controlled trials in the treatment of chronic constipation in adults

QUICK FLICK

8

younger than 65 years, but it was withdrawn from the US market in March 2007 due to an increased risk of serious cardiovascular events (unstable angina, myocardial infarction and stroke). Marketing and sales of the drug was also suspended in Canada. Other prokinetics under investigation for use in chronic constipation include colchicine, the prostaglandin analogue misoprostol, neurotrophins such as neurotrophin-3, and the more selective 5-HT$_4$ agonist prucalopride. Lubiprostone is the only US Food and Drug Administration (FDA)-approved medication for long-term (up to 12 weeks) therapy of chronic idiopathic constipation. It has been proven to significantly increase spontaneous bowel movements compared to placebo and can be used in patients with normal-transit constipation. It is currently available only in the United States, but it is being investigated in Phase III clinical trials in Japan for chronic idiopathic constipation. For patients with opioid-induced constipation, two peripherally active opioid antagonists, methylnaltrexone and alvimopan, are under clinical investigation. Neither of these agents cross the blood–brain barrier, and they are both available in pill form.

Patients with dyssynergic defecation may benefit from biofeedback therapy. The goal of the treatment is to train patients to coordinate the relaxation of pelvic-floor muscles with abdominal manoeuvres to enhance entry of stool into the rectum as well as enhancing rectal sensory perception. This is achieved through a combination of methods to include diaphragmatic muscle training, manometric or electromyographically guided anal sphincter and pelvic-muscle relaxation, and simulated defecation. Up to 67 per cent success rates with this therapy have been reported, depending primarily on patient education and development of rapport with the therapist. If a patient can demonstrate a normal defecation pattern during at least 50 per cent of attempts, as well as improved symptoms on two consecutive training sessions, therapy can be discontinued. The benefits also appear to be long-lasting.

Botulinum type A toxin injection into the puborectalis muscle has been found to be efficacious in small studies, but repeated treatments are required because the effects are transient.

For patients who are refractory to medical therapy, a total colectomy with either an ileorectal asastomosis or ileostomy may be performed. This treatment is usually reserved for patients with slow-transit constipation in contrast to patients with Hirschsprung's disease, where the goal of surgical treatment is to remove or bypass the aganglionic bowel segment only. It is important to exclude pelvic floor disorders, as patients will not respond favourably to surgery if their dyssynergia has not been corrected. A generalised motility disorder must also be excluded by obtaining upper gastrointestinal motility studies. Patients should be advised that a colectomy may not offer relief of abdominal pain or bloating, and that the most common complications related to surgery are small bowel obstruction, diarrhoea and incontinence. Importantly, patients with upper-gut dysmotility or psychiatric co-morbidities have poor outcomes. Furthermore, overall patient satisfaction after colectomy can vary widely, ranging from 39 per cent to 100 per cent. Surgical correction of rectoceles should be reserved for patients whose constipation is relieved by applying digital pressure on the posterior wall of the vagina during defecation. Surgical treatment for dyssynergic defecation is contraindicated, as patients do not receive benefit, and post-operative faecal incontinence is common.

Summary

Chronic constipation is the most common digestive complaint in the general population and has a prevalence between 10 and 20 per cent, depending on country. It is responsible for increased healthcare costs and decreased quality of life.

There are several secondary causes for constipation that can be excluded by obtaining a detailed history and performing a physical examination. For most patients with idiopathic constipation, a trial of fibre with or without added osmotic laxative gives symptom relief. Specialised testing should be reserved for patients with persistent symptoms despite maximal medical therapy, or for those whose initial presentation suggests pelvic floor dyssynergia. Such patients might benefit from biofeedback therapy, but medical management should be continued.

Surgical management should be considered only as a last resort, and when preoperative screening for optimal candidates increases the likelihood of a favourable outcome for them.

Information for patients

What is constipation?

Constipation is a condition defined by infrequent bowel movements, typically fewer than three per week. However, additional symptoms include hard or difficult-to-pass bowel movements, or even the sensation that the bowels are not completely empty.

What causes constipation?

There are many causes for constipation, but often a cause cannot be identified. Several medications as well as certain medical conditions can cause constipation. It is also more common in older people.

QUICK FLICK

8

How is constipation treated?

An initial approach is to develop a consistent pattern of bowel habits. The bowels are most active in the morning after waking and after meals; therefore, stools will pass more easily at these times.

Another option is to increase dietary fibre. The recommended amount is 20–35 grams per day, but to avoid gas and bloating you should slowly increase to that amount. Fibre supplements such as psyllium powder mixed in a glass of water 1 to 3 times a day can be used instead of increasing dietary fibre. Be sure to take these supplements with an extra glass of fluid.

The next step would be the addition of a laxative. The type of laxative chosen depends on how they work, how quickly they provide relief and their safety when taking your medical history into consideration. The broad categories for laxatives are: saline laxatives (magnesium hydroxide, magnesium citrate), osmolar laxatives (lactulose, sorbitol or polyethylene glycol), and stimulant laxatives (bisacodyl, senna).

If your constipation is severe and has not responded to first-line treatments, your physician may elect to perform further testing to rule out other causes of constipation that may be responsive to alternative treatments. Such a treatment is biofeedback, which retrains the muscles of the pelvic floor and anus to relax instead of tightening during defecation.

When should you seek medical attention for constipation?

- If there has been a sudden change in previously normal bowel habits
- If it lasts longer than three weeks
- If over-the-counter laxatives or fibre supplementation have not been successful
- If you have weight loss, blood on the toilet paper, or weakness.

Recommended reading

American Gastroenterological Association Medical Position Statement: guidelines on constipation. *Gastroenterology*. 2000; 119:1761–78.

Bleser SD. Practical symptom-based evaluation of chronic constipation. *J Fam Pract*. 2006; 55:580–4.

Dennison C, Prasad M, Lloyd A, Bhattacharyya SK, Dhawan R, Coyne K. The health-related quality of life and ecomomic burden of constipation. *Pharmacoeconomics*. 2005; 23:461–76.

Drost J, Harris LA. Diagnosis and management of chronic constipation. *JAAPA*. 2006; 19:24–9.

Ghoshal UC, Abraham P, Bhatt C et al. Epidemiological and clinical profile of irritable bowel syndrome in India: report of the Indian Society of Gastroenterology Task Force. *Indian J Gastroenterol*. 2008; 27:22–8.

Higgins PD, Johanson JF. Epidemiology of constipation in North America: a systematic review. *Am J Gastroenterol*. 2004; 99:750–9.

Lacy BE, Levy LC. Lubiprostone: a novel treatment for chronic constipation. *Clin Interv Aging*. 2008; 3:357–64.

Lembo A, Camilleri M. Chronic constipation. *N Engl J Med*. 2003; 349(14):1360–8.

O'Keefe EA, Talley NJ, Tangalos EG, Zinsmeister AR. A bowel symptom questionnaire for the elderly. *J Gerontol*. 1992; 47:M116–21.

Ramkumar D, Rao S. Efficacy and safety of traditional medical therapies for chronic constipation: systematic review. *Am J Gastroenterol*. 2005; 100: 936–71.

Rao S. Constipation: evaluation and treatment. *Gastroenterol Clin North Am*. 2003; 32:659–83.

Talley NJ. Definitions, epidemiology, and impact of chronic constipation. *Rev Gastroenterol Disord*. 2004; 4:S3–10.

Wald A. Pathophysiology, diagnosis and current management of chronic constipation. *Nat Clin Pract Gastroenterol Hepatol*. 2006; 3:90–9.

Wald A, Kamm M, Müller-Lissner SA, Scarpignato C, Marx W, Schuijt C. The BI omnibus study: an international survey of community prevalence of constipation and laxative use in adults. Digestive Disorders Week. 2006; May 20–25. Abstract T1255.

QUICK FLICK

8

Chapter 9: Colorectal cancer

J. Sung (Hong Kong, China)

Key points

▶ While gastric and oesophageal cancers are declining, colorectal cancer is on the rise in Asia.

▶ Always take seriously a complaint of weight loss, bleeding from the gastrointestinal tract, or vague abdominal discomfort in older people, especially if it is a new complaint or one that does not settle rapidly within a few weeks of symptomatic treatment.

▶ In general, surgery offers the best hope of cure.

▶ Conventional barium contrast studies are sensitive diagnostic procedures and delineate the extent of the disease, but histological confirmation is obtained by endoscopic means or by percutaneous biopsy.

▶ Although progress in treating patients with inoperable disease has been slow, major advances have been made in palliation.

▶ Screening and prevention of colorectal cancer should be recommended.

▷ Introduction

Colorectal cancer is the second most common cancer in the West but, in recent years, a rapidly rising trend has also been reported in Asia. Countries such as the United States, Canada and Europe used to have the highest incidence of colorectal cancer, which was associated with obesity, smoking and a family history of colorectal neoplasia and inflammatory bowel disease.

Epidemiology

China, Japan, South Korea and Singapore have witnessed a two- to four-fold increase in incidence in the past decades. The incidences in many Asian countries are in fact on a par with those in the West. Colorectal cancer is now the third most common malignant disease in both men and women in Asia. In Japan, the incidence of colorectal cancer has possibly exceeded that of gastric cancer. The changing epidemiology is very worrying as, unlike statistics in North America and Europe, the rising incidence in Asia has not yet reached a plateau.

Certain ethnic groups in Asia have a substantially higher than average incidence of colorectal cancer. In Singapore, where Malay, Indian and Chinese people share the same environment, the incidence of colorectal cancer is significantly higher among the Chinese. Two recently published studies by the Asia-Pacific Working Group for Colorectal Cancer showed that Japanese, Korean and Chinese populations were also found to have a higher incidence of advanced colonic neoplasia among the symptomatic and asymptomatic groups. Men are more likely to develop colorectal cancer than women. Smoking and obesity are other risk factors identified in colorectal cancers.

▷ Pathophysiology

Most colorectal cancers arise from polyps (Figure 9.1), but only some polyps undergo malignant change.

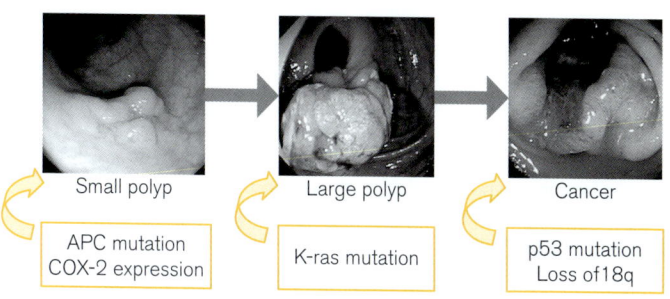

| Small polyp | Large polyp | Cancer |
| APC mutation COX-2 expression | K-ras mutation | p53 mutation Loss of 18q |

Figure 9.1 Colon cancer development

The adenoma–carcinoma sequence

Tubular adenomas have a low malignant potential and comprise 75 per cent of adenomas. Villous (or tubulovillous) adenomas comprise the remainder, with a much higher malignant potential. These adenomas are monoclonal and arise following a single genetic mutation. With time, and as the adenoma becomes bigger, an accumulation of genetic defects occurs which ultimately leads to a carcinoma. There are both environmental and inherited factors that account for these changes. Approximately 30 per cent of cases are known to be related to a genetic predisposition, as characterised by familial hereditary non-polyposis colon cancer and familial polyposis coli, both of which become evident at an early age.

Polyps increase in risk for malignant change as they increase in size (>1 cm), develop a villous component, become sessile, and have frank dysplastic changes in histology. Those at an increased risk include patients who have had a previous colorectal cancer, or who have adenomatous polyps, ulcerative colitis, or one of the familial (polyposis or non-polyposis) cancer syndromes.

Prolonged regular use of aspirin (>325 mg twice weekly) and NSAID is associated with a 30–50 per cent decrease in the incidence of colorectal cancer and adenomas, whereas an increase of dietary fibre is much less effective.

Non-polypoid flat or depressed lesions

While most cases of colorectal cancers are believed to arise from the adenoma–carcinoma sequence, evidence from Asia—Japan in particular—suggests an alternative mechanism. Clinico-pathological studies have shown that there are two groups of colorectal cancers: polypoid tumours and non-polypoid tumours. Non-polypoid tumours are flat lesions with either an elevated or depressed surface. Applying the same techniques as screening for gastric cancer, Japanese endoscopists have reported that some colorectal cancers may be smaller than 1 cm in diameter. These flat or depressed lesions can easily be missed in examination, and are better picked up by new endoscopic modalities such as narrow band imaging (NBI). Compared to colorectal cancers arising from the adenoma–carcinoma sequence, non-polypoid cancers are less likely to have K-ras mutations. It has also been noted that non-polypoid tumours of the colorectal region tend to reach deeper layers of the intestinal wall in the early stage of the disease and with a higher degree of dysplasia, making them more invasive in nature.

◐ Clinical presentation

- Most patients present with passages of bright red blood per rectum, abdominal pain and a change in bowel habit, either constipation or diarrhoea.
- Left-sided lesions tend to present earlier. Right-sided lesions may be brought to the patient's attention only by chronic blood loss leading to anaemia.
- Digital examination of the rectum will permit the diagnosis of most of rectal tumours; a double contrast enema is sensitive for all colorectal tumours. Endoscopy allows a histological confirmation.
- The whole bowel needs to be examined because synchronous tumours are common.
- The level of the serum tumour marker, carcino-embryonic antigen (CEA), is seldom raised in the early stages of disease and is therefore rarely diagnostically useful. If its concentration starts to rise after apparently successful tumour resection, however, it is good evidence that the condition will shortly recur.
- Staging is important in deciding on the appropriate treatment (Table 9.1).

Table 9.1 A simplified outline of staging of colorectal cancer, showing its importance in determining prognosis

Duke's stage	AJCC* stage	Tumour†	Nodes	Metastases	% survival at 5 years
A	I	T1, T2	0	0	85
B	II	T3, T4	0	0	65
C	III	Any T	Present	0	50
D	IV	Any T	Any	Present	<5

*   AJCC = American Joint Committee on Cancer
†   T1: tumour confined to mucosa or submucosa; T2: tumour invades into muscularis propria; T3: tumour invades through the muscularis propria; T4: tumour invades the peritoneal cavity or adjacent organs.

◐ Management

Screening and prevention

Faecal occult blood test, flexible sigmoidoscopy and colonoscopy are recommended options for colorectal cancer screening in US (Table 9.2), Europe and Asia.

Table 9.2 Options for colorectal cancer screening

Tests that detect adenomatous polyps and cancer
Flexible sigmoidoscopy (FSIG) every 5 years
Colonoscopy every 10 years
Double-contrast barium enema (DCBE) every 5 years
CT colonography (CTC) every 5 years
Tests that primarily detect cancer
Annual guaiac-based faecal occult blood test (gFOBT) with high test sensitivity for cancer
Annual faecal immunochemical test (FIT) with high test sensitivity for cancer
Stool DNA test (sDNA), with high sensitivity for cancer, interval uncertain

Stool tests

Annual or biennial screening with faecal occult blood test (FOBT) using a guaiac-based test or an immunochemical test have been shown to reduce both colorectal cancer and related mortality compared to no screening.

Although the sensitivity of a single FOBT is low—in the range of 30–50 per cent—repeated annual testing can detect as many as 92 per cent of colorectal cancer cases. FOBT is regarded as a 'cancer test' rather than a test for polyps or adenoma, and has the advantage that the test can be done at home and it is non-invasive; it needs to be repeated every one or two years, however.

Rehydration of stool sample is not recommended. Although rehydration of the guaiac-based test increases sensitivity, the false positive rate is also raised, leading to the possibility of unnecessary anxiety and performance of invasive tests unnecessarily.

Immunochemical testing obviates the need for dietary restriction. Faecal immunochemical tests for haemoglobin have been shown to be more sensitive than guaiac tests for cancer and adenomas, especially in Asian subjects, probably due to lack of dietary interference.

Faecal DNA tests are under development and may provide more accurate results in future.

Colonoscopy and flexible sigmoidoscopy

These are the only modalities that allow removal of the adenoma and prevent colorectal cancer. Colonoscopy is the 'gold standard' in detecting polyps and diagnosing colorectal cancer. The National Polyp Study has demonstrated a reduced incidence of colorectal cancer and reduced mortality among those who underwent colonoscopy. The effectiveness of colonoscopy depends on the quality of the examination: quality of bowel preparation, skill of the endoscopists and the intubation time are important determining factors.

Flexible sigmoidoscopy has been shown in case-controlled studies to reduce the mortality of colorectal cancer. When an adenoma is found in the left colon, a full colonoscopy is indicated, as proximal lesions may be found. The sensitivity of flexible sigmoidoscopy in detecting advanced neoplasia is reported to be 35–70 per cent, and reduction in cancer risk in rectum and sigmoid by 50–60 per cent.

After a 'normal' test result, colonoscopy should be repeated every 10 years and sigmoidoscopy every five years. The recommendation of five-year interval is based on a cohort study which found that five years after a negative colonoscopy, new advanced neoplasia is rare. The recommended interval between sigmoidoscopy screenings is shorter than for colonoscopy because it is a less sensitive method than colonoscopy, even in the distal colon, due to the quality of bowel preparation, the varied experience of the examiners, and the patient's discomfort which may lead to colonic spasm, in turn affecting the depth of sigmoidoscope insertion and hence adequacy of examination.

Since up to two-thirds of proximal advanced lesions in Asians are found in the absence of distal lesions, the disadvantage of possibly creating a false sense of security using flexible sigmoidoscopy for screening should be noted.

Double-contrast barium enema testing

Double-contrast barium enema testing (DCBE) every five years is listed as one of the options in colorectal cancer screening in national guidelines in North America. The sensitivity of DCBE is lower than that of colonoscopy and it does not permit the removal of polyps or biopsy of cancers. Because of its lower sensitivity, even for large polyps, it is not recommend as a first-line option for colorectal cancer screening.

Radiological imaging

There is increasing evidence that computed tomography (CT) colonography is an accurate screening method for the detection of colorectal neoplasia in asymptomatic, average-risk adults. The sensitivity and specificity of the finding depends on the size of the polyps. High cost, the risk associated with radiation and requirement of bowel preparation are factors inhibiting the use of CT colonography as primary screening at this stage.

In view of the inaccessibility of cutting-edge imaging technology in some Asian countries, CT colonography has not yet been recommended in Asia as a colorectal cancer screening tool. With improvement in technology and increased accessibility, however, CT colonography may become a recommendable tool for colorectal cancer screening in the future.

Treatment and prognosis

All polyps that are detected should be removed and there is now good evidence that this dramatically decreases the subsequent risk of tumour development. Even if there is a focus of malignant change, simple polypectomy is sufficient if the tumour has not invaded through the mucosa.

Once the tumour is established, surgery is the only hope of cure and can be offered to all patients unless there is metastatic disease, extensive local disease, or the patient is otherwise medically unfit. A palliative resection is usually preferred to a bypass procedure for palliation. In those patients undergoing resections with curative intent but in whom regional lymph nodes are involved (Duke's Grade C), post-operative chemotherapy with a 5-fluorouracil-based regimen improves survival to some extent.

Survival is related to the disease stage and ranges from approximately 90 per cent at five years in Duke's A patients, to five per cent in those with metastatic disease (Duke's D: see Table 9.1). Patients with metastatic disease who are in good clinical condition may benefit in terms of survival and quality of life from systemic chemotherapy, although it is never curative. Conventional treatment with 5-fluorouracil (5-FU) and folinic acid leads to a median survival of approximately one year compared with a median figure of six months in the absence of any active treatment.

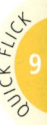
QUICK FLICK 9

Oxaliplatin and irinotecan are important components of treatment for advanced colorectal cancer; in addition, oxaliplatin plus 5-FU outperforms 5-FU alone in the adjuvant treatment of colon cancer, and has been adopted as a standard regimen. New chemotherapeutic agents including TGF-beta and angiogenesis inhibitors have made an important contribution to prolonging survival and improved quality of life in advanced colorectal cancers.

Summary

Colorectal cancer is the second most common cancer in Western countries, and the incidence in many Asian countries is rising to be on a par with the West.

Most colorectal cancers originate with polyps but only a minority of polyps undergo malignant change. Tubular adenomas have low malignant potential and comprise 75 per cent of adenomas. Villous (or tubulovillous) adenomas comprise the remainder and have a much higher malignant potential. In Asia it is reported that flat, depressed small lesions can be easily missed and are better observed using new endoscopic techniques such as narrow band imaging (NBI).

Digital examination of the rectum remains an important component of the clinical examination; however, endoscopic examination is vital since it allows observation of a lesion as well as biopsy, removal and histological examination.

With regard to screening for the prevention of colorectal cancer, faecal occult blood testing, flexible sigmoidoscopy and colonoscopy are the recommended procedures. After a normal result, a colonoscopy should be repeated every 10 years and a sigmoidoscopy every five years. Note, however, that up to two-thirds of proximal advanced lesions in Asians are found in the absence of distal lesions, so that flexible sigmoidoscopy may give a false sense of security.

Surgery is the treatment of choice but in certain circumstances chemotherapeutic agents are used.

Recommended reading

Levin B, Lieberman DA, McFarland B, Smith RA, Brooks D, Andrews KS, Dash C, Giardiello FM, Glick S, Levin TR, Pickhardt P, Rex DK, Thorson A, Winawer SJ. Screening and surveillance for the early detection of colorectal cancer and adenomatous polyps 2008: a joint guideline from the American Cancer Society, the US Multi-Society Task Force on Colorectal Cancer and the American College of Radiology. *CA Cancer J Clin.* 2008; 58:130–60. doi:10.3322/CA.2007.0018.

Sung JJY, Lau JYW, Goh KL, Leung WK for the Asia–Pacific Working Group on Colorectal Cancer. Increasing incidence of colorectal cancer in Asia: implications for screening. *Lancet Oncol*. 2005; 6:871–6. doi:10.1016/S1470-2045(05)70422-8.

Sung JJY, Lau JYW, Young G et al. Asia–Pacific consensus recommendations for colorectal cancer screening. *Gut*. 2008; 57:1166–76. doi:10.1136/gut.2007.146316.

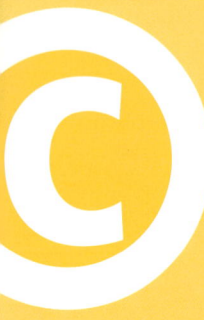

Part C

Diseases of emerging countries making inroads globally

Chapter 10: Gastrointestinal tuberculosis versus Crohn's disease

J. Sollano (The Philippines)

Key points

- The incidence of inflammatory bowel diseases is increasing in regions of the world where tuberculosis is also highly prevalent.
- Gastrointestinal tuberculosis (GI TB) presents with almost identical clinical, radiographic and endoscopic features, such that it is difficult to differentiate it from inflammatory bowel diseases—especially Crohn's disease (CD). Delay in diagnosis and inadvertent administration of inappropriate treatments have serious consequences for the patient.
- In CD, a longer duration of symptoms, chronic and usually bloody diarrhoea, anaemia, perianal disease, longitudinal ulcers, cobblestone appearance of the colonic mucosa, enteric fistulisation and extraintestinal manifestations in younger individuals are common.
- Fever, transverse ulcerations, confluent and large granulomas with caseation necrosis, patulous and rigid ileocaecal valve, concomitant presence of ascites, abdominal lymphadenopathy and pulmonary infiltrates are usually associated with GI TB.
- Therapeutic trials with anti-TB therapy must be avoided and should not be a substitute for strategies for establishing the unequivocal presence of *Mycobacterium tuberculosis*.

○ **Introduction**

The aetiology and pathogenesis of inflammatory bowel diseases (IBD) are not fully understood; therefore there are no specific laboratory tests or clinical features on which to base a reliable diagnosis. Currently, diagnosis combines clinical, laboratory, radiological, endoscopic and pathological features.[1]

Gastrointestinal tuberculosis (GI TB), a form of extrapulmonary tuberculosis, presents with almost identical clinical, radiographic and endoscopic features to inflammatory bowel diseases, especially Crohn's disease (CD), making them difficult to differentiate. GI TB and CD are both granulomatous disorders of the gastrointestinal tract, with similar sites of predilection in the digestive system and other extraintestinal sites. In fact, when Thomas Dalziel first described Crohn's disease in 1913, the diagnostic emphasis was 'chronic interstitial enteritis and not tuberculosis'. Recently, the difficulties encountered in definitively diagnosing CD have been exacerbated by the reported increase in the incidence of IBD in areas of the world where tuberculosis is also prevalent. Tuberculosis and its many clinical variants are also now being reported increasingly in Western countries due to the problems associated with the HIV/AIDS pandemic and rapidly expanding transnational migration.[2–4]

Due to their perplexing clinical presentations, up to 65 per cent of GI TB cases are misdiagnosed as CD in China, and up to 21 per cent in Saudi Arabia. A delay in correct diagnosis of up to seven years has been described in reports coming from Asia and Africa. A recent study in Korea revealed that up to 45 per cent of the patients taking part in a prior therapeutic trial received anti-Koch's TB medications before finally being correctly diagnosed as having CD.[5–8]

Definitive diagnosis of GI TB and CD is important; erroneous or delayed diagnosis can have serious consequences. Furthermore, specific treatments for either disease are associated with morbidities and side effects, so that reckless administration of therapies in the inappropriate patients should be avoided at all times.

Also at issue is the use of a favourable response to the empirical administration of an anti-tuberculous regimen as a diagnostic basis for GI TB. This ill-advised strategy can only lead to multi-drug resistant *Mycobacterium tuberculosis* strains, and further deplete the currently dwindling number of effective anti-Koch's therapies. All these concerns highlight the need to establish the diagnosis of either CD or GI TB unequivocally before starting any form of treatment.

○ **Pathology**

Before the era of pasteurisation, gastrointestinal TB probably developed from ingesting contaminated milk. *M. tuberculosis* may also penetrate the intestinal

mucosa from swallowed infected sputum in those with active pulmonary TB. It can also originate from a haematogenous spread from active pulmonary TB, miliary TB or from silent bacteraemia during primary tuberculosis infection.

Direct extension to the ileocaecal region from adjacent organs is quite rare; however, GI TB has a higher predilection for this segment, probably due to the abundance of lymphoid tissue and relative physiological stasis at this site. The tuberculosis mycobacterium induces an inflammatory cascade which eventually forms granuloma and leads to lymphangitis, endarteritis, caseating necrosis, mucosal ulceration and progressive fibrosis, with resultant narrowing of the intestinal lumen.

Granuloma formation can be seen both in GI TB and CD, but caseation necrosis has been reported only in CD (Table 10.1). The granulomas of tuberculosis are always surrounded by inflammatory cells, and multinucleated (Langhan's) giant cells are usually abundant, whereas the granulomas of CD can occur in otherwise grossly normal mucosa, particularly in the rectum (Table 10.1).[9–11]

Table 10.1 Clinical features to facilitate differentiation between intestinal tuberculosis and Crohn's disease. Note that these diseases may mimic each other in their clinical manifestations.

	Tuberculosis	**Crohn's disease**
Symptoms		
Abdominal pain	Often generalised, including RIF pain	Crampy, often localised to RIF
Weight loss	Often significant	Over a longer period
Pyrexia	Common	± 25%
Diarrhoea	Erratic constipation and diarrhoea	Often, admixed with blood
Perianal Complications	Rare	Can occur in 50%
Endoscopic appearance		
Ulcers	Transverse	Longitudinal
Aphthous ulcers	May be present	More common in TB
Cobblestone appearance	Occasional, <25%	Found in up to 75%

	Tuberculosis	**Crohn's disease**
Histology		
Caseation necrosis	Hallmark	Rare
Granulomas, both large and confluent	Common, up to 75%	Uncommon, 0-25%
Superficial ulceration	Usual	Mucosa to serosa affected
Imaging		
Plain x-ray abdomen	Normal or dilated. Bowel loops, air fluid levels, calcified nodes	Normal or colonic dilation. Bowel loops, air fluid levels, pneumoperitoneum
Barium studies	Strictures, dilated loops, fistulae and sinus tracts are common	Fistulous tracts and strictures are more common
Ultrasound	Mass lesions	Thickened bowel wall
CT	Bowel wall thickening	Absent peristalsis
MRI	Massive lymphadenopathy (with central necrosis)	Perianal disease

Source: Adapted from Almadi et al.[12]

The morphological appearance of the lesions in the ileocaecal region associated with GI TB are usually difficult to differentiate from lesions caused by CD. In the caecum and terminal ileum, GI TB produces three morphological types of lesion which are quite similar to those seen in CD—ulcerative, ulcero-hypertrophic, and fibrous-stricturing. In addition, involvement of the ileocaecal valve (e.g. ulceration, deformity and mucosal nodularities) occurs in both GI TB and CD. A patulous, fibrotic, ileocaecal valve with markedly nodular surrounding mucosa, however, is more likely associated with GI TB.

Clinical presentation

The overlapping clinical presentation of CD and GI TB requires a high index of suspicion among clinicians, and careful consideration and analysis of the patient's clinical, laboratory, endoscopic and other findings if an early definitive diagnosis of either disease is to be achieved (Table 10.1).

Common symptoms of Crohn's disease include abdominal pain, diarrhoea, weight loss, anorexia, fever, night sweats, rectal pain and

QUICK FLICK 10

rectal bleeding; these depend on the location, extent and severity of the inflammation of the involved segment of the colon. Patients with GI TB may present similarly; however, a longer duration of symptoms, chronic, usually bloody diarrhoea, anaemia and extraintestinal features are significantly more common in CD. On the other hand, fever, concomitant presence of ascites, abdominal lymphadenopathy and pulmonary infiltrates are significantly associated with GI TB.[3, 8]

Gastrointestinal tuberculosis has been reported in 10–20 per cent of patients with pulmonary TB, and pulmonary TB has been noted in 20–75 per cent of patients suffering from abdominal tuberculosis.[13, 14]

Other characteristics which indicate a diagnosis of CD are the patient's younger age, aphthoid ulcerations in the colon, perianal disease, enteric fistulisation and extraintestinal manifestations. The almost identical sites of predilection of the extraintestinal manifestations of CD and GI TB, most particularly pyoderma gangrenosum, uveitis, spondyloarthropathy (axial arthropathy) and primary sclerosing cholangitis, make differentiation extremely difficult at the bedside because tuberculous involvement of the joints, eyes, skin and liver also occurs.

While the colon is the most common site of involvement with Crohn's disease, lesions in other regions of the gastrointestinal tract have been described. Likewise, patients suffering from GI TB have been reported to present with lesions in the oesophagus, stomach, duodenum and small bowel, liver, pancreas, appendix, anorectal area and mesenteric and retroperitoneal nodes. In a series of GI TB cases with which the author is familiar, the distribution of GI TB in the oesophagus was 0.14 per cent of patients, in the stomach in 0.60 per cent, duodenum in 2.5 per cent and the colon in 75–90 per cent. In another cohort from China, the ileocaecal region was also the common site of TB involvement in up to 86 per cent of patients.[15–17]

The predilection of GI TB for the ileocaecal area has already been emphasised, but ileocolonic lesions are also common in CD, seen in 22–54 per cent of patients, and isolated colon involvement has been noted in 21–39 per cent.[18–20]

Endoscopic diagnosis

The chronic granulomatous nature of the inflammatory process occurring in both GI TB and CD results in colonic lesions which are difficult to distinguish morphologically. These similarities in endoscopic features are a frequent source of missed and/or erroneous diagnosis (see Table 10.1). Endoscopy, however, allows tissue samples of the colonic lesions to be taken, which can then be tested further for the presence of *M. tuberculosis*.

The colonoscopic examination of 88 Korean patients (44 of whom had GI TB and 44 had CD) revealed that ileocaecal involvement was common in both GI TB (100%) and CD (90.7%). Anorectal lesions, longitudinal ulcers, aphthous ulcers and cobblestone appearance, however, were significantly more common in patients with Crohn's disease. On the other hand, fewer than four segments of the entire colon, a patulous ileocaecal valve, transverse ulcers, and scars or pseudopolyps were more frequently observed to be involved in patients with gastrointestinal tuberculosis than in those with Crohn's disease. It was also observed that longitudinal ulcers had a higher diagnostic value than transverse ulcers for CD in cases where both types of lesions were present in the same patient. A proposed scoring system based on these endoscopic features gave a fairly high diagnostic accuracy of 87.5 per cent. The positive predictive value for GI TB was 88.9 per cent, while the positive predictive value for CD was 94.9 per cent.[19]

In another cohort, ileocaecal involvement was noted in 81 per cent of patients with GI TB and 77 per cent in patients with CD.[8]

A complete ileocolonoscopy and thorough evaluation of the terminal ileum is required in the assessment of patients suspected to suffer from GI TB or CD, since up to 20 per cent of patients may also have lesions in the terminal ileum.

AFB smear and culture, polymerase chain reaction (PCR) assay for *M. tuberculosis*

For the definitive diagnosis of tuberculous infection, unequivocal documentation of *M. tuberculosis* in biopsy/tissue samples is essential. Tuberculosis, however, is a paucibacillary infection so that isolation of the TB bacillus is often difficult. AFB smears are not a reliable test, and have low sensitivity and poor specificity. In one study, only 23 per cent of patients who were eventually diagnosed as GI TB were AFB-positive. Although preparing AFB culture is a more tedious procedure to perform, and the four to six weeks' return time for results is relatively long, in times of multi-drug resistant *M. tuberculosis* AFB culture offers possibilities for antimycobacterial sensitivity testing. Information gathered from these tests, along with the judicious use of both first- and second-line anti-TB drugs, will result in better cure rates.

The more recently developed polymerase chain reaction (PCR) assay for detecting TB bacilli (Mtb-PCR) appears to be both a more rapid and more reliable process for establishing TB infection in sputum and other tissue specimens, with a good accuracy of 82.6 per cent and high specificity of 95 per cent. Compared with mycobacterial culture—BACTEC 460 system and inoculation on Lowenstein-Jensen media—the sensitivity, specificity and positive and negative predictive values of Mtb-PCR are reported to be 79 per cent, 99 per cent, 93 per cent and 98 per cent, respectively. For specimens where the BACTEC 460 system has a positive growth index, the PCR assay has a reported sensitivity of 98 per cent and a specificity of 100 per cent.[11, 21–22]

Other ancillary procedures

Up to 75 per cent of patients with abdominal tuberculosis have concomitant pulmonary tuberculosis; up to 20 per cent of patients with pulmonary tuberculosis may also have GI TB. A chest X-ray finding compatible with pulmonary tuberculosis may further support the diagnosis in patients suspected to be suffering from GI TB.[13–15]

Computed tomography (CT) has helped tremendously in differentiating GI TB from CD. In addition to demonstrating the degree of involvement of the intestinal wall, it can add valuable information about the surrounding structures and organ systems—mesentery, peritoneum, lymph nodes, solid organs and retroperitoneum—abdominal structures which may be involved in either disease.

In the ulcerative form of GI TB, CT may demonstrate preferential thickening of the ileocaecal valve and the medial wall of the caecum. In the hypertrophic or ulcero-hypertrophic form, exophytic masses and nodules may be seen around the ulcers. An inflammatory mass that extends into an adjacent muscle layer suggests GI TB. In the fibrous-stricturing (sclerotic) form, the caecum assumes a conical, shrunken, amputated and/or retracted shape. In contrast, the thickening of the intestinal wall in CD is less severe, more uniform and symmetrical. Several investigators suggest that mural stratification (target sign), vascular jejunisation (comb sign), mesenteric fibrofatty proliferation and advanced skip lesions adjacent to a stricture are seen only in CD. Bowel loop displacement is demonstrable in GI TB and is usually due to associated lymphadenopathy. Intra-abdominal lymph nodes may be enlarged in both disorders, but in GI TB they are larger and may have necrotic centres (Table 10.1).[23]

The use of QuantiFERON®-γ (QFT-G) for diagnosing GI TB has recently been reported. QFT-G and TSPOT.TB are interferon-γ release assays (IGRAs) which have been tested extensively in pulmonary tuberculosis and are currently used as alternatives to the tuberculin skin test (TST) for the detection of latent tuberculosis. Two recent meta-analyses have shown that the specificity of IGRAs for detecting latent tuberculosis is good (>95%), and is unaffected by BCG vaccination status. TSPOT.TB appears to be more sensitive than both QuantiFERON® tests and TST. Further studies on the utilisation of these assays in the diagnosis of GI TB are needed.[24, 25]

◯ Management

In many countries where TB is prevalent, especially where CD is only now being recognised, an empirical trial of anti-TB therapy is used to differentiate TB from CD. In fact, a complete clinical response to this approach without subsequent recurrence in patients with clinical, colonoscopic, radiological and/or operative evidence of intestinal tuberculosis is often used as the final criterion for making the definitive diagnosis of TB.

Therapeutic trial with anti-TB therapy

It should be emphasised that the therapeutic trial strategy is not a substitute for directing early efforts at establishing the unequivocal presence of *M. tuberculosis* before starting any form of treatment. It exposes the patients to unnecessary risks of toxicity attendant to anti-TB medications. It can also delay the administration of the appropriate therapy for patients with CD. When commencing anti-inflammatory and steroid treatment in CD patients where GI TB is extremely difficult to establish, some centres in Asia start with an 'anti-Koch's cover' for a few months while assessing response, as well as the definitive diagnosis during the treatment course. Some routinely perform chest radiography on all IBD patients before initiating any form of immunosuppression, and initiate INH prophylaxis in patients with radiological abnormalities that suggest previous pulmonary TB.

While some reports showed that *Mycobacterium avium* subspecies *paratuberculosis* was isolated more often in CD patients than in controls, currently available evidence does not allow recommending anti-Koch's treatment for Crohn's disease.

According to the Korean guidelines, the obligatory tests for the diagnosis of GI TB are: colonoscopy with biopsy and AFB stain, tissue culture for *M. tuberculosis*, chest X-ray, complete blood count (CBC), erythrocyte sedimentation rate (ESR), blood chemistry, and c-reactive protein (CRP). Some of the optional tests may include tissue TB PCR, tuberculin skin test, interferon-γ assay, small bowel follow-through (enteroclysis), abdominal CT and HIV antibody. For the definitive diagnosis of GI TB, one or more of the following criteria has to be satisfied: (1) presence of caseating granuloma on histology of diseased tissue; (2) demonstration of acid-fast bacilli (AFB) on smear or on histological section; (3) positive culture for AFB; (4) positive TB PCR; (5) histological- or microbiological-confirmed TB at an extraintestinal site.[1,13]

A tentative diagnosis of Crohn's disease is made if at least two of the following criteria are met: (1) clinical history of abdominal pain, weight loss, malaise, diarrhoea, and/or rectal bleeding; (2) endoscopic findings of mucosal cobblestoning, linear ulceration, skip areas, or perianal disease; (3) radiological findings of stricture, fistula, mucosal cobblestoning, or ulceration; (4) macroscopic appearance of bowel-wall induration, mesenteric

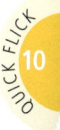
QUICK FLICK 10

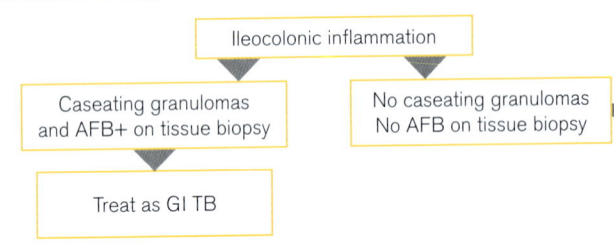

Figure 10.1 Proposed algorithm on the diagnostic work-up of patients with a differential diagnosis of gastrointestinal tuberculosis or Crohn's disease
Source: Modified from Almadi et al.[26]

lymphadenopathy, and creeping fat at laparotomy; (5) pathological findings of transmural inflammation and/or epithelioid granulomas.[26]

For the definitive diagnosis of CD in regions where tuberculosis is highly prevalent the following criteria may be used: (1) presence of at least three different criteria, or the presence of non-caseating granuloma on histology with at least one other criterion; (2) exclusion of TB by histology, negative microbiological and PCR studies; and (3) complete resolution of symptoms and morphological (endoscopic and histological/microbiological) features after one year's treatment with corticosteroid and 5-aminosalicylic acid (5-ASA) preparations (with or without surgery).[11]

Figure 10.1 is a modification of the algorithm proposed in 2009 by Almadi et al. showing a suggested systematic approach to the differential diagnosis of GI TB from CD.[12]

Summary

Tuberculosis of the gastrointestinal tract was a well-described clinical entity long before Crohn's disease but still today, difficulties in the differential diagnosis between the two diseases remain. In the past three decades,

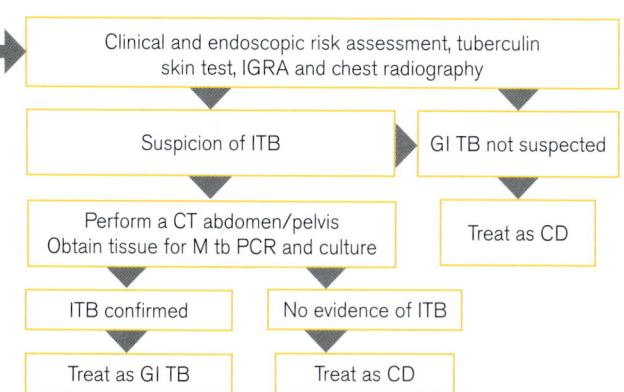

however, there have been major advances in formulating a better description of the clinical and other features of gastrointestinal tuberculosis that distinguish it from Crohn's disease.

In Asia, where CD is still relatively rare, increased awareness and improvement in understanding how to deal with CD has boosted the skills and confidence of physicians who are seeing and treating the disease for the first time. This is an important development which will ensure that CD can be diagnosed and treated properly in areas of the world where gastrointestinal tuberculosis is still prevalent. As better and more efficient diagnostic tests become available for the unequivocal documentation of *M. tuberculosis*, the early and definitive diagnosis of gastrointestinal tuberculosis can only be expected to be even easier.

Clearly, difficulties still remain. However, the diagnostic challenges confronting those who treated these diseases in the past have been reduced substantially. In addition to advances in available therapies and treatment strategies, physicians today are more knowledgeable and better equipped to address the concerns of patients suffering from gastrointestinal tuberculosis or Crohn's disease.

QUICK FLICK 10

Information for patients

What is Crohn's disease?

Crohn's disease (CD) is a chronic, relapsing inflammatory bowel condition characterised by mucosal ulcerations, as well as fistula and stricture formation involving discontinuous segments of the entire gastrointestinal tract, and it may cause rectal bleeding, changes in bowel habits, abdominal pain, loss of appetite and weight loss. Due to the recurring nature of the bowel inflammation it may require long-term, if not lifelong, management.

What is gastrointestinal tuberculosis?

Gastrointestinal tuberculosis (GI TB) is an infection of the intestines by *Mycobacterium tuberculosis*, usually coming from tuberculosis of the lungs, which also causes ulcerations of the intestinal mucosa, producing symptoms that may closely mimic those associated with Crohn's disease. GI TB may present with fever, abdominal pain, loss of appetite, bloody diarrhoea and anaemia. Lymph nodes and fluid in the abdomen (ascites), as well as pulmonary infiltrates, are also prominent findings.

Why is it important to differentiate between gastrointestinal tuberculosis and Crohn's disease?

The signs, symptoms and sites of gastrointestinal tract involvement of GI TB and CD overlap in many ways, making it difficult to tell the difference between them. Definitive diagnosis is important, because wrong or even delayed diagnosis can lead to serious consequences. The specific treatments for both diseases have side effects and adverse reactions, so reckless administration of therapies in inappropriate patients may increase morbidity and/or mortality.

What are the tests that I should undergo so that a clear diagnosis is made before starting treatment?

The more important examinations you may need to undergo to help the doctors make a fairly accurate and reliable diagnosis are colonoscopy and histopathological examination of tissue biopsies taken from the colonic lesions. Stool examination, including tests for intestinal inflammation such as faecal leukocytes, calprotectin and so on are often helpful. If gastrointestinal tuberculosis is suspected, these tissues may also be submitted for acid fast bacilli (AFB) staining, culture and polymerase chain reaction (PCR) assays for *M. tuberculosis*. A chest X-ray, tuberculin skin test, and a computed tomography (CT) scan of the abdomen are helpful. In the appropriate setting, an HIV test may be needed.

When do I need to see a doctor?

If you have recurrent episodes of abdominal pain, bowel changes, blood in the stools, fever, loss of appetite—especially if associated with weight loss or fever—you need to consult your doctor immediately.

Whether or not you have those symptoms, if you are over 50 and, most importantly, if you have a family history of colon cancer, you need to consult your physician and arrange to undergo a colonoscopic examination as soon as possible.

If you have been suffering from Crohn's disease for more than eight to ten years, you need to visit your physician and talk to him/her about screening and surveillance colonoscopy.

References

1. Kim YS, Kim YH, Lee KM, Kim JS, Park YS. Diagnostic guideline of intestinal tuberculosis. *Korean J Gastroenterol*. 2009; 53:177–86.

2. Dye C. Global epidemiology of tuberculosis. *Lancet*. 2006; 367:938–40.

3. Dalziel TK. Chronic interstitial enteritis. *Br Med J*. 1913; 2:1068–70.

4. Ouyang Q. Inflammatory bowel disease in China. *J Gastroenterol Hepatol*. 2000; 15 suppl:S25.

5. Riedel L, Segal I, Mohamed AE, Hale M, Mannell A. The prolonged course of gastrointestinal tuberculosis. *J Clin Gastroenterol*. 1989; 11:671–4.

6. Tonghua L, Guozong P, Minzhang C. Crohn's disease: clinicopathologic manifestations and differential diagnosis from enterocolonic tuberculosis. *Chin Med J*. 1981; 94:431–40.

7. Yang SK. Current status and clinical characteristics of inflammatory bowel disease in Korea. *Korean J Gastroenterol*. 2002; 40:1–14.

8. Gilinsky NH, Marks IN, Kotter RE, Price SK. Abdominal tuberculosis: a 10-year review. *S Afr Med J*. 1983; 64:849–57.

9. Tandon HD, Prakash A. Pathology of intestinal tuberculosis and its distinction from Crohn's disease. *Gut*. 1972; 13:260–9.

10. Surawicz CM, Leisel JL, Ylvisaker T, Saunders DR, Rubin CE. Rectal biopsy in the diagnosis of Crohn's disease: value of multiple biopsies and serial sectioning. *Gastroenterology*. 1981; 81:66–71.

11. Amarapurkar DN, Patel ND, Rane PS. Diagnosis of Crohn's disease in India where tuberculosis is widely prevalent. *World J Gastroenterol*. 2008 Feb 7; 14(5):741–6.

12. Almadi MA, Ghosh S, Aljebreen AMA. Differentiating intestinal tuberculosis from Crohn's disease: a diagnostic challenge. *Am J Gastroenterol*. 2009; 104:1003–12.

13. Wei-Chen S, Leu SY, Hsu H, Lin JK, Lin TC. Trend of large bowel tuberculosis and the relation with pulmonary tuberculosis. *Dis Colon Rectum*. 1992; 35:189–92.

14. Misra SP, Misra P, Dwivedi M. Ileoscopy in patients with ileocolonic tuberculosis. *World J Gastroenterol*. 2007 Mar 21; 13(11):1723–7.

15. Alvarez SZ. Gastrointestinal tuberculosis. *J Gastroenterol Hepatol*. 1998; 3:833–9.

16. Leung VKS, Law ST, Lam CW, Luk ISC, Chau TN, Loke TKL, Chan WH, Lam SH. Intestinal tuberculosis in a regional hospital in Hong Kong: a 10-year experience. *Hong Kong Med J*. 2006; 12:264–71.

17. Oostenbrug LE, van Dullemen HM, te Meerman GJ, Jansen PL, Kleibeuker JH. Clinical outcome of Crohn's disease according to the Vienna classification: disease location is a useful predictor of disease course. *Eur J Gastroenterol Hepatol*. 2006; 18:255–61.

18. Freeman HJ. Application of the Vienna classification for Crohn's disease to a single clinician database of 877 patients. *Can J Gastroenterol*. 2001; 15:89–93.

19. Lee YJ, Yang SK, Byeon JS, Myung SJ, Chang HS, Hong SS, Kim KJ, Lee GH, Jung HY, Hong WS, Kim JH, Min YI, Chang SJ, Yu CS. Analysis of colonoscopic findings for differentiation of intestinal TB and Crohn's disease. *Endoscopy*. 2006; 38:592–7.

20. Alvares JF, Devarbhavi H, Makhija P, Rao S, Kottoor S. Clinical, colonoscopic, and histological profile of colonic tuberculosis in a tertiary hospital. *Endoscopy*. 2005; 37:351–6.

21. Amarapurkar DN, Patel ND, Amarapurkar AD, Agal S, Baigal R, Gupte P. Tissue polymerase chain reaction in diagnosis of intestinal tuberculosis and Crohn's disease. *J Assoc Physicians India*. 2004; 52:863–7.

22. Wobeser WI, Krajden M, Conly J, Simpson H, Yim B, D'Costa M, Fuksa M, Hian-Cheong C, Patterson M, Phillips A, Bannatyne R, Haddad A, Brunton JL, Krajden S. Evaluation of Roche Amplicor PCR assay for *Mycobacterium tuberculosis*. *J Clin Microbiol*. 1996; 34:134–9.

23. Makanjuola D. Is it Crohn's disease or intestinal tuberculosis? CT analysis. *Eur J Radiol*. 1998; 28:55–61.

24. Pai M, Zwerling A, Menzies D. Systematic review: T-cell-based assays for the diagnosis of latent tuberculosis infection: an update. *Ann Intern Med*. 2008; 149:177–84.

25. Epstein D, Watermeyer G, Kirsch R. Review article: the diagnosis and management of Crohn's disease in populations with high-risk rates for tuberculosis. *Aliment Pharmacol Ther*. 2007; 25:1373–88.

26. Loftus EV Jr, Silverstein MD, Sandborn WJ, Tremaine WJ, Harmsen WS, Zinsmeister AR. Crohn's disease in Olmsted County, Minnesota, 1940–1993: incidence, prevalence, and survival. *Gastroenterology*. 1998; 114:1161–8.

Recommended reading

Kirsch R, Pentecost M, Hall P de M, Epstein DP, Watermeyer G, Friederich, PW. Role of colonoscopic biopsy in distinguishing between Crohn's disease and intestinal tuberculosis. *J Clin Pathol*. 2006; 59:840–4.

Ouyang Q, Tandon R, Goh K-L, Ooi CJ, Ogata H, Fiocchi C. The emergence of inflammatory bowel disease in the Asian Pacific region. *Curr Opin Gastroenterol*. 2005; 21:408–13.

Papadakis KA, Tabibzadeh S. Diagnosis and misdiagnosis of inflammatory bowel disease. *Gastrointest Endosc Clin N Am*. 2002; 12:433–9.

Chapter 11: Traveller's diarrhoea

D. Alcid (USA)

Key points

- Traveller's diarrhoea is the most common illness afflicting travellers.
- Depending on the country, it can affect 21–100 per cent of travellers.
- Most cases are self-limited and can be treated supportively.
- Aetiology and symptomatology can be divided syndromically:
  - voluminous diarrhoea, no systemic symptoms, usually due to the toxigenic organisms *Escherichia coli* and *Vibrio cholerae*.
  - dysentery symptoms, small volume stools with systemic symptoms such as fever, chills, blood and mucus in the stools, usually due to invasive pathogens like *Shigella*, *Salmonella* or *Yersinia*.
- The small bowel is the site for toxigenic pathogens, the large bowel for invasive pathogens.
- History and physical examination.
- Stool cultures for invasive pathogens only.
- Blood cultures for invasive pathogens only.
- Most pathogens are self-limited, therefore no antimicrobial therapy.
- Primary therapy is supportive, fluid and electrolyte maintenance.
- An effective vaccine is available for *Salmonella typhi*.
- Prophylactic antibiotics are indicated under special conditions.
- Quinolones are the empiric drug of choice for infections acquired in Asia.
- Patients without systemic symptoms should not be given antibiotics.
- Patients with systemic symptoms and bloody stools, and compromised patients travelling to Asia, should be started on azithromycin.
- Rifaximin for patients without systemic symptoms or bloody stools.
- Methotrexate is effective in steroid-refractive and steroid-dependent Crohn's disease.

◌ Introduction

Depending on the area visited, from 21 to 100 per cent of all travellers will develop an acute diarrhoea, making it the most common infection afflicting travellers. The pathogens implicated are varied (Table 11.1) depending on the area visited.

Table 11.1 Aetiologies of traveller's diarrhoea

	Latin America	**Africa**	**Asia**
Attack rate	20–100%	35–65%	40–60%
Escherichia coli (ETEC, EAEC, EPEC)	28–72%	30–75%	20–57%
Shigella	0–30%	0–15%	4–7%
Salmonella	4%	–	11–15%
Campylobacter	4%	–	2–15%
Vibrio parahaemolyticus	–	–	1–13%
Noroviruses	0–15%	–	4%
Parasites	4%		10%

Symptoms usually develop 3–15 days after arriving in the area; these include malaise, abdominal cramps and watery diarrhoea. Occasionally, some patients develop nausea and vomiting. The illness is usually self-limited, lasting from one to five days. Some patients continue to be sick for up to ten days.

The attack rate depends very much on the travel destination, duration of stay and a wide variety of host factors such as antacid therapy, genetics, duration of stay and lifestyle during travel.

◯ **Pathogenesis**

Enteric pathogens causing traveller's diarrhoea produce disease either by producing enterotoxins (toxigenic). Some toxigenic pathogens produce toxins outside the host, while others produce toxins in the intestinal tract after being ingested.

Other pathogens attach to, penetrate and destroy mucosal and epithelial cells, resulting in tissue destruction and ulceration (invasive). Pathogens like *E. coli* O157:H7, *Shigella* and *Vibrio parahaemolyticus* produce toxins (Shiga toxins or Shiga-like toxins) that are cytotoxic to cultured cell lines (Table 11.2 overleaf). Several strains of *E. coli* (EAggEC, EPEC) can attach to the mucosa and induce secretory diarrhoea through increased intracellular calcium (signal transduction).

Table 11.2 Toxic enteropathogens

Toxin in vivo (enterotoxin)	Invasive	Unknown
Clostridium perfringens	*Salmonella*	Viruses
Bacillus cereus	*Shigella*	*Giardia lamblia*
Escherichia coli (ETEC)	*Campylobacter*	EAggEC
Vibrio cholerae	*Escherichia coli* *Yersinia* *Enterocolitica* *Entamoeba histolytica*	*Cryptosporidium*

Host defence against enteropathogens

Gastric acidity

Most ingested microorganisms never reach the small bowel because of the inhibitory effect of gastric acid (pH <4). Gastric bacterial counts in healthy individuals rarely exceed 10/mL, compared to more than 10 000/mL in achlorhydric patients. Patients with gastric resections, or those on acid suppressive agents, are at increased risk of enteric infection. Antacids decrease the infecting dose of *Vibrio cholerae* (cholera) and *Salmonella* by a factor of 10 000 (from 10^8 to 10^4). Increased susceptibility to *Giardia lamblia* (a protozoan parasite that lives in the small intestine), *Strongyloides stercoralis* (threadworm) and *Diphyllobothrium latum* (broad tapeworm) are also seen in achlorhydric or hypochlorhydric patients.

Intestinal motility

Normal intestinal motility plays an important role in protecting the host against enteric pathogens. *Salmonella* bacteraemia develops in patients given opiates; the severity of symptoms in patients with shigellosis is increased when given lomotil, an antimotility drug. Antimotility agents should be avoided in patients with fever, blood and mucus in their stools.

Intestinal antibodies

Intestinal antibodies, especially IgA, play some role in regulating intestinal colonisation by enteropathogens by inhibiting adherence onto mucosal surfaces by neutralising toxins and viruses. IgA may also be an important defence against parasites like *Giardia lamblia*; patients with selective IgA deficiency or hypogammaglobulinaemia are more susceptible to this parasite.

Genetics

Flores and Okhuysen (2009) reported on the affinity of *Vibrio cholerae* with histo-blood group antigens; genetic polymorphism was found to be associated with an increased risk of diarrhoea and *E. coli* in travellers. Genetic susceptibility to a wide variety of enteropathogens is increasingly being recognised.[1]

Clinical features

Toxigenic

Usually afebrile, non-toxic. Toxigenic pathogens usually affect the small bowel; diarrhoea is usually voluminous with cramping abdominal pain. Illness is self-limited and the patient improves within 3–10 days.

Invasive

Frequently accompanied by systemic symptoms, fever and malaise. The colon is usually involved, with the result that the patient may have tenesmus and urgency, with small but frequent bowel movements. Blood and mucus may be present. The illness is self-limited, but treatment with antibiotics usually decreases the duration of the illness.

◗ Syndromes

Nausea

Toxin produced outside of the GI tract causes vomiting within 1–6 hours. A hallmark of the disease is its short incubation period—the enterotoxins produced by *Staphylococcus aureus* and *Bacillus cereus* strains are already formed before ingestion. The more toxin present, the shorter the incubation period.

The contaminated foods associated with *S. aureus* outbreaks are salads, pies, gravy, cakes and mayonnaise, all seemingly normal in colour, odour and taste. Grains, especially rice, are usually contaminated by *B. cereus* spores that germinate with prolonged heating to produce toxin.

The symptoms for both organisms are identical: nausea, vomiting, headache and, occasionally, mild diarrhoea. The illness is self-limited, usually lasting about 24 hours, and treatment is supportive. It is diagnosed from the patient's history and/or demonstration of the organism from the suspected food or vehicle.

Abdominal cramps

Diarrhoea with low-grade or no fever occurs within 16–72 hours. The major aetiologic agents for this syndrome are *E. coli*, *Vibrio* spp., *B. cereus*, Rotavirus and Norovirus. Symptoms include watery diarrhoea, cramps, no tenesmus or urgency. Vomiting and fever (>102° F, >39° C) occurs infrequently; the presence of vomiting probably excludes these pathogens. Illness usually lasts 24–48 hours and management is primarily supportive: if diarrhoea is not severe, fruit juices or soft drinks are adequate; if severe, oral rehydration salts (ORS) are recommended.[2]

Escherichia coli

Escherichia coli is a most versatile bacterium. Most of what we know about the pathogenesis of enteric infections comes from studies of *E. coli.*

Enterotoxigenic *E. coli* (ETEC)

Similar to *Vibrio cholerae*, ETEC produces a heat-labile (LT) toxin and a heat-stable (ST) toxin. These toxins share a high degree of amino acid sequence identity with cholera toxin (75%) and act in a similar manner through cAMP.[3]

The toxin binds to GM1 gangliosides on the outer membrane surface of host intestinal mucosa cells. Through a complex process, the toxin stimulates the cell's adenylate cyclase enzyme to become continually active. The increased adenylate cyclase results in an abnormally high amount of cyclic adenosine monophosphate (cAMP), which in turn causes the cells to excrete large amounts of chloride ions into the intestines. Water and electrolytes, including Na^+, follow the osmotic and electric gradients created by the excretion of Cl^-. It is this 'pumping' of water and electrolytes that cause the diarrhoea and dehydration seen in the disease.

Enteropathogenic *E. coli* (EPEC)

The mechanism of EPEC-caused diarrhoea is unknown. To date no toxin has been identified. It is believed to be due to signal transduction mediated by *tir* protein causing an increase in intracellular calcium.[4]

Enteroaggregative *E. coli* (EAggEC)

EAggEC produces an ST-like toxin which causes persistent diarrhoea, particularly in children.

Enterohaemorrhagic *E. coli* (EHEC)

Produces Shiga-like toxin (SLT) that is virtually identical to *Shigella dysenteriae* toxin.[5]

Vibrio cholerae

Worldwide in distribution, most cholera pandemics are due to serotype 01; however, recent outbreaks have been due to serotype 0139, an emerging pathogen for which no vaccine is available. The disease is due to the toxin produced intraluminally by the organism. The toxin is an A-B type ADP-ribosylating toxin consisting of an A (enzymatic) subunit and five identical B (binding) subunits. The toxin acts through the cAMP process.

Noroviruses (genus Norovirus, family Caliciviridae)

Previously designated 'Norwalk-like viruses' (NLV), noroviruses are groups of related, single-stranded RNA, no enveloped viruses that cause acute gastroenteritis in humans. The incubation period for norovirus-associated gastroenteritis in humans is usually 12–48 hours.

The disease usually presents as acute-onset vomiting, watery non-bloody diarrhoea with abdominal cramps, and nausea. Low-grade fever also occasionally occurs, and vomiting is more common in children. Symptoms usually last 24–60 hours. Noroviruses are transmitted primarily through the faecal-oral route. They are highly contagious: fewer than 100 viral particles may be sufficient to infect an individual. Noroviruses inhibit gastric emptying, making vomiting a prominent symptom.

A study of norovirus effects found that:

> Among the 232 outbreaks of norovirus illness reported to the CDC [US Center for Disease Control and Prevention] from July 1997 to June 2000, … common settings included restaurants and catered meals (36%), nursing homes (23%), schools (13%), and vacation settings or cruise ships (10%).[6]

▷ Invasive syndromes

Fever, abdominal cramps

The major aetiological considerations for this syndrome, in which diarrhoea occurs within 16–72 hours, are *Salmonella*, *Shigella*, *Campylobacter jejuni*, *Yersinia enterocolitica* and *Vibrio parahaemolyticus*. The incubation period is approximately 16–72 hours; stools may contain mucus and/or blood. Systemic symptoms of fever or malaise are the rule, with vomiting in 35–80 per cent of patients. *Shigella*, *Campylobacter* and *Yersinia* all affect the colon, so patients experience symptoms of tenesmus and urgency. The illnesses usually resolve within 2–10 days without treatment, or less with antibiotic therapy.

Salmonella

The *Salmonella* bacterium is a major cause of foodborne infection worldwide. There are three serotypes: *S. typhi* (one serotype), *S. choleraesuis* (one serotype) and *S. enteritidis* (>2000 serotypes); almost all infections are due to one of the members of the *S. enteritidis* group. Diarrhoea due to *S. enteritidis* is usually self-limited: antimicrobial therapy does not affect the clinical course and may even prolong the carrier state.[7]

Shigella

Shigella spp. are highly infectious, with a dose of only 100–200 organisms required to infect humans. *Shigella* can be spread person-to-person or by vectors such as flies; it is highly resistant to gastric acid. In the colon the organism rapidly enters mucosal cells, divides and spreads laterally to infect adjacent cells. Extensive inflammatory damage occurs, resulting in ulceration.

Campylobacter

Worldwide in distribution, *Campylobacter* spp. are found as commensals in the gastrointestinal tract of cattle, sheep, pigs, dogs, cats, rodents and a wide variety of fowl. Most infected animals become chronic asymptomatic carriers. Infection results either from direct contact with an infected animal or ingestion of poorly cooked, contaminated meat. *Campylobacter* is usually susceptible to macrolides, erythromycin and azithromycin. Many strains of *Campylobacter* isolated from South-East Asia are resistant to quinolones, with some 20 per cent resistance in the USA being reported.[8]

Enteric fever – typhoidal fever

The syndrome is characterised by prolonged fever, headache, abdominal pain, skin rash, relative bradycardia, splenomegaly and bacteraemia. Onset of fever occurs gradually, in a stepwise fashion. The organisms responsible for the syndrome include *Salmonella typhi*, *S. choleraesuis* and *S. paratyphi* A and B.

Because humans are the only reservoir for *S. typhi*, the presence of disease implies a human source. Definitive diagnosis is by isolating the organism from blood, urine, stool or bone marrow. Other organisms that can present in a similar way to 'typhoidal syndrome' include *Yersinia enterocolitica, Brucella* spp. and *Pasteurella tularensis* (typhoidal tularaemia). Vaccine against *S. typhi* is available and is about 70 per cent effective; it is recommended for prolonged travel longer than three weeks. A strain of *S. typhi*, especially from South Asia, is resistant to ciprofloxacin but it continues to be susceptible to ceftriaxone.

Bloody diarrhoea without fever

This syndrome is due to O157:H7, the most common of the pathogenic *E. coli* serotypes (36%), that produces verotoxin, a Shiga-like cytotoxin designated SLT-I and/or SLT-II.[9]

Outbreaks are due to contaminated beef products, contaminated water, and person-to-person contact. Eight per cent of infected patients will develop haemolytic-uraemic syndrome (HUS). Diagnosis is by serotyping sorbitol-negative *E. coli*, or testing the stool for Shiga toxin.

The traveller with AIDS

A traveller with AIDS presents with the unique problem that diarrhoea is usually protracted and difficult to manage and, in some cases, life threatening. The possible enteric pathogens seen in AIDS patients are shown in Table 11.3.

Table 11.3 Enteric pathogens in AIDS patients

Pathogen	Frequency (%)
Cryptosporidium	14–26
Microsporidium	7–33
Cytomegalovirus*	12–45
Shigella spp.	5–10
Mycobacterium spp*.	2–25
Blastocystis hominis	2–15
Entamoeba histolytica	0–15
Salmonella spp.	0–15
Campylobacter spp.	2–11
Giardia lamblia	2–15
Isospora spp.	2–6
Clostridium difficile*	6–7
Strongyloides stercoralis	0–6
One or more pathogen	55–86%

* Can be acquired without travel

Although cure or eradication is difficult for some of these, some do respond to specific therapy and therefore there is a need for specific diagnosis. The use of antiretroviral agents has improved the outcome from of these pathogens. Travellers with AIDS must be extra vigilant regarding food consumption: no uncooked foods, if no bottled drinks available boiled water only, and should be given prophylactic antimicrobial (rifaximin).[10]

Stool cultures

The yield from stool cultures in patients without systemic symptoms or blood in the stool is very low (<6%) since the routine laboratory procedure does not test for ETEC or EPEC, and there is no test available for detecting EaggEC. *V. cholerae* will be missed (unless specifically requested) since it requires special media; also, most toxigenic pathogens are present only within the first 48 hours. Stool cultures are indicated only for patients with fever, bloody stools, tenesmus and urgency. Selective stool cultures increase the yield of diagnoses up to 40 per cent of the samples tested—implying that a routine laboratory test is not able to identify up to 60 per cent of cases.

The test for stool leukocyte tends to be used inappropriately: originally it was designed as a *rapid test* for differentiating invasive from non-invasive pathogens so that therapy could be started immediately. The test should therefore be performed at the point-of-care setting—emergency department, office or clinic—rather than sent to a laboratory where results would typically not be available for at least 24 hours. The stool test for leukocyte lacks sensitivity and specificity, therefore will not differentiate infection from inflammation.

◗ Management

Since most pathogens are self-limited, with more than 95 per cent of patients recovering within 7–10 days, therapy is primarily supportive, including oral rehydrating solutions for severe diarrhoea; otherwise any hydrating solutions will suffice.

A small number of patients might require antimicrobial therapy, depending primarily on the geographic source of the infection. Quinolones are not the first choice for travellers from Asia because of resistance to it: 80 per cent of *Campylobacter foetus* is resistant to quinolone, and the proportion of resistance in *Salmonella* spp. is also increasing.

Empiric antimicrobial therapy should be limited to patients with systemic symptoms, bloody stool with symptoms of dysentery, and patients with positive stool for leukocytes, or those with worsening symptoms at the time of presentation.

Antimotility agents such as loperamide should be avoided in patients with fever or bloody stools.

Azithromycin is the empiric drug of choice, indicated especially for travellers to South-East Asia and for patients with fever, bloody stools, and those with worsening of symptoms at the time of presentation. Rifaximin is a non-absorbable antimicrobial agent recently approved by the US Food and Drug Administration for the treatment of uncomplicated traveller's diarrhoea.

In clinical trials of xifaxan, the cure rate for patients infected with *C. foetus* is 23.5 per cent, similar to placebo; therefore xifaxan should not be used in patients with systemic symptoms (invasive) or in patients travelling to or from South-East Asia.

Prophylaxis is not usually recommended—however there are some instances where it may be indicated: immunocompromised patients including those with AIDS, patients with decreased gastric acidity for any reason (PPI, H_2 blockers, or gastrectomy), and travellers on critically important business. The preferred prophylactic agent is rifaximin.

Summary

Traveller's diarrhoea is a self-limited illness and usually does not require treatment; but if treatment is necessary, empiric therapy is primarily supportive. Empiric antibiotic therapy should be reserved for patients with systemic symptoms, bloody stools or those with worsening symptoms.

Prophylaxis is not usually indicated. Exceptions include immunocompromised patients (e.g. AIDS), patients with decreased gastric acidity (PPI, H_2 blockers, or gastrectomy), or patients on critically important business.

Information for patients

What medical plans should I make for travelling to other countries?

A pre-travel history is advisable. Outline a detailed itinerary in order to determine the risk of exposure to various infectious agents. Also consult your doctor, preferably at least six weeks before departure so that chronic health conditions can be taken into account, and for any necessary immunisations to be arranged.

What medications should I pack?

Travellers should take adequate supplies of their own medications as well as medications for travel-associated diseases. Immunoprophylaxis is available for yellow fever, cholera, hepatitis A, hepatitis B, typhoid, rabies, meningococcal disease, bubonic plague and viral encephalitis.

What food and drink should I be wary of?

Risky foods include uncooked vegetables, meat, seafood, salads, tap water, ice, unpasteurised milk, dairy products and unpeeled fruits.

Unpurified drinking water can be the source of bacterial, viral and parasitic pathogens. Carbonated soft drinks are usually safe, but bottled water may vary in safety standards. Water boiled for five minutes is safe.

Are there any particular health risks that I should be aware of?

Health risks may be related to the type and quality of accommodation that you will live in.

References

1. Flores J, Okhuysen PC. Genetics of susceptibility to infection with enteric pathogens. *Curr Opin Infect Dis*. 2009 Oct; 22(5):471–6.

2. Atia AN, Buchman AL. Oral rehydration solutions in non-cholera diarrhea: a review. *Am J Gastroenterol*. 2009 Oct; 104(10):2596–604; quiz 2605.

3. Thiagarajah JR, Verkman AS. New drug targets for cholera toxin. *Trends Pharmacol Sci*. 2005; 26:172–5.

4. Race PR, Solovyova AS, Banfield MJ. Conformation of the EPEC tir protein in solution: investigating the impact of serine phosphorylation at positions 434/463. *Biophys J*. 2007 Jul 15; 93(2):586–96. doi:10.1529/biophysj.106.101766.

5. Beutin L. Emerging enterohaemorrhagic *Escherichia coli*: causes and effects of the rise of a human pathogen. *J Vet Med B Infect Dis Vet Public Health*. 2006; 53(7): 299–305.

6. Norovirus: Technical fact sheet. National Center for Immunization and Respiratory Diseases: Division of Viral Diseases. [Internet]. Available from: www.cdc.gov/ncidod/dvrd/revb/gastro/norovirus-factsheet.htm.

7. van Duijkeren E, Houwers DJ. A critical assessment of antimicrobial treatment in uncomplicated *Salmonella* enteritis. *Vet Microbiol*. 2000 Apr 4; 73(1):61–73.

8. Smith KE, Besser JM, Hedberg CW, Leano FT, Bender JB, Wicklund JH, Johnson BP, Moore KA, Osterholm MT. Quinolone-resistant *Campylobacter jejuni* infections in Minnesota, 1992–1998. Investigation Team. *N Engl J Med*. 1999 May 20; 340(20):1525–32.

9. Armstrong GL, Hollingsworth J, Morris JG Jr. Emerging foodborne pathogens: *Escherichia coli* O157:H7 as a model of entry of a new pathogen into the food supply of the developed world. *Epidemiol Rev*. 1996; 1(18):29–51.

10. Koo HL, Dupont HL, Huang DB. The role of rifaximin in the treatment and chemoprophylaxis of travelers' diarrhea. *Ther Clin Risk Manag*. 2009; 5:841–8.

Recommended reading

Chen LH, Wilson ME, Davis X, Loutan L, Schwartz E, Keystone J, Hale D, Lim PL, McCarthy A, Gkrania-Klotsas E, Schlagenhauf P, GeoSentinel Surveillance Network. Illness in long-term travelers visiting GeoSentinel clinics. *Emerg Infect Dis*. 2009 Nov; 15(11):1773–82.

Chongsuvivatwong V, Chariyalertsak S, McNeil E, Aiyarak S, Hutamai S, Dupont HL, Jiang ZD, Kalambaheti T, Tonyong W, Thitiphuree S, Steffen R. Epidemiology of travelers' diarrhea in Thailand. *J Travel Med*. 2009 May–Jun; 16(3):179–85.

DuPont HL. Systematic review: the epidemiology and clinical features of travellers' diarrhea. *Aliment Pharmacol Ther*. 2009 Aug; 30(3):187–96.

Dupont HL. Traveling internationally: avoiding and treating travelers' diarrhea. *Clin Gastroenterol Hepatol*. 2010 Jun; 8(6):490–3; quiz e71.

Gautret P, Schlagenhauf P, Castelli F, Brouqui P, von Sonnenberg F, Loutan L, Parola P, GeoSentinel Surveillance Network. Multicenter Euro TravNet/GeoSentinel study of travel-related infectious diseases in Europe. *Emerg Infect Dis*. 2009 Nov; 15(11):1783–90.

Kuhlman FM, Weil GJ. Infectious risk for travelers to the tropics. *Mo Med*. 2009 Jul–Aug; 106(4):263–8.

Shah N, DuPont HL, Ramsey DJ. Global aetiology of travelers' diarrhea: systematic review from 1973 to present. *Am J Trop Med Hyg*. 2009 Apr;80(4):609–14.

Singh E, Redfield D. Prophylaxis for travelers' diarrhea. *Curr Gastroenterol Rep*. 2009 Aug; 11(4):297–300.

Chapter 12: Cholera

H. Paradwala (India)

Key points

- ▶ Cholera is an infectious gastroenteritis caused by enterotoxin-producing strains of the bacterium *Vibrio cholerae*.
- ▶ Transmission occurs through direct faecal–oral contamination or through ingestion of contaminated water and food.
- ▶ It involves the lower part of the small bowel.
- ▶ Cholera probably has its origins in, and is endemic to, the Indian subcontinent.
- ▶ Cholera is mainly transmitted through contaminated water and food and is closely linked to inadequate environmental management. Typical at-risk areas include peri-urban slums and camps for internally displaced people or refugees.
- ▶ The usual incubation period is two to five days, although it can be as short as several hours.
- ▶ Severe cholera is characterised by a sudden onset of profuse, watery diarrhoea accompanied by nausea and vomiting. If left untreated this can rapidly lead to serious dehydration, electrolyte imbalance and circulatory collapse. Over 50 per cent of the most severe cases die within a few hours; with prompt, effective treatment, mortality is less than 1 per cent.
- ▶ Cholera may be asymptomatic or mild in healthy individuals, with diarrhoea as the only symptom.
- ▶ Although signs and symptoms of severe cholera may be unmistakable in endemic areas, the only way to confirm a diagnosis is to identify the bacteria in a stool sample.
- ▶ Rapid cholera dipstick tests are now available.
- ▶ Successful treatment of cholera requires prompt and adequate fluid and electrolyte replacement. Intravenous fluid replacement therapy is necessary for patients with severe dehydration. If vomiting is not prominent, oral replacement is usually adequate.
- ▶ Oral rehydration therapy (ORT) is a simple, cheap and effective treatment for dehydration associated with diarrhoea, particularly gastroenteritis.
- ▶ Oral tetracycline 500 mg every six hours for the first 48 hours shortens the duration of cholera.
- ▶ Children and pregnant women who contract cholera should be treated with ampicillin. Trimethoprim-sulfamethoxazole and furazolidone are also effective.

▶ Measures for preventing cholera consist of providing clean water and proper sanitation to populations potentially affected.

▶ All foodstuffs must be kept covered and vegetables and fruits washed with a solution of potassium permanganate before consumption. Other precautions against this disease include avoiding all uncooked vegetables, thorough washing of hands by all those who handle food, and elimination of all contacts with the disease.

▶ An internationally licensed oral cholera vaccine (OCV) is currently available and is suitable for travellers.

◐ Introduction

Cholera is an extremely virulent disease that affects both children and adults and can be fatal within a few hours. Sometimes known as Asiatic or epidemic cholera, it is an infectious gastroenteritis involving the lower part of the small intestine. It is caused by enterotoxin-producing strains of the short, curved, rod-shaped bacterium *Vibrio cholerae*.

The disease strikes suddenly; it is transmitted by direct faecal–oral contamination, or through ingestion of contaminated water or food. Being a water-borne disease, it is very common during the monsoon season. *V. cholerae* is a Gram-negative bacterium that produces cholera toxin, an enterotoxin whose action on the mucosal epithelium lining of the small intestine causes the disease's most salient characteristic, exhaustive diarrhoea.

The disease is characterised in its most severe form by a sudden onset of acute watery diarrhoea that can lead to death by severe dehydration and kidney failure. The extremely short incubation period—two hours to five days—enhances the explosive pattern of outbreaks, as the number of cases can rise very quickly.

About 75 per cent of people infected with cholera do not develop any symptoms. However, the pathogens remain in their faeces for seven to fourteen days and are shed back into the environment, potentially infecting other individuals. The major reservoir for cholera was long assumed to be humans themselves, but considerable evidence exists that an aquatic environment can serve as a reservoir for the bacteria.

◐ Epidemiology

It is likely that cholera has its origins in, and is endemic to, the Indian subcontinent. Historically, the disease spread by land and sea trade routes to Russia firstly, then to Western Europe, and from Europe to North America. Cholera is now no longer considered a pressing health threat in Europe or North America due to filtering and chlorination of water supplies, but it still heavily affects populations in developing countries.

The disease is now considered to be endemic in many countries and the pathogen causing cholera cannot currently be eliminated from the environment. Cholera remains a global threat to public health and one of the key indicators of social development. While the disease is no longer an issue in countries where minimum hygiene standards are met, it remains a threat in almost every developing country. The number of cholera cases reported to the World Health Organization (WHO) during 2006 rose dramatically, again reaching the level of the late 1990s. A total of 236896 cases were notified from 52 countries, including 6311 deaths, an overall increase of 79 per cent over the number of cases reported the previous year. It is estimated that only a small proportion of cases—less than 10 per cent—are reported to WHO.

Fatality rates are 5 per cent of total cases in Africa, and less than 1 per cent elsewhere. Recent studies suggest that global warming might create a favourable environment for *V. cholerae* and increase the incidence of the disease in vulnerable areas.

Risk factors and vulnerable populations

Cholera is mainly transmitted through contaminated water. Typically, areas at risk include settlements without proper infrastructure for water and sanitation—for example, fringe-area slums or hastily constructed refugee settlements in the wake of war or natural disaster—if the pathogen is present or is introduced.[1]

Both the O1 and O139 (Bengal) serogroups of *V. cholerae* can cause outbreaks, but most are caused by O1. Humans are the main reservoirs, along with brackish water and estuaries, especially when associated with algal blooms. Serogroup O139 has the same virulence factors as O1 and creates a similar clinical picture; the presence of O139 has so far been detected only in South-East and East Asia. Other strains can cause mild diarrhoea but do not develop into epidemics.[2]

Susceptibility

Susceptibility to cholera and other diarrhoeal infections can be affected by blood type: type O individuals appear to be at greatest risk, folowed in order by types A, B and AB, with type AB providing the most resistance.[3, 4]

Susceptibity is increased by immunity deficiency (HIV, for example) and/ or decreased gastric acidity (from using antacids), or by malnourishment.

Transmission

Cholera is rarely spread directly from person to person.

The highly liquid diarrhoea associated with cholera ('rice-water' stool) contains high concentrations of *V. cholerae*. Ingestion of water contaminated by untreated faeces in waterways, in groundwater or in drinking water—and including foods washed with contaminated water, and shellfish living in the affected waterway—can transmit the disease.

The chitinous exoskeleton of zooplankton in fresh, brackish or salt water harbours *V. cholerae*. Both toxic and non-toxic strains of the bacterium exist; non-toxic strains can become virulent through lysogenic bacteriophage action.[5]

In addition, since cholera is a zoonotic disease, disease outbreaks can also occur as the consequence of coastal zooplankton blooms.

�‣ Clinical presentation

A cholera patient is observed to pass through three stages:

1. The patient develops increased peristalsis and a feeling of fullness. Thereafter they develop mild diarrhoea and vomiting, which rapidly worsens. The motions become watery ('rice-water' stool). Abdominal pain and high fever are usually minimal or absent, distinctly disproportionate to the amount of diarrhoea. Electrolyte abnormalities from voluminous diarrhoea may manifest as muscle weakness, severe cramps in the abdominal muscles and limbs, intestinal ileus, or even cardiac dysrhythmia. The temperature rises but the skin is generally cold and blue and the pulse is weak. The intake of water to quench thirst dilutes the body salts still further, and makes the cramps worse.

2. The patient's body becomes colder, the skin dry, wrinkled and purple. Their voice becomes husky and weak. The urine becomes dark, and its formation is less or altogether absent. Mental status changes may also occur due to hypoglycaemia. Without urgent fluid and electrolyte replacement therapy, hypovolemic shock may occur and the patient may die as soon as 24 hours after the onset of the symptoms.

3. Recovery follows in favourable cases and the disease runs its course within two days to a week. All the changes in the patient seem to reverse, fluid loss decreases and there is improvement in the patient's general condition. Even at this stage, however, the patient may relapse or take on a condition similar to typhoid; this may deteriorate over a period of two or three weeks, during which time their temperature may rise and there is a danger of pneumonia.

Important causes of death with cholera in inadequately treated patients are: hypovolemic shock, metabolic acidosis, or uraemia resulting from acute tubular necrosis.

�‣ Diagnosis

In an epidemic, cholera is diagnosed by taking a the patient's history of symptoms together with clinical examination. Treatment is usually started immediately, either before or without confirmation by laboratory tests.

Laboratory findings

Stool and swab samples should be collected at the acute stage of the disease before antibiotics are administered. Direct stool examination is useful for the presumptive identification of *V. cholerae*. The stool tends to lose its faecal odour as the disease progresses and may develop a sweet odour, and becomes watery, turbid and gray, with small flecks of mucus giving the 'rice-water' appearance. Choleric stool does not usually contain blood or neutrophils.

Microscopic examination

Straight or curved bacilli with rapid, darting or 'shooting star' motility suggest *V. cholerae* infection. Inhibition of the motility of the organism by *V. cholerae* O1 antiserum further supports the diagnosis of cholera.

Stool from suspected cholera patients should be cultured on a selective and differential media such as bile salt, gelatin-tellurite-taurocholate agar (GTT agar), or thiosulfate-citrate-bilesalt-sucrose agar (TCBS agar).[6]

On bile salt or GTT agar the organisms typically appear as translucent colonies within 24 hours. On TCBS agar, *V. cholerae* appear at 24 hours as distinct, large, flat, yellow colonies.

Latex agglutination and enzyme-linked immunosorbent assay (ELISA)-based methods have been developed to detect the presence of cholera toxin. These are rapid and may be useful in quickly detecting cholera in patients at the early phases of the disease. Polymerase chain reaction (PCR)-based methods of organism detection have been used successfully to detect *V. cholerae* nucleic acids from choleric stools.

Rapid diagnostic tests for cholera

SMART, Medicos Dip Stick and an Institut Pasteur (IP) cholera dipstick tests can be used. The accuracy of these tests may depend on the skill of the tecnician, however.[7]

Differential diagnosis

Diarrhoeal diseases are caused by other common organisms, including:

- Bacteria: *Salmonella* spp., *Shigella* spp., *Yersinia enterocolitica*, *Campylobacter* spp., *E. coli*
- Viruses: Rotavirus and Norovirus (formerly Norwalk agent)
- Parasites: *Giardia lamblia*, *Cyclospora* and *Cryptosporidium*.

Essentials of diagnosis

- History of exposure, particularly travel to endemic or epidemic locales.
- Acute onset of voluminous, watery diarrhoea with low-grade fever and mild abdominal pain.

- The presence of straight to curved Gram-negative bacilli, with single polar flagellum, in the stool of an infected patient.
- In wet preparation, these organisms demonstrate a characteristic darting or 'shooting star' motility confirmed by motility inhibition with specific antisera.
- Culture of *V. cholerae* from stool with differential media.
- Bacterial growth in nutrient broth, without 1 per cent NaCl supplementation. This characteristic is useful for differentiating between *V. cholerae* and most other *Vibrio* species.
- Detection of *V. cholerae* toxins by latex agglutination or ELISA, or the detection of *V. cholerae*-specific nucleic acid by PCR-based methods.

▷ Management

Successful treatment of cholera requires prompt and adequate fluid and electrolyte replacement, acid-base and glucose management. Intravenous fluid replacement therapy is necessary for patients with severe dehydration (>10 per cent of their body weight) and acidosis (pH <7.2). Lactated Ringer's solution is adequate. Intravenous fluids are initially infused at the rate of 50–100 mL/min until a strong pulse is restored. Subsequently, fluid should be infused in quantities equal to the gastrointestinal losses, sufficient to maintain a normal radial pulse and normal skin turgor. Inadequate or delayed restoration of fluid losses may result in a high incidence of acute renal failure.

Serious hypokalaemic symptoms are rare in adults but may contribute significantly to morbidity in children. If mental status changes are evident, hypoglycaemia should be treated with intravenous glucose infusion (bolus 3–4 mL/kg of a 25% glucose solution, followed by continuous infusion of 10 mg/kg/hr). If vomiting is not prominent, oral replacement is usually adequate.

Management of paediatric patients

Oral rehydration therapy (ORT) is a simple, cheap and effective treatment for dehydration associated with diarrhoea, particularly gastroenteritis caused by cholera or rotavirus. ORT is a solution of salts and sugars which is taken by mouth. It is most important in the developing world, where it saves millions of children a year from death due to diarrhoea—the second leading cause of death in children under five.[8]

Home-made oral rehydration solution (ORS)

To replenish liquid, sugar and sodium being lost from a child's body due to diarrhoea, an ORS can be made by dissolving household salt (1 level teaspoon) and sugar (8 level teaspoons) in 1 litre (approximately 5 cups) of clean or boiled water. One such drink should be given to the child every time a watery stool is passed. Adding orange juice, mashed banana or green coconut water improves the palatability and also provides potassium.

Traditional remedies—breast milk, gruel (cooked cereal diluted with water), carrot soup, or rice water (congee)—are highly effective oral rehydration solutions for preventing dehydration.

If a child demonstrates worsening diarrhoea due to increased serum sodium concentration from the ORS, only small amounts of plain water should be given. This effect may be caused by the slight hypertonicity of the ORS combined with transient partial glucose malabsorption; it can be avoided if water, breast milk or other low-solute drink is given liberally during maintenance therapy with ORS solution, as recommended by the World Health Organization (WHO).[9]

WHO and UNICEF jointly maintain the official guidelines for the contents of reduced osmolarity ORS packets. The reduced osmolarity ORS has a total osmolarity of 245 mmol/L (Table 12.1). The efficaciousness of the reduced osmolarity ORS compared to the standard WHO ORS has been examined in at least one research report.[10]

Table 12.1 Concentrations of ingredients in reduced osmolarity ORS

Ingredient	g/L	Molecule	mmol/L
Sodium chloride (NaCl)	2.6	Sodium	75
Glucose, anhydrous ($C_6H_{12}O_6$)	13.5	Glucose	75
Potassium chloride (KCl)	1.5	Potassium	20
		Chloride	65
Trisodium citrate dihydrate ($Na_3C_6H_5O_7 \cdot 2H_2O$)	2.9	Citrate	10
Total	20.5		245

Source: WHO/UNICEF official guidelines.

Zinc supplementation

Zinc supplementation is also recommended for the management of diarrhoeal disease in addition to ORS, particularly for paediatric patients. For children under five, zinc supplementation significantly reduces the severity and duration of diarrhoea. It is strongly recommended as a supplement to ORS for children who are dehydrated.

Antimicrobial therapy

A dramatic reduction in the duration and volume of diarrhoea and early eradication of *Vibrio* from stool may be effected by antibiotic therapy.

Pregnant women and children who develop cholera should be treated with ampicillin.

Tetracycline and the quinolones are generally not given to children because of potential toxicity; however, in cases in which strains of *V. cholerae* are resistant to other drugs and severe disease is evident, tetracycline or quinolones may be considered. If the patient is allergic to penicillin, trimethoprim-sulfamethoxazole (TMP/SMX) and furazolidone are also effective. In summary:

First choice:

- Ampicillin, 250 mg orally or IV every 6 hours for 5 days.
- Tetracycline 500 mg orally or IV for 5 days (ampicillin during pregnancy).

Second choice:

- TMP/SMX orally or IV (2 months old); YMP, 3–6 mg +SMX 15–30 mg/kg every 12 hours for 5 days.
- Ampicillin 500 mg orally or IV every 6 hours for 5 days.
- Penicillin allergy: TMP/SMX (dosage as above) or furazolidone (liquid 3.33 mg/mL; 1–4 years old, 5–7.5 mL every 6 hours for 5 days.
- Tetracycline (dosage as above) or TMP/SMX orally or IV TMP, 160 mg + SMX 800 mg orally or IV every 12 hours; or furazolidone 100 mg orally every 6 hours for 5 days.

Prognosis

Among people developing symptoms, 80 per cent of episodes are of mild or moderate severity. Of the remaining cases, 10–20 per cent develop severe watery diarrhoea with signs of dehydration.

If untreated, as many as one in two people may die. Under ideal conditions and with prompt and adequate fluid replacement, mortality approaches zero, and significant sequelae are rare. Unfortunately, the prognosis for patients infected during a cholera epidemic is often poor due to lack of basic medical care such as fluid and electrolyte replacement. The success of treatment is significantly affected by the method of treatment and the speed with which it is administered.

If cholera patients are treated quickly and adequately, the mortality rate is lower than 1 per cent, but rises to 50–60 per cent if untreated.

Patients who are not recognised to have an intestinal ileus may fare poorly. They may be misdiagnosed initially or, if recognised to have cholera, may not receive adequate fluid and electrolyte replacement. Prevention and control of cholera outbreaks mostly consist of providing clean water, proper sanitation, health education and good food hygiene.[1]

Potentially contaminated water must be boiled before drinking or being used in cooking. All food must be covered; fruit and vegetables should be washed with potassium permanganate solution; uncooked vegetables should be avoided, and hands thoroughly washed in clean or boiled water by everyone handling food. All contact with the disease must be eliminated.

Once an outbreak is detected, the usual intervention strategy is to ensure prompt access to treatment and to control the disease spreading. Most patients—up to 80 per cent—can be treated adequately through the administration of oral rehydration salts (WHO/UNICEF ORS standard sachet).

Very severely dehydrated patients are treated by administering fluids intravenously, preferably Ringer's lactate solution. Appropriate antibiotics can be given to severe cases to diminish the duration of diarrhoea, reduce the volume of rehydration fluids needed and reduce the duration of *Vibrio* excretion.

Oral cholera vaccines

Oral cholera vaccines (OCV) are currently available and are suitable for travellers. They are safe and effective (85–90 per cent after six months in all age groups, declining to 62 per cent after one year among adults). They are available for individuals from the age of two years, and are administered in two doses taken 10–15 days apart.[1]

The schedule is given in Table 12.2.

Table 12.2 Cholera vaccine schedules

Age	Primary course	Reinforcing doses
Adults and children from 6 years and older	2 doses with an interval of at least one week between them. If more than 6 weeks have elapsed between doses, the primary course should be restarted.	Single dose after 2 years. If more than 2 years have elapsed since initial course, the entire course should be repeated.
Age 2 to 6 years	3 doses with an interval of at least one week between doses. If more than 6 weeks have elapsed between doses, the primary course should be restarted.	Single dose after 6 months. As with adults and children over 6 years, if more than 2 years have elapsed, the whole course should be repeated.

Source: Chen-qui: The world of micro-organism, www.dowell-netherlands.com/p/cholera.html.

Contraindications
- Hypersensitivity to active substances or excipients of the vaccine.
- Current acute gastrointestinal illness or febrile illness.

Adverse events
In clinical trials, adverse events were uncommon; those most frequently reported were gastrointestinal, including abdominal pain, diarrhoea, abdominal cramps and general discomfort.

Travel and trade
Countries no longer require proof of cholera vaccination as a condition for entry. The International Certificate of Vaccination no longer provides a specific space for recording cholera vaccinations. Experience has shown that quarantine measures and embargos on movements of people and goods—especially food products—are unnecessary.

Summary

Cholera is an infectious gastroenteritic disease caused by the bacterium *Vibrio cholerae*. Fatality rates are 5 per cent of total cases in Africa, and less than 1 per cent elsewhere. Transmission can occur by faecal–oral contamination, but it is mainly transmitted through contaminated water and food, and is closely linked to inadequate environmental management.

The usual incubation period is two to five days. It may cause sudden profuse, watery diarrhoea, vomiting and nausea, which can lead to dehydration, electrolyte imbalance and circulatory collapse. In more than half of the worst cases, patients die within hours. Prompt treatment reduces mortality to below 1 per cent.

Healthy people may experience only mild diarrhoea. Identifying the bacteria requires a stool sample test; rapid cholera dipstick tests are available.

Treatment of dehydration from diarrhoea requires prompt fluid and electrolyte replacement, usually orally if there is no vomiting. Oral rehydration therapy (ORT) is a simple, cheap and effective treatment. Intravenous fluid replacement may be needed for patients with severe dehydration and acidosis.

Oral tetracycline 500 mg every 6 hours for the first 48 hours will shorten the duration of cholera. Ampicillin should be used to treat children and pregnant women.

Oral cholera vaccines are available.

Information for patients

What is cholera?

Cholera is a diarrhoeal infection caused by the *Vibrio cholerae* bacterium. Infection usually only causes mild diarrhoea or no symptoms at all. In 5–10 per cent of cases, however, patients develop very severe watery diarrhea and vomiting. This causes the loss of large amounts of fluids, which can rapidly lead to severe dehydration. If left untreated, the patient can die within hours.

How does cholera spread?

By drinking contaminated water or eating contaminated food: raw or poorly cooked seafood, raw fruit or vegetables, or other foods that are contaminated during storage or preparation. Cholera can spread rapidly in places where sewage and drinking water supplies are inadequately treated.

Where do outbreaks occur?

Cholera is a constant risk in many countries, especially Africa, Asia and parts of the Middle East. New outbreaks can occur wherever unsafe water supplies, sanitation or food are found, or where hygiene is inadequate, such as in overpopulated communities and refugee settings. For information about cholera in a particular area, contact your health care provider or travel health centre.

What is the risk for travellers?

Extremely low for most travellers—about 0.2 per 100 000. For long-stay travellers where outbreaks occur, the rate may be as high as 500 cases per 100 000 people.

Can cholera be prevented?

Yes: by following a few commonsense rules of good hygiene and safe food preparation—careful hand washing before handling or eating food, thorough cooking of food and eating it while it's hot, treating or boiling drinking water, and using sanitary facilities.

Things to avoid include untreated or unboiled water, ice and ice blocks, raw seafood, other raw foods (except fruit and vegetables you have peeled yourself), partly cooked food, cold cooked food, unpasteurised milk unless it has been boiled, and ice cream.

Drinks that are usually safe include hot tea or coffee, wine, beer, carbonated water or soft drinks, and bottled or packaged fruit juices.

What treatments are available for cholera?

The most important is prompt rehydration to replace the water and salts lost through severe diarrhoea and vomiting, by drinking large quantities of a solution of oral rehydration salts. Early rehydration saves the lives of almost all cholera patients. Patients who become severely dehydrated may need to receive fluid intravenously.

Packets of oral rehydration salts are available from most city pharmacies and health care facilities. The World Health Organization recommends that travellers include these in their medical kits.

If you have diarrhoea—especially if it severe—and you are in an area where there is cholera, seek treatment immediately from a physician or other trained health care provider.

What about antibiotics and other drugs?

Treatment with oral tetracycline 500 mg every 6 hours for the first 48 hours will reduce the duration of cholera. Ampicillin should be used to treat children and pregnant women. For someone allergic to penicillin, trimethoprim-sulfamethoxazole or furazolidone can be used.

Antidiarrhoeal medicines such as loperamide are not recommended and should never be given.

Do vaccines confer protection?

Oral cholera vaccines provide good protection for up to three years for travellers. These do not provide 100 per cent protection, however, so that basic hygienic precautions should always be followed. (Nations no longer require proof of cholera vaccination as a condition for entry, and even the International Certificate of Vaccination no longer provides a space for recording cholera vaccination.)

References

1. International Classification of Diseases, 6th ed, 9th revision, Clinical Modification (ICD-9-CM): Cholera. [Internet]. Available from: www.allcountries.org/health/cholera.html.

2. Questions and answers on acute diarrhoea and cholera. [Internet]. Available from http://medicaltutors.com/FEATURED/featured_article_detail.aspx?itemid=359&categoryid=13.

3. Sack DA, Sack RB, Nair GB, Siddique AK. Cholera. *Lancet*. 2004 Jan; 363(9404):223–33.

4. King AA, Ionides EL, Luckhurst J, Bouma MJ. Inapparent infections and cholera dynamics. *Nature*. 2008 Aug; 454(7206):877–80.

5. Archivist. Cholera phage discovery. *Arch Dis Child*. 1997; 76:274. doi:10.1136/adc.76.3.274.

6. Centers for Disease Control and Prevention. Laboratory methods for the diagnosis of epidemic dysentery and cholera. Atlanta, GA. 1999.

7. Kalluri P, Naheed A, Rahman S, Ansaruzzaman M, Faruque AS, Bird M, Khatun F, Bhuiyan NA, Nato F, Fournier JM, Bopp C, Breiman RF, Nair GB, Mintz ED. Evaluation of three rapid diagnostic tests for cholera: does the skill level of the technician matter?. *Trop Med Int Health*. 2006 Jan; 11(1):49–55.

8. UNICEF. The state of the world's children 2008: child survival. New York: UNICEF. 2007 Dec; p. 8. Available from: www.unicef.org.

9. WHO, UNICEF. Oral rehydration salts: production of the new ORS. [Internet]. Available from http://libdoc.who.int/hq/2006/WHO_FCH_CAH_06.1.pdf.

10. el-Mougi M, el-Akkad N, Hendawi A, Hassan M, Amer A, Fontaine O, Pierce NF. Is a low-osmolarity ORS solution more efficacious than standard WHO ORS solution?. *J Pediatr Gastroenterol Nutr*. 1994 Jul; 19(1):83–6.

Chapter 13: Malaria

H. Paradwala (India)

Keypoints

- Malaria is transmitted by the bite of the infected female *Anopheles* mosquito.
- It is a parasitic disease caused by the protozoan parasite *Plasmodium* species: *P. falciparum* (severe infection), *P. vivax* (most cases), *P. ovale*, *P. malariae* and *P. knowlesi*.
- *P. falciparum* has the highest morbidity rates. It is generally the only species that causes death in humans. Some strains of the bacterium resist all commonly used antimalarial drugs.
- *P. vivax* malaria rarely causes complications. It responds to chloroquine; resistance to it has been reported only in a few cases.
- Peripheral blood smear is the 'gold standard' test. Clinically impossible to differentiate *P. vivax* from *P. falciparum*.
- Early diagnosis and prompt treatment are basic to malaria control, shortening the disease duration, preventing complications, further transmission and even preventing deaths.

Introduction

Malaria is one of the most dangerous human diseases. It is both preventable and curable. Approximately 300–500 million people are infected, and somewhere between 1.5 and 2.7 million lives are lost to malaria each year.

Epidemiology

Malaria is the most significant tropical parasitic disease in the world. It kills more people than any other communicable disease except tuberculosis. In many developing countries, especially Africa, malaria exacts large costs in lives, medical treatment and lost labour. More than 90 per cent of all malaria cases occur in sub-Saharan Africa; most deaths occur among young children, especially in remote rural areas with poor access to health services. Other high-risk groups are pregnant women, non-immune travellers, and refugees and displaced persons and labourers entering endemic areas.

In malaria-endemic parts of the world, the risk of malaria can be heightened as the unintended result of overpopulation, economic activity or agricultural policy that changes the use of land (e.g. building dams, irrigation schemes, commercial logging and deforestation).

Cyclic climatic events such as El Niño may also play a role in increasing the risk of malaria if associated weather disturbances influence mosquito breeding sites, and therefore the transmission of the disease. Many areas have experienced dramatic increases in the incidence of malaria during extreme weather events correlated to El Niño. Moreover, outbreaks may not only be larger, but more severe, as the affected populations may not have high levels of immunity. Table 13.1 shows the life cycle of the malarial parasites.

Table 13.1 Life cycle of malarial parasites

Plasmodium parasites have a complex life cycle, which is shared between a vertebrate host and an insect vector

Malaria is a protozoan disease transmitted by the female *Anopheles* mosquito

Causes: *Plasmodium* spp.: *P. falciparum* (severe infection), *P. vivax* (most cases), *P. ovale, P. malariae, P. knowlesi*

◑ Pathology

P. falciparum is the most dangerous species, with the highest morbidity rates, and generally is the only species that causes death in humans. It flourishes and overwhelms *P. vivax* where transmission conditions are most intense. Under harsher conditions, however, *P. falciparum* is less robust than *P. vivax*, which then tends to be the main species found.

As malaria control measures become more effective, *P. vivax* is likely to become the species that must be dealt with. In most locations where *P. falciparum* malaria is rampant there are major failures to provide effective health services, but this is less true for *P. vivax* malaria, which can persist in less favourable conditions.

The resistance of the malarial parasite (mainly *P. falciparum*) to common antimalarial drugs such as chloroquine, and the decreasing effectiveness of quinine and the resistance of mosquitoes to insecticides have resulted in a resurgence of malaria in many parts of the world.

Chloroquine is the treatment of choice for *P. vivax*.

Presentations

Uncomplicated acute malaria

Acute malaria that does not lead to complications is the most common presentation: in 70 per cent of cases it is due to *P. vivax*, in the remainder *P. falciparum*. The incubation period is 8–14 days. Symptoms are initially malaise, fatigue and headache, followed by a typical malarial paroxysmal fever with a hot phase, cold phase and wet phase. Both species cause tertian malaria, in which fever recurs every 48 hours. The only physical findings may be anaemia, splenomegaly and mild icterus. Uncommonly there may be cough, diarrhoea and/or herpes labialis (Table 13.2). Clinically it is not possible to distinguish between infection by *P. vivax* and *P. falciparum*.

Table 13.2 Clinical features

Sequential fever, chills, sweating (hot phase → cold phase → wet phase)
Nausea, vomiting, diarrhoea, headache, muscle pain, pallor, mild jaundice, breathlessness, cough, oliguria, altered sensorium, convulsions, coma, bleeding manifestations
Physical findings: fever, anaemia, jaundice (usually mild), hepatosplenomegaly, purpura, petechial haemorrhages

Severe or complicated malaria

Approximately one in a hundred of *P. falciparum* patients may develop severe malaria leading to failure of various organ systems. Microcirculatory obstruction may occur. *P. vivax* infects only young red blood cells. *P. falciparum* can infect red cells at all ages, producing heavier parasitaemia.

Severe malaria can present as cerebral malaria, severe anaemia, renal failure, pulmonary oedema, hypoglycaemia, shock, disseminated intravascular coagulopathy (DIC), acidosis, convulsions, jaundice and haemoglobinuria.

Chronic malaria

Symptoms are progressive splenomegaly. Patients with persistent hepatic *P. vivax* infection may develop partial immunity, which permits asymptomatic low-grade parasitaemia.

Transfusion malaria

There is no incubation period. The disease may be severe in debilitated and critically ill patients. The hepatic phase is absent as erythrocytic infection is directly transmitted.

Mild jaundice may be due to haemolysis, but a large rise in bilrubin is usually associated with hepatic dysfunction. (See Table 13.3)

Mortality is increased significantly when high bilrubin values are associated with acute renal failure and cerebral malaria. Clinical signs of liver failure with hepatic encephalopathy are rare.

Hepatic dysfunction may lead to altered handling of antimalarial drugs.

Other investigations (See Table 13.3)

Blood smear examination is the 'gold standard'. Ideally blood should be collected for testing when the patient's temperature is rising.

A thick film blood smear test should be the first step, since 3 to 40 times more parasites can be seen than in a thin film smear; however, these may be distorted, making species identification difficult. Once a parasite is seen in thick film, species should be confirmed by examining a thin film.

A thin film smear test is also useful for detecting mixed infections, determining parasite count, red blood cell morphology and platelets.

Diagnosis of malaria rests on demonstration of asexual forms of parasite in a peripheral smear. If negative, a repeat smear should be made where there is high degree of suspicion. Gametocytes may remain evident for several days after treatment, so unless trophozoites are also visible, drug resistance is not occurring.

The relationship between parasitaemia and prognosis is complex. In general, patients with >10 000 000 parasites per microlitre are at increased risk of dying, but non-immune patients may die with much lower counts; semi-immune persons may tolerate parasitaemia levels many times higher with only minor symptoms. In severe malaria, a poor prognosis is indicated by a predominance of more mature *P. falciparum* parasites—that is, more than 20 per cent of the parasites have visible pigments, or circulating schizonts are present in the peripheral blood film.

Newer methods of diagnosis

- Quantitative buffy coat analysis, immunological tests to detect malarial antigens such as the *P. falciparum* histidine-rich protein (pf-HRP)
- RNA and DNA probe CR techniques: these are useful for detecting infection when repeated peripheral smear examination is negative
- Dipstick tests are available.

◗ Management

- A blood schizonticidal drug and primaquine should be administered to all types of malaria to alleviate symptoms of blood forms of the parasite: chloroquine, quinine, pyrimethmine/sulfadoxine, artemisinin.
- To prevent relapse due to hypnozoites of *P. vivax* and *P. ovale*: tissue schizonticidal drugs, e.g. primaquine.

- To prevent spread which is through the gametocytes: gametocytocidal drugs—primaquine for *P. falciparum* and chloroquine for all other types.
- Symptomatic and supportive treatment for fever, gastritis, vomiting and hypoglycaemia.

Clinical situations

- Clinically strong suspicion of malaria but peripheral smear for *Plasmodium* is negative. Treat as *P. falciparum* malaria.
- Clinically strong suspicion of malaria but peripheral smear for *Plasmodium* and malarial antigen test both negative. Treat as *P. vivax*, as negative malarial antigen test rules out *P. falciparum*.
- Smear positive for *P. vivax* malaria. Treat with chloroquine plus primaquine.
- Smear positive for *P. falciparum* malaria. Use quinine, pyrimethmine/sulfadoxine, artemisinin, mefloquine plus primaquine.
- Smear positive for both *P. vivax* and *P. falciparum* malaria. Treat as *P. falciparum* and prophylaxis as with *P. vivax* malaria.

Presumptive treatment

Presumptive treatment must be practised in all cases as an early cure and to prevent the spread of *P. vivax* malaria.

The first loading dose of chloroquine should be administered immediately after collecting the blood specimen, without waiting for the test report. If the fever is indeed malaria, this treatment alleviates symptoms early and helps to prevent the spread of malaria by destroying *P. vivax* gametocytes (the most common form of malaria).

In areas with high transmission of *P. falciparum* malaria, chloroquine alone as presumptive treatment may not be enough as it does not sterilise the gametocytes of *P. falciparum* and will not prevent its spread. In these areas a single dose of primaquine with chloroquine is recommended.

In areas with confirmed resistance to chloroquine, a presumptive therapeutic dose of pyrimethamine/sulfadoxine can also be administered.

Treatment of *P. vivax* malaria

P. vivax malaria is usually more common than *P. falciparum* malaria and rarely causes any complications. Most cases of *P. vivax* malaria respond to chloroquine; resistance has been reported only in sporadic cases. Therefore, *P. vivax* malaria should be treated with chloroquine and primaquine *only*.

NOTE: Do not give chloroquine at the time of high fever.

In areas where *P. falciparum* malaria is also seen in significant numbers, however, a mixed infection is possible. Further, in some cases, the tests for malarial parasite may reveal only *P. vivax* infection. Therefore, all cases of *P. vivax* malaria should be carefully observed during initial stages of treatment: if there are no signs of improvement or deterioration, a possible co-infection with *P. falciparum* should be considered.

After six days of treatment, a repeat test for malarial parasites should be done to confirm clearance of parasitaemia.

Patients should be monitored for vomiting for one hour after the administration of any oral antimalarial drug. Dehydration and hypoglycaemia are common problems with malaria. In such cases, use IV fluids to avoid hospitalisation.

Drugs for treatment of uncomplicated malaria

All cases of *P. vivax* malaria and uncomplicated cases of *P. falciparum* malaria are treated with oral drugs.

Chloroquine is the only drug used for *P. vivax* malaria because it is almost unknown to resist chloroquine. Most cases of *P. falciparum* malaria can also be treated with chloroquine alone; however, in areas with known resistance to chloroquine, it is safer to combine chloroquine with another oral antimalarial drug such as pyrimethamine/sulfadoxine. Primaquine should be used in both types of malaria for radical treatment.

The first dose of chloroquine should always be larger to obtain sufficient blood levels, in view of the large volume of distribution.

Treatment of complicated/chloroquine-resistant *P. falciparum* malaria

Different treatment is required for *P. falciparum* than for other types of malaria, depending on the severity of the infection, the status of the patient and the drug sensitivity pattern in the locality. It is safest to regard cases of severe *P. falciparum* malaria as being resistant to chloroquine. Two drugs should be used: one rapid-acting and one slower-acting. In severe malaria, oral antimalarials should not be used: vomiting, poor general health, poor compliance, erratic gastrointestinal absorption due to splanchnic vasculopathy and similar conditions reduce the reliability of the drug. Severe cases should always be treated with parenteral antimalarials to ensure adequate treatment. (See Table 13.4)

P. falciparum malaria is the cause of all mortality and most of the morbidity in malaria. It can present with atypical features and can cause dramatic complications; treatment may be rendered difficult due to its resistance to antimalarial drugs.

Blood schizonticidal drugs such as chloroquine are sufficient to give a radical cure, and the gametocytocidal drug primaquine should be administered to all patients to help prevent the spread of the disease; however, primaquine should not be used concurrently with quinine or mefloquine.

Table 13.4 Referral for hospital admission

1.	If smear is positive but patient does not respond to chloroquine or quinine
2.	If patient cannot take oral medications and requires parenteral therapy
3.	If there is evidence of complications (e.g. jaundice, oliguria, dyspnoea, haemoptysis, purpura, altered mentation, hypoglycaemia and/or bleeding from any site
4.	If smear shows high parasitaemia
5.	If patient is pregnant
6.	If there are co-morbid conditions

QUICK FLICK

13

Primaquine is also contraindicated in pregnancy and lactation, and for infants under one year. In these two categories, chloroquine should be given every week as a suppressive chemoprophylaxis to prevent relapse of *P. vivax* malaria.

For malaria known to be resistant to chloroquine, quinine plus doxycycline or tetracycline or artemether or clindamycin or artisunate or mefloquine can be used. Both sulfa and primaquine can precipitate haemolytic crisis in patients with glucose 6-phosphate dehydrogenase deficiency.

All antimalarial drugs have a narrow safety range and an excess dosage may produce adverse effects. Mefloquine or halofantrine should only be used concurrently with quinine when tests prove drug-resistant malaria. In addition, artemisinin derivatives can be used in cases of hyperparasitaemia or life-threatening complications because they clear the parasitaemia more rapidly than other antimalarial drugs.

Primaquine should not be used in patients who have severe systemic illness likely to cause leukopaenia (severe rheumatoid arthritis, systemic lupus erythematosus (SLE) and similar). It should not be used with other drugs likely to cause bone marrow depression. Concurrent administration of primaquine and mefloquine can increase blood concentrations of mefloquine and may increase its adverse side effects.

In all cases of *P. falciparum* malaria, follow-up malaria parasite tests should be done on the 6th day after treatment to assesses clearance of parasitaemia, and on the 28th day to identify recrudescence:

• 6th day smear: if the parasite is sensitive to the drugs that have been used, then the parasitaemia should clear within seven days. However, gametocytes may be found on the smear but this does not require any treatment; if primaquine has not yet been given, it can be given at this time. Persistence of ring forms of the parasite indicates incomplete clearance and drug resistance. These cases should then be re-treated with other antimalarial drugs.

- 28th day smear: if the parasite is not completely eradicated due to its partial resistance to the drug, then the 28th-day smear will be positive. All such cases should be re-treated with other antimalarial drugs. Primaquine should be re-administered in these cases to destroy freshly formed gametocytes.

Special clinical features and management of severe malaria in pregnancy (See Table 13.4)

Women developing malaria during pregnancy or postpartum are at higher risk of developing severe complications than non-pregnant women, and mortality is twice to 10 times higher.

The clinical manifestations of malaria in pregnancy may vary greatly depending on the patient's level of immunity. Non-immune pregnant women are more likely to develop cerebral and other complications, particularly hypoglycaemia and acute pulmonary oedema. They have an increased risk of abortion (in severe malaria), stillbirth, premature delivery and low infant birth weight. Uterine contractions may be induced, the frequency and intensity of which appear to be related to the height of the fever.

Several factors make pregnant women more vulnerable to malaria and its complications, including mortality:

- Malaria parasites are preferentially sequestered in the placenta.
- Acquired immunity against malaria is known to decline during pregnancy.
- During the second half of pregnancy a transient immunosuppression occurs due to high levels of adrenal steroids, chorionic gonadotropin, alpha-foetoprotein and depression of the role of lymphocytes. Therefore the incidence of malaria relapses, recrudescence and severe malaria is more common.
- Frequency of heavy parasitaemia is greater during pregnancy than in the non-pregnant state.
- Primigravidae are at higher risk of morbidity and mortality from malaria.

Management of malaria during pregnancy

Pregnant women with severe malaria should be transferred to an intensive care unit for careful monitoring. The safety of antimalarials during pregnancy is as follows:

- Quinine (both intravenous and oral) can be safely used in all trimesters of pregnancy. It does not cause abortion in therapeutic dose.
- Artesunate and artemether should not be used in the first trimester.
- Chloroquine is safe throughout pregnancy.

- Mefloquin and lumefantrine-artemether are safe in the second and third trimesters.
- Drugs containing sulfa, tetracyclines and primaquine are contraindicated.

Resistance of malaria parasites to antimalarial drugs

Drug resistance occurs selectively in the species *P. falciparum*. The other species have no documented resistance apart from regional resistance of *P. vivax* to choroquine, observed in Papua New Guinea and Irian Jaya.

How to detect drug resistance

Resistance has developed to all classes of antimalarial drugs except the artemisinin derivatives. The World Health Organization has developed a simple scheme for estimating the degree of resistance. The parasitaemia is studied over a 28-day period following treatment, involving smear tests on days 2, 7 and 28. If there is normal response to the drug, the patient's parasite count falls to 25 per cent of the pre-treatment value by day 2, and the smear should be negative by day 7.

Chemoprophylaxis for malaria

As there is no vaccine against malaria, chemoprophylaxis can offer protection. Chemoprophylaxis is not recommended for residents of an endemic area. Fever occurring within three months of leaving a malaria-endemic area is considered a medical emergency and should be investigated urgently.

Recommendations for travellers to malaria-endemic areas

All travellers to malaria-endemic areas are at risk of contracting malaria and being non-immune. *P. falciparum* infection in these cases can be severe. Therefore, all travellers to malaria-endemic areas are advised to use an appropriate chemoprophylaxis and personal protection measures to prevent malaria. Malaria can still be contracted, however, regardless of the methods employed. Symptoms can develop as early as eight days after initial exposure in a malarious area, and as late as several months after leaving the area. The risk varies with the region visited, the length of stay, the season, type of activity, protection taken against mosquito bites, and compliance with chemoprophylaxis.

Pregnant women, infants, young children and people who have undergone splenectomy are at higher risk of severe malaria. If travel is unavoidable, they should take strict precautions to avoid mosquito bites and take adequate chemoprophylaxis without fail.

Types of prophylaxis

- Primary prophylaxis: Use antimalaria drugs at recommended doses. Primaquine and proguanil are effective (primaquine is not yet recommended for general use).

- Suppressive prophylaxis: Use of blood schizonticides suppresses the blood forms of the malaria parasite and thus protects against clinical illness; however, *P. vivax* and *P. ovale* may cause relapses from the hypnozoites. To prevent this, terminal prophylaxis may be needed.

Chemoprophylaxis regimen

Chemoprophylaxis is preferably started one or two weeks before travelling to a malarious area. As well as ensuring adequate blood levels of the drug, this regimen allows any potential side effects to be evaluated. Chemoprophylaxis should continue while in the malarious area and for up to four weeks after leaving.

The following factors should be considered when choosing an appropriate chemoprophylactic regimen:

- the travel itinerary: determine whether the traveller will actually be at risk of acquiring malaria
- the risk of acquiring chloroquine-resistant *P. falciparum* malaria (CRPF)
- any previous allergic or other reaction to the antimalarial drug
- accessibility of medical care during travel.

In areas where chloroquine-sensitive *P. falciparum* is found:

- start chloroquine one week before exposure
- continue while in the area
- continue for the next four weeks.

In areas with low-degree, localised chloroquine-resistant *P. falciparum*:

- start chloroquine one week before exposure
- continue as above
- start proguanil 1–2 days before exposure
- continue as above.

In areas with high-degree, widespread chloroquine-resistant *P. falciparum*:

- chloroquine plus proguanil as above, OR
- mefloquine, OR
- doxycycline, OR
- atovaquone plus proguanil.

Prophylaxis during pregnancy

Malaria infection in pregnant women may be more severe than in non-pregnant women. Prophylaxis with chloroquine or hydroxychloroquine is not contraindicated; however, because no chemoprophylactic regimen is completely effective in areas with CRPF, women who are pregnant or likely to become so should avoid travel to such areas.

Chloroquine and proguanil are the preferred chemoprophylactic drugs against malaria in the first trimester. Mefloquine can be given during the second and third trimesters if the situation demands.

Mefloquine and doxycycline can be used by non-pregnant women with child-bearing potential, but pregnancy should be avoided for three months after using mefloquine, and for one week after using doxycycline. However, in cases of unplanned pregnancy, malaria chemoprophylaxis is not considered to be an indication for terminating the pregnancy.

Doxycycline, which is a tetracycline, is generally contraindicated. Adverse effects in the foetus include discolouration and severe dysplasia of the teeth and inhibition of bone growth. Tetracyclines would be indicated only if required to treat life-threatening infections due to multi-drug-resistant *P. falciparum*.

Primaquine should not be used during pregnancy because the drug may be passed transplacentally to a G6PD-deficient foetus and cause life-threatening haemolytic anaemia in utero.

Whenever radical cure or terminal prophylaxis with primaquine is indicated, chloroquine should be given once a week until delivery, at which time the decision to give primaquine may be made.

Prophylaxis while breast feeding
Very small amounts of antimalarial drugs are secreted in the breast milk of lactating women, but is not thought to be harmful to the nursing infant.

Chemoprophylaxis for children
Children of any age can contract malaria. WHO advises against taking babies and young children to malarious areas, in particular where *P. falciparum* is found. Malaria can rapidly cause complications in children: any child suffering from fever after returning from a malarious area should be considered to have malaria until proved otherwise.

Since it may be difficult to administer drugs to children and since paediatric formulations and accurate dosage may not be available, it is best to protect babies and children against mosquito bites.

- The indications for prophylaxis are identical to those described for adults.
- Doxycycline is contraindicated for children under eight.

NOTE: Overdose of antimalarial drugs can be fatal.

Chemoprophylaxis for long-term travellers
Long-term travellers intending to stay for more than one to three months should seek the advice of a local healthcare professional regarding malaria.

The risk of serious side effects associated with long-term use of chloroquine and proguanil are low; however, anyone who has taken

300 mg of chloroquine (as base) weekly for over five years and requires further prophylaxis should have twice-yearly screening to detect early retinal changes. If changes are observed, an alternative regimen should be considered.

Mefloquine and doxycycline should be reserved for those at greatest risk of infection. There appears to be no increased risk of serious side effects with long-term use of mefloquine. The risk associated with long-term use of doxycycline is unknown.

Chemoprophylaxis for frequent travellers

Frequent travellers should reserve chemoprophylaxis for high-risk areas only. They should maintain rigorous self-protection against mosquito bites and carry a course of antimalarials as stand-by.

In areas of Thailand near the borders with Cambodia and Myanmar, and in western Cambodia, *P. falciparum* infections do not respond to chloroquine or pyrimethamine-sulfadoxine, and sensitivity to quinine is reduced. Treatment failures of over 50 per cent are also reported. In these areas, chemoprophylaxis with doxycycline is recommended. Doxycycline is contraindicated in children below the age of 8 years and pregnant women, and they should avoid travelling to these areas.

Information for patients

Which are the countries with malaria risk?

Travellers to sub-Saharan Africa have the greatest risk of both getting malaria and dying from their infection. However, all travellers to countries with malaria risk may get this potentially deadly disease. Malaria is transmitted in:

- large areas of Central and South America
- the island of Hispaniola in the Caribbean
- Africa
- Asia (including the Indian subcontinent and South-East Asia)
- the Middle East
- Eastern Europe
- the South Pacific.

When do symptoms start to appear?

Symptoms of malaria tend to appear between 10 days and 4 weeks after the initial bite. However, in some cases, depending on the type of parasite you are infected with, it can take a year before your symptoms start to show.

How can I prevent mosquito bites?

To help prevent being bitten by mosquitoes while travelling in countries where there is a risk of malaria:

- Use insect repellent on your skin and in sleeping environments. The most effective repellents contain diethyltoluamide (DEET). These are available as sprays, roll-ons, sticks, plug-in devices and creams. Some sun protection lotions contain insect repellents.
- Men and women should wear long trousers and long-sleeved shirts or tops, especially in the early evening and at night when mosquitoes prefer to feed.
- Stay in accommodation that has screens on doors and windows, and sleep under a mosquito net that has been treated with insecticide.

QUICK FLICK 13

Who is at risk of getting malaria?

Anyone can get malaria. Most cases occur in countries with malaria risk. It is possible to get malaria through a blood transfusion, although this is very rare. Also, an infected mother can transmit malaria to her infant before or during delivery.

Is malaria contagious?

No. Malaria is not spread from person to person like a cold or the flu, and it cannot be sexually transmitted. You cannot get malaria from casual contact with malaria-infected people, such as sitting next to someone who has malaria.

How do I know if I have malaria?

At the beginning of the disease, most people have fever, sweats, chills, headaches, malaise, aching muscles, nausea and vomiting. Malaria can very rapidly become a severe and life-threatening disease. The surest way to check if you have malaria is to have a diagnostic test—a drop of your blood is examined under the microscope for the presence of malaria parasites. If you are sick and it could possibly be malaria—for example, if you have recently been in a malaria-risk area—the test should be performed without delay.

Is there a malaria vaccine?

No.

Should infants and children be given antimalarial drugs?

Yes, but not all types of malaria drugs. Children of any age can get malaria. They should be on an antimalarial drug if they are going to a malaria-risk area. However, some antimalarial drugs are not suitable for children.

Is it safe for me to breastfeed if I am taking an antimalarial drug?

Not much is known about the safety of antimalarial drugs while breastfeeding, but the amount of the drug that you transfer to your baby is not thought to be harmful.

What determines my risk of getting malaria?

All visitors to malaria-risk areas can get malaria; however, many factors determine individual risk, such as:

- being unaware of malaria-risk areas
- how much malaria is in the area
- the time of year
- the type (species) of malaria parasite in the area
- night-time exposure to mosquito bites
- preventative measures taken
- your immunity, or lack of immunity, to malaria.

I live in an area where malaria is a problem. How can I prevent my family and myself from getting sick?

There are several things you can do:

- Use insect repellent to keep mosquitoes away, especially at night.
- Wear long trousers or jeans and long sleeves when you are outdoors at night.
- Take antimalarial drugs.
- Spray insecticides on the walls of your home to kill any mosquitoes that come inside.
- Sleep under mosquito nets—especially effective if they have been treated with insecticide.

Recommended reading

Centers for Disease Control and Prevention. Travelers' health. [Internet]. Available from: wwwnc.cdc.gov/travel.

Malaria Foundation International. [Internet]. Available from: www.malaria.org.

SanJoaquin MA, Murray CK, Bennett JW. Rapid diagnosis of malaria. *Interdiscip Perspect Infect Dis*. 2009; Article ID 415953. doi:10.1155/2009/415953.

Van den Eede P, Van HN, Van Overmeir C, Vythilingam I, Duc TN, Hung LX, Manh HN, Anné J, D'Alessandro U, Erhart A. Human *Plasmodium knowlesi* infections in young children in central Vietnam. *Malar J*. 2009; 8:249. doi:10.1186/1475-2875-8-249.

Wells TNC, Alonso PL, Gutteridge WE. New medicines to improve control and contribute to the eradication of malaria. *Nat Rev Drug Discov*. 2009 Nov; 8:879-91. doi:10.1038/nrd2972.

World Health Organization Media Centre. Fact sheets. [Internet]. Available from: www.who.int/mediacentre/factsheets/en.

World Health Organization. Prevention. [Internet]. Available from: www. who.int/about/en.

World Health Organization and Tropical Diseases Research. Malaria database. [Internet]. Available from: www.wehi.edu.au/ MalDB-www/who.html.

QUICK FLICK 13

Chapter 14: Leptospirosis

H. Paradwala (India)

Key points

- Leptospirosis is a disease caused by the bacterium *Leptospira*.
- It is also known as Weil's disease, mud fever, trench fever, ricefield fever, cane cutter's fever, swamp fever, flood fever, autumnal fever and many other names.
- An important transmissible infectious disease with a worldwide distribution.
- Severe disease forms can be fatal.
- Causes high degree of severe pulmonary haemorrhage syndrome.
- There is a lack of an adequate diagnostic test and effective control measures.

Introduction

Leptospirosis is a major health problem in China, Brazil and some parts of India. Future challenges will be to translate research advances into public health measures for developing countries. The results of poverty, such as poor sanitation, are often responsible for transmission.

Epidemiology

Leptospirosis has been documented worldwide, including the USA, the Caribbean islands, Central and South America, South-East Asia, the Pacific islands and India.

In the USA, for example, the prevalence of the disease in Hawaii has been reported to be approximately 128 cases per 100 000 persons; the major risk factors include the use of water catchment systems, wild pig hunting, and the presence of skin wounds. Approximately 30 per cent of children in urban Detroit and 16 per cent of adults in Baltimore have demonstrated serologic evidence of past infection.

Leptospira infects many types of mammals—rats, dogs, cats, cattle, pigs, squirrels, raccoons, mongooses and bandicoots. The host animals of leptospiral species and serogroups vary from region to region, and individual animals may carry several serovars. Humans are the end-point hosts of the bacterium in all cases.

◐ Pathology

The genus *Leptospira* belongs to the Leptospiraceae family of the order Spirochaetales. The traditional system divides the genus into two species: the pathogenic *Leptospira interrogans* and the non-pathogenic *Leptospira biflex*. Within these species, leptospires are further grouped by serogroups, serovars and strains, on the basis of microscopic agglutination testing (MAT).

Humans usually become infected when the eyes, nose, mouth or broken skin come in contact with water or damp soil contaminated with the urine of infected animals. The disease can also be spread by direct contact with urine or tissues of infected animals, or by eating urine-contaminated foods.

Rats are the most common source of infection for humans worldwide. In the USA, the most significant sources of infection for humans are dogs, livestock, rodents and wild mammals.

Leptospira live in warm, wet environments. In favourable conditions, leptospires can survive in fresh water for as long as 16 days, and in soil for up to 24 days. Many published case studies have focused on seasonal outbreaks and leptospirosis acquired occupationally or recreationally.

Leptospirosis is a disease of recreation. Recreational activities that present some risk include:

- travelling to tropical areas
- canoeing, hiking, kayaking
- fishing, windsurfing, swimming
- waterskiing, wading, riding trailbikes through puddles
- white-water rafting

and other outdoor sports played in contaminated water. Camping and travelling in endemic areas also add some risk.

Leptospirosis may be spread in epidemic proportions throughout large populations in conditions of widespread flooding in urban areas, especially when heavy rainfall increases the risk of water-borne infection, and drives rodents into urban dwellings.

People who work with animals or in warm, moist environments (farmers, abattoir workers, veterinarians, military troops, rice and sugarcane field-workers, sewer workers) are at increased risk of contracting the disease.

Clinical features

Virulence factors include hyaluronic acid and burrowing motility. Entry of the organism leads to leptospiraemia and spreads to all organs, inflicting damage to the capillary endothelium to cause vasculitis, which is responsible for most of the manifestations of the disease.

Leptospires mainly infect the kidneys and the liver, but any organ in the body may be affected. In the kidneys it causes interstitial nephritis and tubular necrosis, and hypovolumia due to dehydration or altered capillary permeability. In the liver, centrilobular necrosis associated with a proliferation of Kupffer cells may be caused. Pulmonary involvement occurs due to haemorrhage.

Skeletal muscle invasion leads to swelling, vacuolation of myofibrils and focal necrosis.

When antibodies are formed, leptospires are eliminated from all the sites except the eyes, renal tubules and brain, where they may persist for weeks or months. Persistence of the organism in the eyes may cause recurrent uveitis. Cardiac complications such as myocarditis and coronary arteritis may also occur.

The incubation period of leptospirosis varies from two to 20 days.

Mortality/morbidity

In 10 per cent of cases, leptospirosis has severe manifestations including renal failure, hepatitis or pulmonary haemorrhage; mortality rates of 10 per cent may occur.

Gender

Leptospirosis is most common among adult males, probably resulting from occupational and recreational exposures.

Age

Outbreaks have been reported in which more than 40 per cent of patients were younger than 15 years, a reversal of traditional prevalence rates.

Human infections with *Leptospira* are broadly classified as either icteric (10% of cases) or anicteric (less severe; 90% of cases).

Symptoms and signs

Leptospirosis follows a bi-phasic course. In the early non-specific bacteraemic phase there is acute febrile illness with chills, headache, myalgia, back pain, anorexia, nausea, vomiting and sore throat. Symptoms may sometimes be severe, with haemoptysis, dyspnoea and vomiting. This stage lasts from four days up to a week, and is followed by remission lasting for two days. During this phase *Leptospira* can be cultured from blood and colony-stimulating factor (CSF), but not from urine. Serological tests are negative at this stage.

Wide dissemination of the organism can cause meningeal irritation, myalgia, muscular tenderness and hepatomegaly. Purpura can occur because of the decreased platelet count.

In the second (immune) phase, the patient has by now developed antibodies to the organism and meningeal and hepatorenal manifestations are prominent. Bleeding can occur into the skin, mucous membranes and lungs.

Jaundice and hepatomegaly occurs, followed by oliguric renal failure, shock and myocarditis. The patient can develop pulmonary oedema and subpleural haemorrhage with haemoptysis, and significant gastrointestinal haemorrahge can occur.

In some patients there is no remission between the two phases and severe infection can occur within one week. Recovery can take months, and mortality can approach 20 per cent if liver/renal compromise is not treated aggressively.

Renal failure is the main cause of death; other causes include myocarditis, adrenal failure, haemorrhage and cerebral artery thrombosis.

Late complications

In the central nervous system, meningitis and cerebral arteritis are unusual late complications.

In the eyes, subconjunctival haemorrhage can occur during an acute attack. Invasion of the eye by the organism may be followed by uveitis after weeks or months. Retinal haemorrhage and intravascular coagulation can occur.

Pulmonary involvement in leptospirosis has reportedly increased in the past few years, and may be the main cause of death in some countries. Respiratory symptoms may become severe and progress to acute respiratory distress syndrome (ARDS), requiring intubation and mechanical ventilation.

Leptospirosis occurring during pregnancy can bring about spontaneous abortion and perinatal death can occur.

○ Diagnosis

Important clues for early diagnosis include occupational or recreational exposure. If there is an outbreak of the disease, fever, myalgia, intense headache, subconjuctival haemorrhage, jaundice with renal failure and lymphocytic meningitis can occur.

Tests at the early stage, blood and CSF can be subjected to microscopy examination and culture: blood culture is positive if done within 1–4 days of onset of the illness. After that the positive yield rapidly falls. Urine should be examined for *Leptospira* only after 10 days.

Diagnostic tests
- White blood cell counts are generally more than 10 000.
- Urinalysis is frequently abnormal.
- Elevated creatine kinase is found in approximately 50 per cent of patients.
- About 40 per cent of patients have minimal to moderate elevation of liver enzymes. Diagnosis is most frequently made by serologic (antibody) testing.

- Bacteria are best visualised by dark-field microscopy, silver stain or fluorescent microscopy.
- *Leptospira* can be grown from blood, urine and CSF.
- The organism can be isolated from the blood in 50 per cent of cases.
- Urine cultures become positive from about day 10 to day 30 of the illness.
- For rapid diagnosis, a dipstick, a lateral flow test and a latex agglutionation test have been developed.

Differential diagnoses include (in alphabetical order) bronchopneumonia, brucellosis, dengue, encephalitis, enteritis meningitis, infectious mononucleosis, malaria, measles, pneumococcal pneumonia, poliomyelitis, salmonellosis, streptococcal pharyngitis, viral hepatitis and viral meningitis, among others.

◌ Management

The combination of fever, jaundice, renal failure and meningeal signs are only seen in leptospirosis. If leptospirosis is suspected, treatment should be started as early as possible using the anti-spirochaetal antimicrobial drugs amoxicillin, ampicillin, erythromycin, penicillins, streptomycin or tetracyclines (doxycycline) (see Table 14.1).

Table 14.1 Treatment and chemoprophylaxis of leptospirosis

Purpose	Level of disease	Drug regimen
Treatment	Mild	Doxycycline
	Moderate to severe	Penicillin G: 2 mega units IV or Ampicillin IM 6-hourly for 7–10 days or Amoxicillin IM 6-hourly for 7–10 days For penicillin-allergic patients: tetracycline or erythromycin
Chemoprophylaxis		Doxycycline 200 mg orally once a week

Intensive care support is required for very ill patients. Patients with ARDS require mechanical ventilator support and may need haemodialysis or haemoperfusion. Peritoneal dialysis can also be done. Patients with Weil's syndrome may need whole blood or platelet transfusion. Tetracyclines such as doxycycline have the merit of eliminating the organism from the kidneys.

The treatment can provoke a Jarisch-Herxheimer reaction, which may persist for 24 hours.

Prognosis

The fatality rate is usually low, but it can be as high as 30 per cent depending upon the serovar.

In the early stages of illness, vascular collapse, myocardial disease or gastrointestinal haemorrhage may cause death.

In the second week of the disease, renal and hepatic complications may cause death. Patients surviving this critical period enter convalescence which is often complicated by the recurrence of fever, myalgia, headache and malaise for a few days.

Thereafter most patients make a complete recovery.

Prevention

Doxycycline is an effective prophylaxis. Leptospirosis can also be prevented by:

- avoiding drinking untreated water, and avoiding swimming or wading in water that might be contaminated with animal urine
- wearing protective clothing (aprons, gloves and boots) if there is risk of exposure to infected animals or contaminated water or soil
- eliminating rodents
- vaccinating dogs and farm animals.

On average, 10 per cent of all freshwater sites can be assumed to be infectious. The probability is higher for sites which host rats (urban ponds, slow-moving rivers and canals, lakes near farm buildings). The risk is less for rapidly flowing streams or very large estuaries or river deltas as rodent urine will be diluted by the greater flow. Water treated with chlorine or UV-sterilisation is safe. The bacteria cannot survive in seawater or in tidal saltwater regions of rivers.

In general, in the developed countries there is a wariness of open water sites for general cleanliness reasons. In developing countries the risks are greater due to higher rat populations and also the widespread use of untreated water for drinking and washing, and the association between hygiene risks and open water is rarely made.

Summary

Leptospirosis is caused by *Leptospira* bacteria, which have a worldwide distribution. It causes epidemics in poor urban slum conditions. Mortality is high in severe forms of the disease. Treatment with anti-spirochaetal antimicrobial drugs should be started as soon as possible after symptoms are recognised. Leptospirosis infects many types of animals, with humans as the end-point hosts.

A possible key to correct diagnosis is a thorough history focusing on the patient's travel history, activities, and exposure to animals.

Recommended reading

Croda J, Ramos JGR, Matsunaga J, Queiroz A, Homma A, Riley LW, Haake DA, Reis MG, Ko AI. *Leptospira* immunoglobulin-like proteins as a serodiagnostic marker for acute leptospirosis. *J Clin Microbiol*. 2007 May; 45(5):1528–34. doi:10.1128/JCM.02344-06.

Dolhnikoff M, Mauad T, Bethlem EP, Carvalho CR. Leptospiral pneumonias. *Curr Opin Pulm Med*. 2007 May; 13(3):230–5.

Leptospirosis Information Center. [Internet]. Available from: www.leptospirosis.org.

National Institute of Communicable Diseases, Zoonosis Division. Guidelines for prevention and control of leptospirosis. [Internet]. Available from: www.whoindia.org/en/section3/section217_1291.htm.

Palaniappan RU, Ramanujam S, Chang YF. Leptospirosis: pathogenesis, immunity, and diagnosis. *Curr Opin Infect Dis*. 2007 Jun; 20(3):284–92.

Chapter 15: Listeriosis

H. Paradwala (India)

Key points

▶ Listeriosis is a rare but potentially lethal food-borne infection caused by the bacterium *Listeria monocytogenes*.

▶ The bacterium is found in soil, stream water, sewage, plants and food.

▶ Infections are either asymptomatic, or produce a mild influenza-like disease.

▶ Pregnant women are affected during the third trimester. They account for 27 per cent of all cases.

▶ Others affected include newborns, and adults with weakened immune systems.

▶ *Listeria* can be found in uncooked meats, uncooked vegetables, unpasteurised milk, foods made from unpasteurised milk, and processed foods. The bacterium is killed by pasteurising or cooking.

▶ The disease may be a self-limited gastrointestinal tract illness or a more severe central nervous system infection or bacteraemia.

▶ Listeriosis is diagnosed by culture of the organism from blood, cerebrospinal fluid or other sterile body fluid.

▶ Intravenous antibiotics ciprofloxacin, linezolid and azithromycin must be started immediately when the diagnosis is suspected or confirmed.

◖ Introduction

Named after Joseph Lister (1827–1912) who pioneered antiseptic surgery, *Listeria* is a bacterial genus comprising six species. *L. monocytogenes* is the species that causes listeriosis.

◖ Aetiology, epidemiology and pathology

The term 'listeriosis' encompasses a wide variety of disease symptoms that are similar in animals and humans.

The case fatality rate for those with a severe form of infection may approach 25 per cent. Until about 1960, *L. monocytogenes* was thought to be associated almost exclusively with infections in animals, and only rarely in humans. At least 42 species of wild and domestic mammals and 17 avian species, including domestic and game fowl, can harbour listeriae.

L. monocytogenes is reportedly carried in the intestinal tract of 5–10 per cent of the human population without any apparent symptoms. The infection can spread to the central nervous system and cause meningitis. *Listeria* occurs often in newborns, having infected the foetus by penetrating the endothelial layer of the placenta.

Listeriae can contaminate ready-to-eat foods because contamination can occur after cooking and before packaging.

◐ Clinical forms and diagnosis

The two main clinical manifestations are sepsis and meningitis. Unusually for bacterial infections, the meningitis is often complicated by encephalitis.

Microscopically, *Listeria* spp. appear as small, Gram-positive rods, which are sometimes arranged in short chains. In direct smears they may be coccoid, so they can be mistaken for *Streptococcus*.

Most *Listeria* bacteria are targeted by the immune system before they cause infection. Those that escape the immune system's initial response, however, spread though intracellular mechanisms and are therefore guarded against circulating immune factors (AMI).

The list of foods that have caused outbreaks of listeriosis includes hot dogs, processed meats, unpasteurised milk, cheeses—particularly soft-ripened cheeses such as feta, brie, camembert, blue-veined, or Mexican-style *queso blanco*—raw and cooked poultry, raw meats, ice cream, raw vegetables, raw and smoked fish and the green lip mussel.[1]

Seventy per cent of all non-perinatal infections occur in immunocompromised patients. People at most serious risk of contracting listeriosis are:

- pregnant women are some 20 times more likely than other healthy adults to get listeriosis; about one-third of listeriosis cases occur during pregnancy; newborns rather than their mothers suffer the serious effects of infection contracted during pregnancy
- persons with weakened immune systems, cancer, diabetes or kidney disease, and the elderly
- people with AIDS are almost 300 times more likely to get listeriosis than people with normal immune systems
- persons who take glucocorticosteroid medications.

Frequency

The true incidence of listeriosis in humans is not known because infections are usually asymptomatic, or at most produce a mild influenza-like disease. In the USA, for example, the frequency of *L. monocytogenes* infection is 9.7 cases per million population; 2500 cases are reported annually, with higher incidence rates during the summer months.

Mortality/morbidity

The overall mortality rate of *L. monocytogenes* infection is 20–30 per cent. Of all pregnancy-related cases, 22 per cent result in foetal loss or neonatal death, but mothers usually survive.

With the exception of pregnant women, no gender predilection is recognised. Women of childbearing age are commonly affected. Neonates and elderly individuals are at risk.

Pathophysiology

L. monocytogenes is a Gram-positive bacillus with aerobic and anaerobic characteristics. Under light microscopy it has a characteristic tumbling motility. It grows best at neutral to slightly alkaline pH, at temperatures ranging from 1 to 45 °C. It is beta-haemolytic and has a blue-green sheen on blood-free agar. It is difficult to isolate in mixed cultures and may be mistaken for *Streptococcus* or contaminants such as *Corynebacteria*. The incubation period is from two to six weeks.

Most listeriosis infections occur following oral ingestion, with access to the systemic circulation after intestinal penetration. Protection against *Listeria* is mediated via lymphokine activation of T cells on macrophages, and by the interleukin-18 protein.

Infection of the central nervous system may manifest as meningitis, meningoencephalitis, or abscess; endocarditis is another possible presentation. Localised infection may manifest as septic arthritis, osteomyelitis or, occasionally, pneumonia.

Clinical

Symptoms can include fever, myalgia, arthralgia, back pain and headache. The clinical features depend on the organ system involved.

During pregnancy, listeriosis usually occurs during the third trimester. *Listeria* can proliferate in the placenta and cause infection when the mother's immunity is at its lowest. Symptoms may mimic those of a flu-like illness and may be mild and self-limited. Infection of the central nervous system in pregnant women is very rare, although it is observed frequently in other compromised hosts. Preterm labour and/or delivery is common, and abortion, stillbirth and intrauterine infection can occur.

Neonatal infection (granulomatosis infantisepticum)

This occurs in one of two forms:

- Early-onset sepsis, with *L. monocytogenes* infection in utero via transplacental transmission, resulting in premature birth. Listeriae can be isolated in the placenta, blood, meconium, ears, nose and throat, among other sites, and can manifest as abscesses and/or granulomas.

- Late-onset meningitis is acquired through vaginal transmission, and has also been reported associated with caesarean deliveries.

Listeriosis in non-pregnant adults

Sepsis is the most common presentation. *L. monocytogenes* can produce a febrile gastroenteritis evoking a food-borne diarrhoeal disease, which is typically non-invasive. The incubation period is one or two days, with diarrhoea lasting anywhere from one to three days. The prevalence of diarrhoeal illness is high in individuals exposed to inocula of *Listeria*.

Patients who present with fever, myalgia and diarrhoea recover with supportive care.

In central nervous system infection, the brain parenchyma, especially the brain stem and meninges, are affected. Mental status changes are common. Focal and generalised seizures appear in at least 25 per cent of patients. Cranial nerve deficits may be present, and stroke-like syndromes with hemiplegia may occur, but nuchal rigidity is less common. Tremor, myoclonus and ataxia may occur.

Patients may present with encephalitis, especially of the brainstem.

Meningitis is possible.Ventriculitis, particularly of the fourth ventricle, may develop. Cervical myelitis has been reported.

Brain abscess is an uncommon complication associated with high mortality, occuring in 10 per cent of central nervous system infections. It is often located in the thalamus, pons and medulla.

The possibility of endocarditis is magnified in people with previously damaged or prosthetic valves, frequently with systemic embolisation.

Focal infections such as endophthalmitis, osteomyelitis and abscess can occur.

◐ Differential diagnosis

The following differential diagnoses are listed on the eMedicine website http://emedicine.medscape.com/:

Cryptosporidiosis, bacterial gastroenteritis, viral meningitis, sarcoidosis, Streptococcus Group B infections, toxoplasmosis, Wegener granulomatosis, meningeal carcinomatosis, lymphomatous meningitis, multiple sclerosis, vasculitis, viral encephalitis or meningitis, fungal meningitis, brain abscess, bacterial meningitis, septic abortion, pyelonephritis in pregnancy.[3]

◐ Laboratory studies

The following appears on the eMedicine website http://emedicine.medscape.com:

- Blood cultures should be performed. Blood culture results are positive in 60–75 per cent of patients with central nervous system (CNS) infections.

- *Listeria* demonstrates 'tumbling motility' in wet mounts of cerebrospinal fluid (CSF). *Listeria* organisms are motile in wet mounts of CSF.
- CSF Gram stain results are positive in less than 50 per cent of patients. CSF analysis reveals pleocytosis, and CSF protein levels are moderately elevated. CSF glucose levels may be low, and if so, are associated with a poor prognosis.
- Laboratory results that show diphtheroids should prompt heightened awareness for the possibility of *Listeria* infection, particularly in immuno-compromised patients.
- CSF culture findings are positive in nearly 100 per cent of patients.
- Serologic testing is not reliable.
- Stool cultures are neither sensitive nor specific.[3]

Imaging studies

The following information appears on the eMedicine website http://emedicine.medscape.com/:

- MRI is superior to CT scan for demonstrating CNS disease, especially in the brainstem.
- Transoesophageal echocardiography should be performed if endocarditis is suspected.[3]

○ Management

Isolation precautions are not necessary since person-to-person contagion does not occur.[4]

Antibiotics effective against *Listeria* spp. include penicillin G, ampicillin, vancomycin, ciprofloxacin, linezolid, gentamycin, cotrimoxazole, tetracycline and azithromycin. Combination therapy is necessary for maximal listericidal therapy. Cephalosporins should not be used.

The following advice is contained on the KidsHealth website http://kidshealth.org:

> *Listeriosis is usually treated with antibiotics administered in the hospital through an intravenous catheter (IV). Typically, treatment lasts for about 10 days but that can vary depending on the body's ability to fight off the infection.*
>
> *Children whose immune systems are compromised by illness or infection, such as cancer or HIV, are more likely to develop severe listeriosis infections and may require additional treatment.[5]*

The following advice is contained on the eMedicine website http://emedicine.medscape.com:

> *Bacteraemia should be treated for 2 weeks in the immunocompromised patient. Longer [antibiotic] courses may be required in the immunocompromised patient. Meningitis should be treated for 3 weeks; endocarditis, for 4–6 weeks;*

Todar K. Todar's online textbook of bacteriology: *Listeria monocytogenes* and listeriosis. University of Wisconsin-Madison Department of Biology. 2003. [Internet]. Available from: http://textbookofbacteriology.net/Listeria.html.

University of Florida Medical School. More about *Listeria*. [Internet]. Available from: www.med.ufl.edu/biochem/DLPURICH/morelist.html.

WrongDiagnosis.com. Statistics about *Salmonella* food poisoning. [Internet]. Available from: www.wrongdiagnosis.com/s/salmonella_food_poisoning/stats.htm.

Chapter 16: Amoebiasis

O. Shrivastav (India)

Key points

▶ The epidemiology of amoebiasis concerns the carrier state, invasive disease, the global traveller, and annual mortality.

▶ The disease is enteroinvasive, involving erythrocyte ingestion, oxygen tension and iron sulfur proteins.

▶ Transmission may be through contaminated water or food. Humans are the definitive host. Pathophysiology includes mucosal migration, inflammatory cytokines, contact-dependent cell killing, lectin, amoebapore, cysteine proteinase, electron-dense granules, calcium modulated protein (calmodulin), complement-mediated lysis.

▶ The clinical spectrum covers the carrier state, liver disease, colonic disease, extra-hepatic disease, multiple abscess, toxaemia and encephalopathy.

▶ Laboratory diagnosis involving operator-dependency, antigen detection, ELISA, PCR, pyaemia and riboprinting.

○ Introduction

Among the earliest writings about a pathological process involving fever and dysentery were by Hippocrates (460–377 BC) and in the Old Testament (140–87 BC). A far greater understanding of a process of disease that presents with liver abscess and colitis came in the nineteenth century. Amoebas were first observed in a stool sample in 1865, and in 1925 a landmark observation by Brumpt established the parasite *Entamoeba histolytica* as the only pathogenc amoeba. Several crucial developments in the understanding of cell biology and pathogenesis since that time have led to a far deeper knowledge of the parasite.

○ Epidemiology

The spectrum of disease caused by the protozoal parasite *Entamoeba histolytica* ranges from a mild carrier state to life-threatening emergencies involving various organs. Documented clinical experience of invasive amoebiasis comes largely from endemic areas. Most cases in the historical literature have been reported from the developing world, but the advent of both global travel and increased migration have skewed this data considerably. Since 1933, invasive amoebiasis has been reported in some 3000 patients in the United States. Another estimate suggests 50 million cases of diarrhoea annually worldwide, with or without dysentery, and with an annual mortality of 100 000 people.

◔ Pathophysiology

Among the eight species of *Entamoeba* that inhabit the human gut, only *E. histolytica* is capable of being enteroinvasive and causing disease. Other species of amoeba include *E. dispar*, *E. moshkovskii*, *E. coli*, *E. hartmanni*, *E. polecki*, *Dientamoeba fragilis Iodamoeba bütschlii* and *Endolimax nana*. Whether *E. polecki*, *D. fragilis* and *I. bütschlii* cause clinically significant disease in humans is still being debated.

It is well known that amoebas ingest erythrocytes, but the cellular mechanism that triggers macrophages is not as well understood. Carbohydrates and cholesterol increase the progression of the disease, and proteins inhibit it.

Metabolic pathways and increased oxygen tension are cytotoxic to amoebiasis. Its metabolism requires anaerobic conditions to flourish. An iron-sulfur protein, ferredoxin, acts as an electron transfer ion when the concentration gradient turns a non-toxic element into a toxic one. It is for this reason that metronidazole works so well.

There are probably several other elements to the pathogenesis of *E. histolytica* that are only partly understood; and further inroads into the cell biology of the disease process are needed.

Studies of amoeba–host interaction have demonstrated that amoebas gain access to the submucosal area by inducing damage in mucosal cells and migrating between mucosal cells. The damage may be caused in part by released cytotoxins; however, this appears to be a non-specific protease effect, and is likely to be inhibited rapidly by protease inhibitors. The major pathogenic effect of amoebas is contact-dependent cell killing (Figure 16.1).

Adherence of the trophozoite to the colonic epithelial surface involves a complex interplay of many factors, some of which are still poorly understood (see Figure 16.2).

Independent of the factors in Figure 16.2, the proteinases degrade host factors and suppress complement, thereby promoting adherence. Pathogenic isolates are resistant to complement-mediated lysis, a property critical for survival in the bloodstream. In contrast, non-pathogenic species such as *Entamoeba dispar*—which is non-invasive—is rapidly lysed by complement, and is therefore restricted to the bowel lumen. Immunohistochemistry

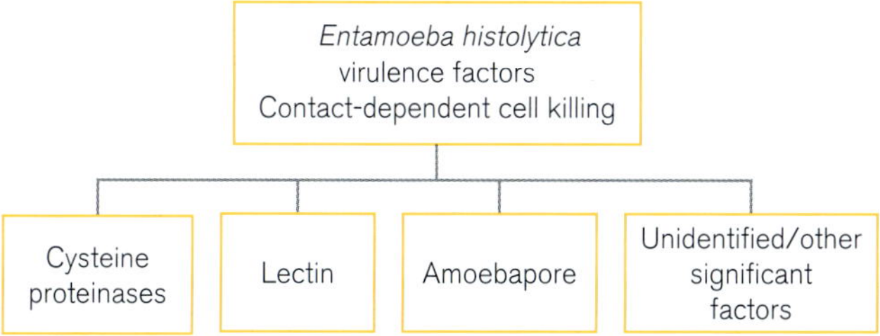

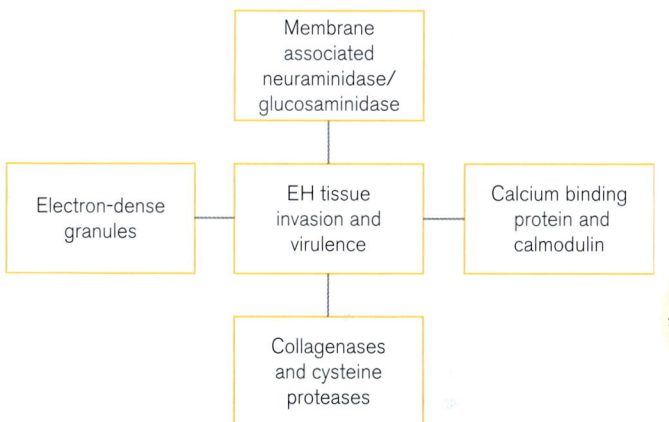

Figure 16.1 Contact-dependent virulence factors of *Entamoeba histolytica*

Figure 16.2 Factors involved in adherence of the trophozoite to the colonic epithelial surface

observations consider the localisation of the antigenic molecule of *E. histolytica* trophozoites, and of molecules such as intercellular adhesions molecule 1 (ICAM-1), ICAM-2 and von Willebrand's factor, in activated endothelial cells.

Alkaline phosphatase level is the most reliable and consistent biochemical indicator of acute liver abscess, usually doubling or quadrupling in patients with the disease. Katzenstein et al. (1982) suggested that the alkaline phosphatase level is correlated to the duration of the disease. The level is normal in acute cases, and patients with a chronic history may have an abnormal alkaline phosphatase, usually more than twice the normal serum level.[1]

Serum bilirubin is raised mildly and transiently in a small number of patients. Severe hyperbilirubinaemia, though unusual, carries a grave prognosis.

○ Life cycle

Humans are the definitive host for *E. histolytica*, and transmission in the vast majority of cases is through ingesting contaminated water or contaminated food. In a smaller subset of the population, men having sex with men are infected due to faeco–oral contamination during penetrative sex.

In various small but significant studies, the role of zoonotic transmission has been evaluated. Clinically significant strains of *E. histolytica* have been reproduced in laboratory animals, most likely from transmission due to close proximity with humans.

Arthropods such as cockroaches are known to harbour infected cysts of *E. histolytica*, as are some animal reservoirs (pigs and monkeys), but they constitute a very small population contributing to clinical events.

The life cycle of *E. histolytica* has two distinct stages: a trophozoite stage and an infected cyst stage. Cysts in themselves are not infective or invasive; they can remain viable for weeks in certain environments, especially under moist, damp conditions. As the trophozoite progresses through the colon, it changes from its single-nucleus precyst state into a tetranucleated state (having four nuclei); in the process it loses other elements of the cell, such as food vacuoles and ribosomes. It is at the tetranucleated stage that clinically significant events are initiated in affected individuals.

○ Clinical spectrum

Asymptomatic carrier state

Since most authentic studies in the past have been based on microscopic identification of *E. histolytica* (which was often *E. dispar*, but incorrectly identified), the precise incidence of *E. histolytica* is difficult to determine. Patients are often asymptomatic or have mild symptoms, with an unremarkable stool examination, and the infection may only be recognised by serology.

Clinically significant disease may manifest in no more than 10 per cent of patients after *E. histolytica* becomes enteroinvasive. Even though patients may be asymptomatic, treatment should be offered since disease progression is by the faeco–oral route which has implications for public health.

Liver disease

In 1947, Warren Bostick and colleagues gave a remarkable description of liver abscess:

> These areas of amebic histolysis are not simple cavities, but consist instead of honeycombed channels of digested liver cells that are transversed by irregular strands of liver connective tissue which is more resistant to amebic digestion and therefore remains behind.
>
> Microscopically, the liver abscesses are characterised by the presence of the central brown, autolyzed liver and blood tissues ('anchovy paste'), by an irregular margin of viable but injured liver cells among which active ameba are wandering. The characteristic tissue reaction is again evident in that leukocytes are infrequent, lysis is evident and pyogenic reactions predominant only when secondary bacterial invasion occurs.[2]

Acute liver abscess rarely affects children, and most commonly affects adults between 20 and 60 years of age. Males are affected eight to ten times more than females. The disease is particularly seen in chronic alcoholics and in diabetics in this age range.[3]

Multiple abscesses may manifest as toxaemia, deep jaundice, and encephalopathy. Ascites developing in a patient with acute liver abscess suggests development of inferior vena cava obstruction, and a cough with copious expectoration of reddish-brown 'anchovy sauce' pus suggests rupture into the right lower lobe bronchus.

During the course of the illness, one-third of all patients may develop clinical jaundice. Severe icterus may be due to a large abscess, or multiple abscesses, or an abscess situated at the porta hepatis. An abscess larger than 10 cm in the superior part of the right lobe may be associated with complications (rupture in the pleural space or right lower lobe bronchus). The left lobe abscess may rupture in the pericardium or may extend into the perisplenic space and pouch of the Douglas region.

While fever may be conpiciously absent in more than 60 per cent of patients with colonic involvement, abdominal discomfort and fevers typify liver involvement with *E. histolytica*; this can manifest significantly in the acute phase.

There may be an undiagnosed or partially treated subacute phase that simmers, with symptoms of weight loss, lack of appetite, mild leukocytosis and unremarkable stool examination.

Extrahepatic involvement

Unusual sites or complications of extraintestinal amoebiasis include direct extension from the liver to the pleura and/or pericardium, brain abscess, and genitourinary amoebiasis.

QUICK FLICK 16

Colonic disease

The most common features are abdominal discomfort and diarrhoea with mucus and blood, where patients may sometimes have up to ten motions per day. *E. histolytica* may mimic several conditions, particularly non-infective colitis, and therefore it is vital for the clinician to make a correct diagnosis to avoid patients' being erroneously commenced on disease-modifying agents such as steroids.

Laboratory diagnosis

Historically, demonstration of *E. histolytica* in stool samples under microscopy or stool culture has been the standard for diagnosis, but the introduction of enzyme-linked immunosorbent assays (ELISAs) and more recent molecular diagnostic techniques have made rapid and significant inroads towards far greater yield not only in diagnosis, but also in differentiating non-pathogenic from pathogenic strains.

The difficulty with stool culture is that it cannot regulate the growth of only pathological species, and dominance of a species other than *E. histolytica* may lull the interpreter into a false sense of security; additionally, a negative stool culture does not necessarily exlude the presence of *E. histolytica*.

A less desirable outcome of such techniques is that some tests may continue to remain positive for up to four years after the acute infection has resolved, and therefore the interpretation of such results should be made in the context of demonstrating active disease (gel diffusion precipitin test detecting antibodies).

The yield of visual *E. histolytica* under the microscope increases with three or more stool samples. The importance of visualising a fresh stool sample within four hours cannot be overstated; the presence of ingested red blood cells within *E. histolytica* trophozytes in a patient with dysentery is still considered a 'gold standard' in diagnostics. Some authorities place importance on the linear movement of *E. histolytica* trophozytes (rather than a zigzag movement), the staining techniques of a wet mount (fixed with alcohol, staining of the nucleus with iodine makes it prominent and visible) or the presence of eosinophilic degradation products (Charcot-Leyden crystals); however, the percentage of recognition of such features depends directly on the skills and experience of the operator.

Antigen-based detection studies

This is the most sensitive diagnostic modality for *E. histolytica* in stool samples. Because of their high sensitivity and specificity, they are sound and reliable, besides being able to differentiate *E. histolytica* from *E. dispar*. The other valuable aspect of their application is in epidemiological studies and outbreaks.

These assays have been further refined to identify several antigens of *E. histolytica* that promote the disease process (monoclonal antibodies against sereine, lectin, lysine and unspecified antigens). Detection of antigen is limited to the examination of fresh or frozen samples, since the presence of alcohol used as a fixing agent impedes all antigen-based detection techniques.

Antibody detection

Antibody detection techniques are restricted by one major limitation: they cannot differentiate a current infection from past exposure. Therefore it is necessary to employ them in conjunction with either antigen detection or polymerase chain reaction (PCR)-based assays to yield significant diagnostic rates.

During acute infections, up to 85 per cent of patients will demonstrate antibodies to *E. histolytica*. Several modalities for diagnosis have been employed, including electrophoresis, indirect haemagglutination (IHA), gel diffusion techniques, complement fixation and latex agglutination, but outcomes of significant results require stringent laboratory standards and significant operator skills.

Among other modalities, ELISA is now considered more reliable and sensitive than counterimmunoelectrophoresis (CIE) or IHA. It has a sensitivity of 95 per cent or more to serum antilectin immunoglobulin G (IgG) antibodies present in patients with amoebic colitis and acute liver abscess within one week of the onset of symptoms. The interpretation of serum antilectin immunoglobulin M (IgM) is more complex, since travellers to endemic areas may require a different interpretation from inhabitants of that area.

Some authors endorse CIE as being more specific in invasive amoebiasis, but it has low sensitivity in intestinal amoebiasis. ELISA-based studies have poorer rates of diagnosis in the first week of acute infections, but the success rate rises significantly between two and three weeks. Titres reflect neither response to therapy nor severity of disease.

Polymerase chain reaction (PCR)-based assays

PCR-based techniques possess high specificity and sensitivity, but are limited by cost and the time taken to obtain results, and the requirement for highly skilled operators. The method is particularly useful in establishing *E. histolytica* in pyaemic samples. With current techniques of DNA extraction, a single trophozyte of *E. histolytica* can be identified in a milligram of sample.

Riboprinting, the restriction site polymorphism analysis method involving amplification followed by restriction fragment length polymorphism (RFLP) analyses of the small and large subunit rDNA, is a very useful tool for evaluating different *Entamoeba* species.

QUICK FLICK
16

◑ **Management**

Most patients with dysentery or liver abscess respond sufficiently to conservative medical therapy within 48 hours of commencing imidazole treatment. Metronidazole (500–750 mg tds for 10–14 days) crosses the blood–brain barrier, making it the drug of choice in disseminated amoebiasis.

If at the end of four days of therapy the patient's response is suboptimal or clinically worsening, bacterial complications (such as co-infection of liver abscess with bacterial pathogen), viral complications (hepatitis A or hepatitis E co-infection) or drug resistance should be considered. *E. histolytica* has several features in common with the multidrug resistance phenotype described in mammalian tumour cells, including cross-resistance to unrelated drugs, increased efflux and decreased accumulation of radiolabelled drugs, reversal of resistance by calcium channel blockers such as verapamil, and overexpression of 4.5 kb long mRNAs homologous to the mammalian P-glycoprotein.

Other therapies—diiodohydroxyquin, paromomycin, emetine and chloroquine—have also been used as alternative drugs; however, emetine is rarely used because of its toxicity. Diloxanide furoate is the main drug for treating asymptomatic cyst carriers. Chloroquine can be used along with metronidazole/emetine in cases of hepatic amoebiasis. Metronidazole, tinidazole and other 5-nitroimidazole agents that kill the trophozoites by causing alterations in the protoplasmic organelles of the amoeba are ineffective in treating cyst passers. Chloroquine, however, acts on the vegetative forms of the parasite and kills it by inhibiting DNA synthesis, and emetine kills the trophozoites mainly by inhibiting protein synthesis. Table 16.1 details the drug dosages for adults.

Table 16.1 Treatment of amoebiasis

Drug	Dosage	Comments
Paromomycin	Adult: 25–35 mg/kg/d PO divided tid for 7 d	Pregnancy: Foetal risk revealed in studies in animals but not established or not studied in humans; may use if benefits outweigh risk to foetus Precautions: Because of narrow therapeutic index and toxic hazards associated with extended administration, not for long-term therapy; caution in renal failure, hypocalcaemia, myasthaenia gravis, and conditions that depress neuromuscular transmission; adjust dose in renal impairment; may cause abdominal cramping, nausea, emesis and diarrhoea; malabsorption, ototoxicity and nephrotoxicity can occur if administered in high doses or in ulcerative colitis

Drug	Dosage	Comments
Diloxanide	Adult: 500 mg PO tid for 10 d	Dichloroacetamide derivative. Amoebicidal against trophozoite and cyst forms of *E. histolytica*
Metronidazole (Flagyl)	Adult: 500–750 mg PO tid for 10 d	Drug of choice for intestinal amoebiasis and liver abscesses
Tinidazole (Fasigyn)	Adult: Intestinal amoebiasis: 600 mg PO bid for 5 d alternatively, 2 g PO qd for 3 d with food. Hepatic amoebic abscess: 2 g PO qd for 3–5 d with food	Useful as alternative therapy for adult intestinal amoebiasis and amoebic abscesses
Iodoquinol	Adult: 650 mg PO tid for 20 days	Amoebicidal against *E. histolytica*. Considered effective against trophozoite and cyst forms

Summary

Amoebiasis is caused by the protozoal parasite *Entamoeba histolytica*. The spectrum of the disease ranges from a mild carrier state to life-threatening emergencies involving various organs. Of the eight species of *Entamoeba* that inhabit the human gut, only *E. histolytica* is capable of being enteroinvasive and causing disease. Humans are the definitive host for this parasite, and transmission in the vast majority of cases is by way of contaminated water or food.

The life cycle of *E. histolytica* has two distinct stages: a trophozoite stage and an infected cyst stage. The tetranucleated stage is the key to initiating clinically significant events in affected individuals. The major pathogenic effect of amoebas is contact-dependent cell killing.

Alkaline phosphatase level is the most reliable and consistent biochemical indicator of acute liver abscess, asymptomatic carrier state, liver disease, colonic disease and extrahepatic involvement. Note that an abscess size greater than 10 cm in the superior part of the right lobe may be associated with complications. Abdominal discomfort and fevers are the main symptoms of liver involvement with *E. histolytica*. The importance of visually examining a fresh stool sample within four hours cannot be overstated.

Drugs used for management include metronidazole, diiodohydroxiquin, paramomycin, emetine and chloroquine.

QUICK FLICK **16**

References

1. Katzenstein D, Rickerson V, Braude A. New concepts of amebic liver abscess derived from hepatic imaging, serodiagnosis, and hepatic enzymes in 67 consecutive cases in San Diego. *Medicine (Baltimore)*. 1982 Jul; 61(4):237–46.

2. Bostick W, Johnstone HG, Anderson HH. Amebiasis: pathology, diagnosis and recent developments in therapy. *Calif Med*. 1947 Oct; 67(4):245–8.

3. Mathur S, Gehlot RS, Mohta A, Bhargava N. Clinical profile of amoebic liver abscess. *J Indian Acad Clin Med*. 2002; 3(4):367–73.

Recommended reading

Adams EB, MacLeod IN. Invasive amebiasis. II. Amebic liver abscess and its complications. *Medicine (Baltimore)*. 1977; 56:325–34.

Fritsche TR, Smith JW. Medical parasitology. In: Henry JB, editor. Clinical diagnosis and management by laboratory methods. Philadelphia: The W.B. Saunders Co. 2001; pp 1196–239.

Mandell JI. Interaction between *Entamoeba histolytica* and human polymorphonuclear neutrophils. *J Infect Dis*. 1981; 143:83–93.

Ravdin JI. *Entamoeba histolytica* (amebiasis). In: Mandell GL, Bennett JE, Dolin R, editors. Mandell, Douglas and Bennett's principles and practice of infectious diseases. 5th ed. Philadelphia: Churchill Livingstone, Inc. 2000; pp 2798–810.

Chapter 17: Schistosomiasis: global impact

S. Fedail (Sudan)

Key points

- ▶ Schistosomiasis is found in Africa, South America and South-East Asia.
- ▶ It is the third most prevalent parasitic infection in the world. Some 200–300 million people are infected, mostly in sub-Saharan Africa.
- ▶ There are five species of schistosome infecting humans. The commonest is *Schistosoma mansoni*.
- ▶ The pathological changes are caused by intense inflammatory reaction around trapped schistosome eggs in the body.
- ▶ Clinical presentations depend upon species. The greatest morbidity is caused by chronic complications of portal hypertension and urinary tract involvement.
- ▶ Praziquantel is the main drug of choice, used both for treatment and for mass prevention of schistosomiasis.

◗ Introduction

Schistosomiasis is also known as bilharziasis, named after the German physician Theodore Bilharz, who was the first to identify the parasite in Egypt in 1852. Schistosomiasis is caused by infection with a helminthic blood parasite of the genus *Schistosoma*. Schistosomiasis causes serious morbidity and mortality in endemic areas. It is second only to malaria as a global health problem in terms of public health and economic impact. It is the third most prevalent parasitic infestation in the world. There are 200–300 million people affected worldwide, more than two-thirds of whom live in Africa. It is estimated to cause 280000 deaths per year in sub-Saharan Africa. Schistosomiasis is endemic in 76 countries. It is not a single disease but a complex of diseases caused by the eggs of the five principal *Schistosoma* species. *Schistosoma mansoni* is the most prevalent, being endemic in 54 countries, most of them in Africa.

◗ Life cycle

The life cycle of schistosomes requires both an intermediate host (snail) and a final host (human). The adult worm is approximately 1–2 cm long. The male schistosome is folded, forming a gynaecophoric canal or 'schist' where the female resides. Depending on species, the female produces hundreds to thousands of eggs per day. When humans discharge schistosome eggs in water, each egg releases a ciliated miracidium larva which seeks a snail, the intermediate host (see Table 17.1). The miracidium enters the snail to undergo asexual reproduction, and undergoes a series of developmental changes until the final larval stage of the parasite, the cercaria, is produced and is ejected into the water by the snail. Snails once infected are infected for life; they act as a 'photocopier', producing thousands of cercariae daily. The cercariae are less than 1 mm long with a bifurcated tail. They are attracted to humans by certain chemicals found in human skin. The cercariae penetrate the human skin, shed their forked tail and transform into pre-adult schistosumula which migrate from the skin into blood and lymph vessels. They eventually reach the liver where they live temporarily for 1–4 weeks while they mature into adult worms. The mature worms pair in the liver and remain in a constant state of copulation.

Table 17.1 Five principal *Schistosoma* species

Species of *Schistosoma*	Endemic areas	Organ of the body where it lives	Location of *Schistosoma* eggs spine	Intermediate host snail genus
S. mansoni	Africa, South America, Caribbean	Intestine	Lateral spine	*Biomphalaria*
S. japonicum	China, Philippines, Thailand, Indonesia	Intestine	Inconspicuous spine	*Oncomelania*
S. haematobium	Africa, Middle East, Turkey	Urinary tract	Terminal spine	*Bulinus*
S. intercalatum	West Africa	Intestine	Terminal spine	*Bulinus*
S. mekongi	Laos, Cambodia	Intestine	Inconspicuous spine	*Tricula*

The adult worms migrate against portal blood flow to different organs in the human body as follows:

1. The mesenteric vessels of the colon—*S. mansoni* and *S. intercalatum*
2. The mesenteric vessels of the small intestine—*S. japonicum* and *S. mekongi*
3. The vesical venous plexus—*S. haematobium*.

What guides the adult schistosomes to their respective final destination in various organs is unknown. The adult worms remain in these blood vessels for life, adhering to the vessel wall by their suckers. Worms usually survive 5–10 years, but survival up to 30 years has been reported. The adult schistosome does not replicate within the host; within 1–3 months of reaching their final residence, the female worm produces eggs which travel from the vessels through host tissue to the lumen of the intestine or urinary bladder, or are carried by blood to other sites. Only *S. japonicum* has a definite animal reservoir.

▷ Pathogenesis

The adult worms do little damage to the host and cause no symptoms unless they settle in an unusual location such as the brain or spinal cord. The major pathogenesis is caused by schistosomal eggs trapped in tissues, which leads to fibrosis and scarring of affected tissues. The eggs induce granuloma formation in a delayed type of hypersensitivity reaction. In the bowel, eggs cause ulceration and scarring, leading to blood in stool. In the urinary bladder papillomatous lesions appear, ulcerate and bleed, causing haematuria. The surface of the urinary bladder roughens and sandy patches are seen. Calcium is deposited in the wall of the urinary bladder, producing calcifications in the bladder wall with fibrosis, leading eventually to ureteric obstruction and hydronephrosis. It is accepted that the changes in the urinary bladder predispose to the development of carcinoma of the urinary bladder.

Eggs carried by portal blood flow to the liver wedge in the presinusoidal radicals of the portal vein; this elicits a fibrotic reaction that eventually blocks the venous blood flow of the liver. The characteristic pathology is periportal or 'pipe-stem' fibrosis which may occur 5–15 years after onset of the infection; it is the most critical, most dreaded and costly complication of schistosomiasis. The presinusoidal blockage leads to severe portal hypertension and formation of portosystemic collaterals and varices at the oesophagus, stomach and other sites, causing recurrent gastrointestinal bleeding. Unlike liver cirrhosis, the hepatocytes are not affected because liver cell perfusion is preserved, the nodular architecture of the liver is maintained and nodular regenerative hyperplasia does not occur. Most of the disease burden is caused by infection with *S. mansoni*, *S. haematobium* and *S. japonicum*.

▷ Clinical features

Acute schistosomiasis

Most acute infections in endemic areas are asymptomatic.

Swimmer's itch

This is a skin reaction at the site of cercaria entry, typically on the lower legs and feet, which occurs two or three days after the cercaria penetrates the skin. It causes a transient pruritic maculopapular rash. This is usually a self-limiting condition, and symptoms rarely last more than a week. It is most common with *S. japonicum*. The condition is particularly seen when humans are exposed to avian schistosomes.

Katayama fever

Katayama fever occurs in areas of high transmission rates. History of contact with contaminated water two to eight weeks earlier is usual. It is thought to be a systemic hypersensitivity reaction against the migrating parasite, most frequently *S. mansoni* and *S. japonicum*. Katayama fever is a serum-sickness-like syndrome with fever, generalised lymphadenopathy and hepatosplenomegaly. The symptoms usually resolve spontaneously over a period of few weeks, although aseptic meningitis and death have been reported. The diagnosis of Katayama fever relies on obtaining an appropriate history of exposure in addition to the clinical features. Eggs are rarely found; most patients have positive serological tests. Marked eosinophilia is an important surrogate marker.

Chronic infection

The main clinical findings of chronic schistosomiasis are species-dependent; the severity of the disease depends upon wormload.

Intestinal schistosomiasis

Caused by *S. mansoni*, *S. japonicum*, *S. intercalatum*, *S. mekongi*, it presents with intermittent bloody diarrhoea, tenesmus and colicky lower abdominal pain. Chronic fatigue from anaemia is often complained of. On examination, the patient may be pale, and lower abdominal tenderness is frequently elicited. Complications of longstanding intestinal schistosomiasis include colonic ulcers, stricture and colonic polyps. Colonic polyps may present as inflammatory masses which may even mimic cancer. In rare cases, colonic polyposis results in protein-losing enteropathy.

Hepatic schistosomiasis

This commonly occurs in *S. mansoni* but can occur with all other types, but very rarely in *S. haematobium*. The patient develops haematemesis from oesophageal or gastric varices or, very rarely, from ectopic varices. The haematemesis is usually of sudden onset without prodromal symptoms but, rarely, it is preceded by dizziness, fatigability and epigastric discomfort. Melaena can be the first symptom, but usually follows haematemesis.

The liver is shrunken, left lobe may be enlarged; the spleen is usually palpable but after severe bleeding becomes palpable only after resuscitation. Ascites is very rare except with massive bleeding due to hepatocellular ischaemia. Jaundice and features of chronic liver disease or hepatic encephalopathy are rare, as the hepatocytes are normal in these patients. Some may have symptoms of anaemia due to chronic blood loss from varices, portal hypertension gastropathy or hypersplenism. Dragging left hypochondrial pain from gross splenomegaly is reported by some patients.

The differential diagnosis includes visceral leishmaniasis, tropical splenomegaly syndrome, blood disorders and liver cirrhosis.

Genitourinary schistosomiasis

Caused by infection by *S. haematobium*. Early in the disease, more than 80 per cent of infected patients have haematuria, dysuria and urinary frequency. Patients usually have terminal haematuria. As the disease advances, fibrosis and calcification of the bladder and ureters occur, resulting in hydroureter and hydronephrosis; secondary bacterial infection is frequent. *S. haematobium* infection causes genital disease in approximately one-third of infected women, sometimes in the form of vulval or perineal disease. In men, the epididymis, testis, spermatic cord or prostate can be involved.

Other clinical types of schistosomiasis

- Pulmonary schistosomiasis producing pulmonary hypertension
- Neuroschistosomiasis causing epilepsy
- Paediatric schistosomiasis causing substantial growth retardation.

Recurrent bacteraemia due to *Salmonella* may lead to recurrent attacks of enteric fever. The bacteria seem to colonise the adult worm that act as a reservoir of infection. Eradication of the adult worm is essential in order to get rid of the recurrent bacteraemia.

▷ Diagnosis

Microscopy

Schistosoma eggs can easily be detected in stool and urine and identified by microscopy due to their size, shape and their typical lateral or terminal spine. It is the diagnostic 'gold standard': the cheapest and most widely used method of diagnosing schistosomiasis in endemic areas. The diagnostic yield can be maximised by sedimentation or filtration of urine. Schistosome eggs are found in stool specimens; in field studies the Kato-Katz concentration method is a rapid, simple and inexpensive method of quantifying the quantity of eggs in stool. Schistosome eggs may also be seen in tissue biopsy specimens from the rectum, intestine, liver and urinary bladder.

Serology

Serologic tests are available that can detect antischistosomal antibodies in the serum, mostly enzyme-linked immunosorbent serologic assay (ELISA)-based. No test can distinguish between a past infection and a currently active disease, however. Antibody tests also cross-react with other helminths. Serology is a more specific test for travellers who are not otherwise expected to have schistosomal antibodies. Seroconversion generally occurs within four to eight weeks after infection. A positive serologic test may be diagnostic in patients in whom there are no eggs in excreta, such as those with Katayama fever. Serology is also helpful in the difficult central nervous system schistosomiasis for which eggs cannot be recovered. Most tests have positive results for at least two years after cure and in many cases much longer.

Other tests

Anaemia may be found in chronic cases due to blood loss. Pancytopaenia due to hypersplenism is common in endemic areas. Routine white cell count may show eosinophilia in infected patients. Liver function tests are usually normal, as the hepatocytes are well preserved.

Ultrasound is very valuable in showing the classical periportal fibrosis. Computed tomography (CT) and magnetic resonance imaging (MRI) also show classical features of periportal fibrosis but they are expensive and usually unavailable in endemic areas; they give no more information than unltrasonography which is cheap and available—although CT or MRI might be useful for evaluating central nervous system disease. Ultrasound is also useful in urinary schistosomiasis since it shows the urinary bladder changes or kidney changes. Plain X-rays of abdomens may show calcifications of the urinary bladder wall. Intravenous urography may show hydronephrosis.

Gastroscopy will show oesophageal, gastric or duodenal varices. Sigmoidoscopy or colonoscopy show patchy erythema and shallow ulcers; sometimes diffuse erythema can resemble ulcerative colitis.

Cystoscopy demonstrates the sandy patches inside the urinary bladder and allows biopsies to be obtained. Liver biopsy is rarely done; ultrasound testing has replaced it.

◗ Management

Swimmer's itch

Clears up in few days without treatment. Anti-itching creams such as calamine lotions help. In severe cases, oral antihistamines can be given to reduce itching.

Katayama fever

Primarily treated with corticosteroids to suppress the hypersensitivity reaction. Praziquantel is given initially and after six weeks, to eradicate the mature worms at onset of the illness and the worms that will mature later.

Treatment of chronic schistosomiasis

Praziquantel is now almost exclusively used to treat schistosomiasis. It is a pyrazino-isoquinoline derivative which is effective against all five major species of human schistosomiasis; it is given orally at a single dose of 40 mg/kg body weight. The exact mechanism of its action is unknown but it is thought to produce paralysis of the adult worm, resulting in its detachment from the vein wall. It is well tolerated and causes few side effects—mainly nausea, vomiting, malaise and abdominal pain, most of which are thought to be caused by immune response to the dying worms. It is safe for treatment in pregnancy, lactation, and in young children, and has also been reported to reduce fibrotic changes in the liver. Praziquantel has little or no effect on schistosome eggs or immature worms. There is increasing concern about the development of resistance to praziquantel, however.

The drug oxamniquine, which is effective against *S. mansoni* only, was used extensively in Brazil at one time but has now been replaced by praziquantel.

Treatment of chronic complications of schistosomiasis

The chronic complications are the main cause of morbidity and mortality and reduction of productivity, and are the most expensive to treat. Bleeding oesophageal varices is the main presenting symptom of hepatic schistosomiasis, requiring blood transfusion. Blood products are always in short supply since almost everyone in the village has varices and cannot donate.

Iron supplement is given regularly. The varices need to be treated in hospitals with endoscopy facilities to inject them with sclerosants, or to band ligate them. Endoscopic treatment of varices is very effective in cases of hepatic schistosomiasis, but the patient initially needs treatment monthly until the varices are eradicated, followed by a lifetime of one- or two-yearly check-ups and treatment of new varices.

Non-selective beta-blockers, mainly propranolol, are used as primary prophylaxis for those with large varices that have never bled, and as secondary prophylaxis if no endoscopic facilities are available, or in addition to endoscopy when available. Tolerance to beta blockers is very good, and few patients stop the treatment because of side effects. The response to beta blocker plus endoscopic treatment is excellent, as liver functions are well maintained. Some patients are reported to undergo regular sclerotherapy and band ligation for over 25 years.

QUICK FLICK

17

Sengstaken-Blakemore tubes are useful for temporary arrest of bleeding; for transfer of patients to endoscopy units, inflation of the gastric balloon alone is enough. Terlipressin is very effective but also very expensive, and is used only rarely, when a patient continues to bleed after endoscopic therapy.

Transjugular intrahepatic portosystemic shunt (TIPS) is very expensive treatment and is used in very few cases since it is difficult to introduce the stent as the liver is fibrotic and hard.

Portal hypertension gastropathy is sometimes encountered, and responds to beta blocker therapy.

Gastric vascular ectasia is very rare; it is treated with argon plasma coagulation therapy.

Surgery is used when there is hypersplenism, to remove the spleen. Urological complications may need surgery.

◖ Control of schistosomiasis

The World Health Organization recommends schistosomiasis population control based on indefinite yearly treatment with praziquantel, as there is little natural immunity to re-infection in the exposed population.

Schistosomiasis can be controlled by health education, behavioural changes, provision of safe water and sanitation, and eradication of poverty. Proper planning and innovative management of water resource schemes for power generation and irrigation are very important. The Sennar Dam in the Blue Nile in Sudan in 1925 introduced schistosomiasis for the first time in central Sudan and has resulted in immense suffering of the population until the present day. More recently the erection of Diama Dam in Senegal in 1986 introduced schistosomiasis to Senegal and Mauritania, and by 1994 virtually the whole population of northern Senegal was infected with schistosomiasis.

Summary

Schistosomiasis, or bilharziasis, is a water-based disease caused by a worm of the genus *Schistosoma*. The transmission cycle involves an intermediate host—a snail—and a definite host, a human. The three most important species causing human disease are *S. mansoni*, *S. haematobium* and *S. japonicum*. Schistosomiasis is endemic in 76 countries—more than 200–300 million people are infected worldwide.

The chronic complications of schistosomiasis are responsible for much loss of life and loss of productivity. The most important complication is the development of portal hypertension from hepatic schistosomiasis, which leads to bleeding oesophageal varices needing special resources, and is expensive to treat. Praziquantel is the drug treatment of choice, and is also used in population-based chemotherapy to control schistosomiasis. No vaccine is as yet available.

Information for patients

What is schistosomiasis?

Schistosomiasis, sometimes called bilharziasis or bilharzia, is a disease caused by a blood parasite—a worm called *Schistosoma*. It can cause serious liver fibrosis leading to vomiting of blood, or urinary bladder infection and renal impairment.

How do I get schistosomiasis?

If you come in contact with water infected with the schistosome larvae. They penetrate the skin and develop into adult worms inside your body.

How do I avoid getting schistosomiasis?

Avoid bathing, wading, washing and swimming in freshwater lakes, ponds, irrigation canals or near banks of slowly running rivers in endemic areas. Schistosomiasis occurs in Africa, South America, South-East Asia and the Middle East.

Untreated piped water coming directly from freshwater sources may contain the larvae—to help eliminate the risk of infection, filter the water using a paper coffee filter, or heat the water to 50 °C (122 °F) for five minutes, or allow the water to stand for at least 48 hours before use.

Schistosomiasis can't be acquired from salt water in oceans or seas. Chlorinated swimming pools are considered safe.

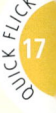

What are the symptoms of schistosomiasis?

You can get an immediate skin rash with itching known as swimmer's itch when you are infected with the *Schistosoma* larvae. You may get a febrile illness known as Katayama fever, with enlargement of your lymph nodes, four to six weeks after being infected.

After several months, or even years, you can get either (a) intestinal schistosomiasis which causes diarrhoea, lethargy, abdominal pain and blood in faeces, or (b) urinary schistosomiasis manifested by painful urination with blood at the end of urination.

After years of infection, the parasite can damage the liver, intestines, lungs and urinary bladder.

Is there a satisfactory treatment for schistosomiasis?

To avoid swimmer's itch, rinse the exposed skin with fresh water immediately after leaving the suspect water. Vigorously dry your skin with a towel or apply alcohol to the exposed area. If you have severe itching, use an anti-itching cream such as calamine lotion.

If you have Katayama fever you should see a doctor, as you may need hospital admission and treatment with corticosteroids.

If you have urinary or intestinal schistosomiasis the medication is a drug called praziquantel. The dose is calculated according to body weight. It is safe for children and pregnant women.

Is there a vaccine?

No.

Recommended reading

Gryseels B, Polman K, Clerinx J, Kestens L. Human schistosomiasis. *Lancet*. 2006; 368:1106–18.

Mahmound AAFM, editor. Schistosomiasis. Tropical diseases: Science and practice; vol. 3. Singapore: Imperial College Press; 2001.

Ross AGP, Bartley PB, Sleigh AC, Olds GR, Li Y, Williams GM, McManus DP. Schistosomiasis. *N Engl J Med*. 2002; 346:1212–20.

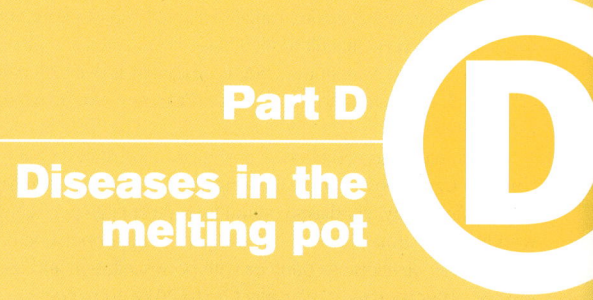

Part D

Diseases in the melting pot

Chapter 18: Giardiasis, cryptosporidiosis and cyclosporiasis

D. Alcid (USA)

Key points
- Similar symptomatology for all three diseases.
- Metronidazole is used to treat giardiasis.
- Sulfa/trimethoprim is used to treat cyclosporiasis.
- Azithromycin is used to treat cryptosporidiosis.
- Pregnant women with giardiasis are treated with paromomycin.
- The three diseases represent a global problem.

Introduction

These three protozoan diseases have identical clinical presentations and epidemiology. The different treatment modalities are discussed in detail for each organism.

The symptoms of all three are identical: weight loss, bloating, flatulence, belching, stomach cramps, nausea, vomiting, myalgia, low-grade fever, fatigue, malaise and loss of appetite.

Giardiasis

Giardiasis in humans is an infection caused by the intestinal protozoan *Giardia lamblia*. It occurs worldwide; there is a prevalence of 20–30 per cent in developing countries, but it is also found in certain areas of developed countries. *Giardia* has a wide range of human and other mammalian hosts, thus making it very difficult to eliminate. The Centers for Disease Control and Prevention report that, in the USA, *Giardia* infects over 2.5 million people annually. It is also the most commonly diagnosed enteric parasite in the United States.[1]

The disease was named after Professor A. Giard in Paris and Vilem Lambl, a Czech physician. Lambl originally named the organism *Cercomonas intestinalis*. Today, giardiasis continues to affect large populations of people worldwide. Giardiasis infects 2–5 per cent of the population of developed countries; in developing countries with poor sanitation and contaminated food or water sources, it may affect up to 20 or 30 per cent of the population.

Epidemiology

Giardiasis is caused by ingesting infective cysts. There are many ways in which the disease can be transmitted: person-to-person, water-borne, and through sexual (faecal–oral) contact. Giardiasis is most often transmitted from one person to others and, not surprisingy, transmission is usually associated with poor hygiene, insanitary conditions and inadequate water supply arrangements.

In the United States, giardiasis epidemics are commonly associated with the ingestion of contaminated water. Food-borne epidemics of giardiasis have occurred following contamination of food by infected food-handlers. Liu and Nevins (2009) discussed the high rate of infection as follows:

> *High infection rates occur in hikers and backpackers in the United States. Giardiasis is a common infection in active outdoors populations because of their exposure to areas inhabited by infected wild animals and ingestion of free-flowing water which may contain cysts. Furthermore, giardiasis is common in tourists and business travellers to developing countries, especially Mexico, South-East Asia, western South America and [Central and Eastern Europe]. An increased prevalence of giardiasis among homosexual men has been reported by a number of studies. Lastly, because infection may be caused by poor hygiene, giardiasis has high infection rates in daycare centres and nursing homes, though the groups most at risk for infection are overseas travellers and hikers.*[2–5]

Life cycle

Infection begins when the host ingests cysts from contaminated food, water, fomites or faecal matter. Mature cysts are resistant to acid, so they survive the digestive acids in the stomach and migrate to the small intestine.

The parasites multiply and colonise the small intestine by attaching to the intestinal mucosa. Trophozoites do not invade other organs but may penetrate the secretary tubules of the mucosa to the gallbladder and biliary drainage.

Gastrointestinal infection

Most infected people are asymptomatic cyst carriers. In some there is abrupt onset of abdominal cramps with explosive, watery diarrhoea, vomiting, foul flatus and fever which may last for three or four days before subsiding to a less acute phase. There may be dysentery-like symptoms of tenesmus, urgency and bloody stools.

Stool examination

Multiple specimens of freshly passed stools are tested for trophozoites; these disintegrate rapidly but can be present in fresh, watery stools. At least three stools taken at two-day intervals are examined for ova and parasites. Cysts are found in soft and semi-formed stools. Test kits for detecting *Giardia* antigen are commercially available. These have a sensitivity of 85–90 per cent and specificity of 90–100 per cent. Kits are also available for detecting both *Giardia* and *Cryptosporidium* with similar sensitivity and specificity.

Management

The current drug of choice is metronidazole (flagyl), 250 mg administered three times a day for five days. Other drugs are:

- tinidazole (fasigyn): Adult dose: 2 g given as a single dose
- paramomycin (humatin), a non-absorbable aminoglycoside:
  - adult dose: 25–35 mg/kg of body weight three times a day for seven days
  - paediatric dose: 25–35 mg/kg of body weight three times a day for seven days.
  - it is also the drug of choice for treating *Giardia lamblia* during pregnancy.

Cryptosporidiosis

Cryptosporidiosis is a zoonotic infection—one of the most common causes of infectious diarrhoea. One of the largest outbreaks in humans occurred in Milwaukee (Wisconsin, USA) where almost 500 000 individuals were infected.

Dairy calves are high-risk hosts; other livestock, pets and humans are also important. *Cryptosporidium hominis* (formerly *C. parvum* genotype 1) is the species responsible for most human cases in the United States, sub-Saharan Africa and Asia. In Europe, and particularly in the United Kingdom, *C. parvum* is responsible for most of the cases in humans.

Although it is a self-limiting infection in a normal host, *Cryptosporidium* can cause significant morbidity in immunocompromised patients, specially those with AIDS. Before antiretroviral therapy was available, *Cryptosporidium* infection was difficult to eradicate. It is highly infectious, requiring only 10^1–10^3 oocysts to cause disease. These are immediately infectious after they pass into the environment.

The life cycle of *Cryptosporidium* includes an autoinfection stage. Because the oocyst is acid-resistant and an autoinfection stage occurs in the host, the infective dose remains low. Oocysts that are excreted by the infected carrier are resistant to chlorine at levels used for routine municipal treatment, with the result that contamination of municipal water systems is common.

Cryptosporidium causes diarrhoea by increasing intestinal permeability, chloride secretion, and malabsorption, probably the host's immune response to the infection. In otherwise healthy individuals the infection is usually limited to the small intestine. The biliary tract may be affected in people with AIDS or other immunodeficiencies.

Management

Cryptosporidiosis can be difficult to treat. In an otherwise healthy host the disease is self-limiting but antiparasitic drugs are indicated for immuncompromised patients, especially those with AIDS. Drugs such as nitazoxanide can decrease the frequency of diarrhoea. Azithromycin may be given together with nitoxanide. The main approach to treating these patients is antiretroviral agents to improve immune function.

⊙ Cyclosporiasis

Unlike *Giardia* and *Cryptosporidium*, *Cyclospora* must sporulate outside the host for days or weeks before it becomes infective. Cyclosporiasis is not transmitted from person to person, unlike the other two diseases.

Stool examination

Stool examination for oocysts is the standard procedure for diagnosing *Cyclospora cayetanensis*. Intestinal aspirates and duodenal or jejunal biopsy samples may also contain oocysts. Since standard laboratory procedures for ova and parasites do not identify *Cyclospora*, the laboratory must be notified that they are to test specifically for *Cyclospora*. Kinyoun acid-fast stain may be useful in *Cyclospora* testing.

Management

The only effective treatment for cyclosporiasis is trimethoprim-sulfamethoxazole (bactrim-septra). Dosage is one double-strength tablet orally, twice a day for seven to ten days. There are apparently many ineffective drugs, based on anecdotal and non-randomised studies.

For patients who are allergic to sulfa and who have significant morbidity, a referral to an allergist for desensitisation against sulfa may be beneficial.

Summary

Giardiasis, cryptosporidiasis and cyclosporiasis have identical presentation in normal patients. In immunocompromised patients, such as those with AIDS, the clinical course can be prolonged.

The testing for *Cyclospora* may be difficult. The laboratory must be notified that a specialised test such as AFB smears may need to be performed.

In all three diseases, patients with AIDS require antiretroviral drugs to improve immune function.

References

1. Centers for Disease Control and Prevention. *Giardia*. [Internet]. Available from: www.cdc.gov/parasites/giardia.

2. Liu J, Nevins S. Stanford University ParaSites Project: Giardiasis. 2009. [Internet]. Available from: www.stanford.edu/group/parasites/ParaSites2009/NevinsANDLiu_Giardiasis/NevinsANDLiu_Giardiasis.htm.

3. Brodsky RE, Spencer HC Jr, Schultz MG. Giardiasis in American travelers to the Soviet Union. *J Infect Dis*. 1974 Sep; 130(3):319–23.

4. Peters CS, Sable R, Janda WM, Chittom AL, Kocka FE. Prevalence of enteric parasites in homosexual patients attending an outpatient clinic. *J Clin Microbiol*. 1986 Oct; 24(4):684–5.

5. Schrader B. Giardiasis. eMedicine. [Internet]. Available from: www.emedicinehealth.com/giardiasis/article_em.htm.

Recommended reading

Abubakar I, Aliyu SH, Arumugam C, Usman NK, Hunter PR. Treatment of cryptosporidiosis in immunocompromised individuals: systematic review and meta-analysis. *Br J Clin Pharmacol*. 2007; 63(4):387–93.

Centers for Disease Control and Prevention. Patient information. [Internet]. Available from: www.cdc.gov/crypto/, www.cdc.gov/ncidod/dpd/parasites/giardiasis/factsht_giardia.htm/, www.cdc.gov/ncidod/dpd/parasites/cyclospora/default.htm.

Herwaldt BL. *Cyclospora cayetanensis*: a review, focusing on the outbreaks of cyclosporiasis in the 1990s. *Clin Infect Dis*. 2000; 31(4):1040–57.

Pennardt A. Giardiasis. eMedicine. [Internet]. Available from: http://emedicine.medscape.com/article/782818-overview.

Shlim DR. *Cyclospora cayetanensis. Clin Lab Med*. 2002; 22(4):927–36.

QUICK FLICK 18

◘ **Introduction**

The 2009 report of the Joint United Nations Programme on HIV and AIDS (UNAIDS) estimated that 33.4 million people were living with HIV infection in 2008, of whom 31.3 million were adults. There were 2.7 million newly infected people in 2008 alone. Sub-Saharan Africa contributed 71 per cent of new infections. The increase in the number of people living with HIV infection is due to high rates of new infection and prolonged survival in those on HAART. The epidemic appears to have stabilised in most regions, although the prevalence continues to rise in Eastern Europe and Central Asia, and in other parts of Asia, due to a high rate of new HIV infections. These epidemics have moved from transmission among injection drug users to sexual transmission.

Gastrointestinal and hepatobiliary disorders are extremely common in patients with HIV infection. Evaluation of these conditions should be based on the degree of immunosuppression, which can be seen in clinical features such as oral thrush, and CD4 count if available. More than one infection may account for the symptoms. The extent of investigation depends on availability of resources and on the severity of illness. People with HIV infection may also have conditions brought on by the usual causes in the immunocompetent population.

◘ **Gastrointestinal disorders**

Oesophagitis

Symptoms include dysphagia and odynophagia. There is usually no fever. The commonest cause is oesophageal candidiasis (Table 19.1). Oral candidiasis is usually, but not always, present and can present in four ways. Pseudomembranous candida is the best recognised form, with white painless plaques that can be easily scraped off, leaving an erythematosus base. Next most common is an erythematosus form with smooth red spots which may coalesce to form larger red areas. Least common are angular cheilitis, and fourth, a hyperkeratotic form—usually on the tongue—which cannot be scraped off and which, in other parts of the mouth, may mimic oral hairy leukoplakia.

Other causes of oesophagitis in which odynophagia is most prominent are ulcerations caused by *Cytomegalovirus* (CMV) infection (often with fever) and aphthous or idiopathic oesophageal ulcers and, least commonly, herpes simplex. There may also be ulceration with acute HIV infection. Oesophagitis due to *Candida* and herpes simplex are usually seen with a CD4 $<200/mm^3$ and CMV and idiopathic ulcers below $50/mm^3$.

Malignancies such as Kaposi's sarcoma, lymphoma or squamous cell carcinoma can very occasionally be the cause, as can opportunistic infections at CD4 $<200/mm^3$, including tuberculosis, *Mycobacterium avium* and

Table 19.1 Oesophageal disorders in patients with HIV infection

Cause	Clinical features	Diagnosis	Treatment	Duration
Candida	Dysphagia Odynophagia Pain Oral thrush (70%)	Responds to empiric therapy	Fluconazole 200 mg daily or 200 mg stat and 100 mg daily Itraconazole 200 mg daily Amphotericin B 0.3–0.5 mg daily.	7–14 days
Cytomegalovirus (CMV) infection	Odynophagia Dysphagia Pain Fever often	Endoscopy and biopsy (intranuclear inclusions) CMV antigen (pp65) in blood often negative	Ganciclovir 5 mg/kg/dose bid Valganciclovir Foscarnet	14–21 days
Idiopathic ulcers	Odynophagia Dysphagia Pain	Endoscopy and biopsy	Prednisone 40 mg daily orally and taper down by 10 mg weekly Thalidomide 200 mg daily	4 weeks
Herpes simplex virus	Odynophagia Dysphagia Pain Oral ulcers often	Endoscopy and biopsy	Acyclovir 400 mh tid orally or 200 mg 5x/day orally or 5 mg/kg/dose ivi tid. Valacyclovir 1 gm bid orally Famciclovir 500 mh bid orally	10–14 days

histoplasmosis. Non-HIV-related conditions including reflux oesophagitis with heartburn and possibly regurgitation may also be evident.

Management

An empirical approach to patients with dysphagia and odynophagia is reasonable and involves treating for *Candida* oesophagitis, by far the most common cause, which responds rapidly to treatment within a few days. It may recur after treatment.

QUICK FLICK 19

If the symptoms do not resolve, ideally endoscopy with biopsy should then be performed. If endoscopy cannot be done, then treatment can be directed empirically at resistant candidiasis with amphotericin B, at idiopathic ulcers with prednisone, and at herpes simplex with acyclovir. If ganciclovir is available, then CMV infection can also be targeted.

Diarrhoea

Diarrhoea occurs in more than half of all patients with AIDS and causes significant morbidity and mortality. With sufficient investigation, a specific cause can be found in up to 80 per cent of patients (Table 19.2). Chronic

Table 19.2 Common causes of AIDS-associated diarrhoea

Infections
Bacterial
Salmonella *Shigella* *Campylobacter* spp. *Clostridium difficile* MAC bacteraemia *Mycobacterium tuberculosis*
Protozoal
Cryptosporidium *Isospora belli* Microsporidium *Cyclospora* *Entamoeba histolytica* *Giardia*
Viral
Cytomegalovirus HIV (idiopathic) Herpes simplex
Neoplasms
Lymphoma Kaposi's sarcoma
Drugs
Lopinavir/ritonavir

or persistent diarrhoea becomes more common as the CD4 count drops to low levels. Chronic diarrhoea is important in people starting HAART as it may cause malabsorption of the antiretroviral drugs and increase virological failure. Basic investigations are detailed in Table 19.3.

Table 19.3 Investigation of AIDS-associated diarrhoea (> 5 days)

Specimen	Investigation	Cause of diarrhoea
Stool	Bacterial culture	*Salmonella*, *Shigella*, *Campylobacter*
	Microscopy with wet mount	*Isospora* and *Entamoeba*
	Microscopy with modified acid-fast stain	*Cryptosporidia* and *Cyclospora*
	Microscopy with modified trichrome stain	Microsporidia
	Clostridium difficile toxin	*Clostridium difficile*
Blood	Culture for bacteria and mycobacteria	Non-typhoidal *Salmonella*
	Culture for mycobacteria	MAC
Biopsy for histopathology	Colonoscopy	*Cytomegalovirus* and exclude lymphoma and Kaposi's sarcoma

Treatment is tailored to specific causes. There are alternative drugs for a number of the causes (see Table 19.4 overleaf). Cryptosporidial infection may cause fulminant diarrhoea and has no consistently successful therapy, although it is usually self-limited at CD4 counts >100/mm^3. Immune reconstitution by initiating HAART is therefore essential, while providing supportive therapy and using antiperistaltic agents such as loperamide or atropine diphenoxylate. *Cytomegalovirus* colitis may be complicated by haemorrhage and perforation.

Other infectious causes of perforation include typhoid and tuberculosis. Although *Salmonella, Shigella* and *Campylobacter* usually cause acute diarrhoea, they may be persistent in patients with low CD4 counts. *Mycobacterium avium* complex (MAC) bacteraemia presents with systemic illness characterised by fever, weight loss and profound diarrhoea. Lopinavir/ritonavir causes mild-to-moderate diarrhoea, usually self-limiting, in 15–25 per cent of people at initiation. In areas where investigation will delay therapy or is rationed, it seems reasonable to initiate empiric treatment with ciprofloxacin and metronidazole (Table 19.4) while sending stool specimens for ova and

Table 19.4 Treatment of AIDS-associated diarrhoea

Cause	Medication
Shigella, Salmonella, Campylobacter, Isospora belli	Ciprofloxacin 500 mg bid
Clostridium difficile, Entamoeba, Giardia	Metronidazole 400–500 mg tid
Microsporidia (*Encephalitozoon intestinalis*)	Albendazole 400 mg bid x 21 days
Cytomegalovirus	Ganciclovir, valganciclovir or foscarnet
MAC bacteraemia	Clarithromycin or azithromycin with ethambutol and a third agent
Isospora belli, Cyclospora	Trimethoprim-sulfamethoxazole
Enterocytozoon bieneusi	Fumagillin (60 mg/day)
Cryptosporidium, microsporidia	HAART

parasite testing. If the diarrhoea still does not resolve, albendazole and anti-peristaltic agents can be added while awaiting mycobacterial culture results. In very severe chronic diarrhoea, codeine 30 mg orally 4–6 times a day or tincture of opium 0.6 ml orally 3–4 times per day can be used to control it.

Biliary tract disorders

AIDS cholangiopathy and acalculous cholecystitis are relatively uncommon and are overshadowed by non-HIV-related conditions (Table 19.5). AIDS-related cholangiopathy is seen in late-stage patients and may be a presenting condition. It is associated in more than 50 per cent of patients with infections such as *Cryptosporidium, Cytomegalovirus*, microsporidia, *Cyclospora* and MAC, but treatment of the underlying infection does not alter the prognosis.

The clinical presentation is variable. The more common manifestations include right upper quadrant pain and fever associated with a markedly raised alkaline phosphatase level more than eight times normal. The transaminases may be raised two or three times normal. Jaundice is not common. Diarrhoea may be present due to the associated infection. Sonography frequently suggests strictures of the biliary tract, leading to ERCP. There are four patterns seen on ERCP, namely papillary stenosis with sclerosing cholangitis (50%), sclerosing cholangitis (20%), papillary stenosis (10%), and extrahepatic strictures. Endoscopic sphincterotomy may provide symptomatic relief. The median survival is nine months, which improves with HAART.

Table 19.5 Other conditions of the gastrointestinal system affected by AIDS

Condition	Causes
Pancreatitis	Drugs: didanosine, stavudine, lamivudine (children), ritonavir, lopinavir/ritonavir, pentamidine, cotrimoxazole Infections: *Cytomegalovirus*, MAC, tuberculosis, *Cryptosporidium*, toxoplasmosis, *Cryptococcus*. Hypertriglyceridaemia may be part of lipodystrophy drug side effect
Hepatitis	Drugs: HAART, especially nevirapine; efavirenz, delavirdine; stavudine, didanosine, zidovudine; all protease inhibitors; many other drugs including acyclovir, ganciclovir, foscarnet, isoniazid, rifampicin, pyrazinamide, cotrimoxazole, fluconazole
Peliosis hepatis	Infections: especially bacillary angiomatosis due to *Bartonella* Malignancy: Hodgkin's lymphoma, Castleman's disease, leukaemia Drugs: steroids
Ascites	Infections: tuberculosis, MAC, histoplasmosis, toxoplasmosis, *Cryptococcus* Malignancy: Primary effusion lymphoma (flow cytometry)

Acalculous cholecystitis, which is linked to infection with *Cytomegalovirus* and *Cryptosporidium*, is managed by cholecystectomy.

Immune reconstitution inflammatory syndrome

Immune reconstitution inflammatory syndrome (IRIS) is the term used for the atypical clinical deterioration that has been noted in people with HIV infection after introduction of HAART and immune recovery. The condition occurs within days to months of starting HAART and is due to the restoration of pathogen-specific immune responses, which cause immunopathology. It is estimated that 10–25 per cent of unselected adults who start HAART experience this syndrome. It may involve unmasking of previously undiagnosed infections or a paradoxical deterioration, often involving florid inflammatory responses. The abdomen may be involved by both *Mycobacterium tuberculosis* and MAC. Lymphadenopathy occurs, which may be necrotic, along with splenic microabscesses. Histology reveals granulomata, and local culture is frequently positive for the organism.

There may be flares of hepatitis B and C. Another cause of hepatitis B flares is induced resistance to the antiviral agents lamivudine, emtricitabine and/or tenofovir, or severe toxicity if the drugs are abruptly stopped because of virologic failure, and a new regimen substituted. In such cases, these

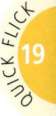

antiviral agents should be continued if possible and included in the salvage antiretroviral regimen.

Sexually transmitted infections (STIs) of the GIT

There has been an increase in STIs of the rectum and anus in men who have sex with men and in women who have receptive anal intercourse. The STIs increase the risk of acquisition of HIV infection. The usual presentation is with proctitis (Table 19.6).

Table 19.6 Features of proctitis

Symptoms	Anorectal pain
	Rectal bleeding
	Rectal discharge
	Tenesmus
	Pruritus
	Vary in severity; may be asymptomatic
Signs	Inflamed mucosa
	Ulcerations
	Exudate

Examination should include inspection of the skin and mucous membranes and palpation of lymph nodes. Palpation for fissures and masses, with anoscopy and sigmoidoscopy, if necessary, should ideally be performed. Basic investigations are a rectal swab for gonorrhoea, chlamydia and herpes simplex, and serologic blood testing for syphilis. Empiric treatment for gonorrhoea and chlamydia should be given when these infections are suspected (Table 19.7). Partners should be considered for treatment. Enteric pathogens can also cause proctocolitis. Fissures, warts and perianal abscesses also occur. Patients with lymphogranuloma venereum often develop unilateral lymphadenopathy or buboes when the evanescent ulcer has disappeared. In patients with AIDS, it is necessary to add *Cytomegalovirus*, MAC, *Cryptosporidium*, microsporidia, *Isospora* and Kaposi's sarcoma to the differential diagnosis.

Human papillomavirus (HPV) is a risk factor for anal neoplasia and anal carcinoma, in a similar way to cervical neoplasia. The risk is increased in HIV-infected people with low CD4 counts who have anal intercourse. Anal Pap smears are recommended. HAART does not seem to improve the outcomes of anal neoplasms.

Table 19.7 Causes, investigation and treatment of sexually transmitted infections of the anorectal region

Cause	Infection	Test	Treatment
Bacteria	Gonorrhoea	Culture or NAAT*	Ceftriaxone 250 mg im stat or cefixime 400 mg orally stat
	Chlamydia (non-LGV)	NAAT*	Doxycycline 100 mg bid for 1 week
	Lymphogranuloma venereum (LGV)	NAAT*	Doxycycline 100 mg bid for 3 weeks
	Shigellosis	Stool culture	Ciprofloxacin
	Syphilis	Serology or dark field microscopy	Benzathine penicillin 2.4 mU im x1; doxycycline 100 mg bid for 14 days
Viruses	Herpes simplex	NAAT* or viral culture	Acyclovir or famciclovir or valacyclovir
Parasites	Amoebiasis	Stool microscopy	Metronidazole

* NAAT: nucleic acid amplification test.

Summary

It has been estimated that 33.4 million people were living with AIDS in 2008. Although sub-Saharan Africa has the highest prevalence, we are witnessing a great increase in Asia and Eastern Europe. The major impact of AIDS on the digestive system is in the oesophagus, where candidiasis has the major effect. Other infections are CMV and idiopathic herpes simplex virus.

Diarrhoea is a common AIDS symptom with many possible causes. It causes significant morbidity and mortality. A specific cause may be found in 80 per cent of patients.

Biliary tract disorders include AIDS-related cholangiopathy in which ERCP is the diagnostic 'gold standard'. HAART has improved survival.

An immune reconstitution inflammatory syndrome may result in the unmasking of undiagnosed opportunistic diseases. It can occur days or months after starting HAART.

Sexually transmitted infections (STIs) increase the risk of acquiring HIV. Human papillomavirus (HPV) is a risk factor for anal carcinoma.

QUICK FLICK 19

▶ The palliation of patients with advanced non-resectable oesophageal cancer involves treatment modalities such as endoscopic insertion of self-expandable metallic stents, endoscopic ablation, radiotherapy and chemotherapy.

◌ Introduction

Oesophageal cancer is the eighth most common cancer worldwide. It is also the sixth most common cause of cancer mortality. Globally there is a striking geographic variation in the incidence rates, with a 20-fold variation between high-risk China and low-risk western Africa. The two main histological subtypes are squamous cell carcinoma (SCC) and adenocarcinoma (AC). SCC occurs mainly in the middle and distal oesophagus, whereas AC arises from the distal oesophagus. Despite progress in diagnostic and therapeutic techniques, the prognosis of oesophageal cancer remains poor, with overall five-year survival rates of 10–16 per cent reported in Europe and the United States.[1] This chapter discusses the epidemiology, diagnosis and treatment of SCC and AC.

◌ Geographic variations in epidemiology

There is a striking geographic variation in the incidence rates of oesophageal cancer (see Table 20.1). The age-standardised incidence rate (ASR) in males and females is 27.4/100 000 and 12/100 000 in China, 5.8/100 000 and 1.3/100 000 in North America, and 1.3/100 000 and 0.3/100 000 in western Africa.[1] SCC was the predominant type of oesophageal cancer worldwide.

Over the past two decades, a marked increase of AC has been observed in Western developed countries such as the United States, United Kingdom, Scandinavia, France, Switzerland, Denmark, Italy, Australia and New Zealand, making it the predominant oesophageal cancer subtype in these regions. In the United States, for example, AC now accounts for 60 per cent of oesophageal cancer cases and is believed to be related to the rising incidence of Barrett's

Table 20.1 Age-standardised incidence rates of oesophageal cancer

Country	Males: ASR (/100 000)	Females: ASR (/100 000)
Africa		
Southern Africa	19.7	7.0
Eastern Africa	19.1	8.0
Northern Africa	2.1	1.4
Central Africa	1.5	0.2
Western Africa	1.3	0.6

Country	Males: ASR (/100 000)	Females: ASR (/100 000)
Asia		
China	27.4	12.0
Japan	10.0	1.3
South-Central Asia	8.1	5.9
Australia/New Zealand	5.5	2.3
South-East Asia	3.1	1.2
Western Asia	3.0	2.0
Europe		
Northern Europe	7.9	3.3
Western Europe	7.6	1.4
Eastern Europe	6.2	0.9
Southern Europe	4.6	0.8
America		
South America	7.1	2.0
North America	5.8	1.3
Central America	2.2	0.9

Source: Parkin DM, Bray F, Ferlay J, Pisani P. Global cancer statistics, 2002. *CA Cancer J Clin.* 2005; 55:74–108.

oesophagus (BE).[1] Asian countries have a high incidence of SSC, with the ASR often exceeding 100/100 000 in northern and central China, north-eastern Iran, and in the region between these two countries.[1]

○ Risk factors

The main risk factors associated with SSC are cigarette smoking and alcohol consumption (see Table 20.2 overleaf). Both current smokers (hazard ratio 9.27) and past smokers (hazard ratio 4.35) have an increased risk of SCC compared to non-smokers.[1] The risk is dose-related, with patients who smoke 80 or more packets of cigarettes per year being at significantly higher risk than those smoking 40–80 packets per year (odds ratio of 16.9 vs 5.2). Excessive alcohol (more than three drinks daily) reportedly causes a three to five times increase in the risk of SCC.[2] Cigarette smoking is also an important risk factor for AC, with

Table 20.2 Risk factors for oesophageal cancer

Risk factor	ESCC	EA
Tobacco	++++	++
Alcohol	+++	
Achalasia	+++	
Caustic injury	++++	
Tylosis	++++	
Plummer-Vinson syndrome	++++	
History of head/neck cancer	++++	
History of radiotherapy for breast cancer	+++	+++
Barrett's oesophagus		++++
Weekly reflux symptoms		+++
Obesity		++

Source: Modified from American Joint Committee on Cancer. AJCC cancer staging manual. 6th ed. New York: Springer; 2002. Esophagus; pp. 91–8.

an increased risk for both current smokers (hazard ratio 3.7) and past smokers (hazard ratio 2.8).[1]

The main risk factor associated with AC is BE, producing an overall 30–50-fold increase in risk. AC arises from BE at an estimated incidence rate of 0.4–0.7 per 100 patients/year. BE without dysplasia and with low-grade intraepithelial neoplasia (LGIN) generally produces slow rates of disease progression. A recent study has shown that 27 per cent of patients with LGIN developed either high-grade intraepithelial neoplasia (HGIN) or AC over a period of eight years. HGIN produces a definite risk of disease progression, with rates exceeding 10 per cent per year.[3]

Significant risk factors for AC in BE are male gender, Caucasian race, the presence of reflux and a high body mass index (BMI). Other risk factors associated with oesophageal cancer include a prior history of caustic injury to the oesophagus, achalasia, tylosis and genetic predisposition. A summary of known risk factors sorted according to histological subtype is shown in Table 20.2.[4]

◉ Clinical features

Early oesophageal cancers can be asymptomatic. In the context of AC associated with BE, patients may have longstanding reflux symptoms. The onset of oesophageal symptoms is inevitably associated with an advanced disease stage; they include dysphagia, odynophagia and weight loss. Dysphagia arises as a consequence of circumferential involvement of the oesophagus causing luminal stenosis, whereas pain is due to invasion of adjacent structures.

◯ Diagnosis

Evaluation of symptomatic patients

Endoscopy is indicated as the first-line diagnostic test, as it can exclude other differentials and allow tissue to be obtained for histological examination. Barium swallow is an alternative to endoscopy and can reveal a stenosed oesophageal lesion. When it is not possible to pass an endoscope across the stricture, a barium swallow is useful for assessing the anatomical extent.

Cancer staging

Table 20.3 Staging of oesophageal cancer

TNM definitions		
Primary tumour (T)	Regional lymph nodes (N)	Distant metastasis (M)
TX: Primary tumour cannot be assessed	NX: Regional lymph nodes cannot be assessed	Overall: MX: Distant metastasis cannot be assessed
T0: No evidence of primary tumour	N0: No regional lymph node metastasis	M0: No distant metastasis
Tis: Carcinoma in situ	N1: Regional lymph node metastasis	M1: Distant metastasis
T1: Tumour invades lamina propria or submucosa		Definition based on tumour site: 1. Tumours of the lower thoracic oesophagus:
T2: Tumour invades muscularis propria		M1a: Metastasis in coeliac lymph nodes
T3: Tumour invades adventitia		M1b: Other distant metastasis 2. Tumours of the midthoracic oesophagus:
T4: Tumour invades adjacent structures		M1a: Not applicable
		M1b: Non-regional lymph nodes and/or other distant metastasis
		3. Tumours of the upper thoracic oesophagus:
		M1a: Metastasis in cervical nodes
		M1b: Other distant metastasis

continued

Table 20.3 *continued*

TNM definitions
AJCC stage groupings
Stage 0: Tis, N0, M0
Stage I: T1, N0, M0
Stage IIA: T2, N0, M0 or T3, N0, M0
Stage IIB: T1, N1, M0 or T2, N1, M0
Stage III: T3, N1, M0 or T4, any N, M0
Stage IV: Any T, any N, M1 (Stage IVA: Any T, any N, M1a; Stage IVB: Any T, any N, M1b)

Source: American Joint Committee on Cancer. AJCC cancer staging manual. 6th ed. New York: Springer; 2002. Esophagus; pp. 91–8.

Computed tomography

Computed tomography (CT) is used to look for local disease infiltration and invasion within the mediastinum, regional and distant nodal involvement, and distant metastases to the lungs and liver.

Endoscopic ultrasound

This is useful in T-staging, and documentation of lymph node involvement. Endoscopic ultrasound guided fine needle aspiration may also be used to confirm the presence of malignant lymph nodes histologically.

Surveillance of asymptomatic patients

Early oesophageal cancer may be a chance finding during endoscopy. To systematically detect early oesophageal cancer, endoscopic screening and surveillance would be required in asymptomatic individuals. The cost-effectiveness of surveillance for high-risk patients has yet to be proven and the decision to perform surveillance has to be individualised.

Image enhanced endoscopy, with or without optical magnification, has been reported to improve the detection rate of early cancer. With Lugol's iodine chromoendoscopy, the normal oesophageal squamous epithelium is stained brown, whereas dysplastic areas will be unstained. Limited studies conducted in high-risk subjects, such as those with a past history of head and neck cancer, have shown that endoscopic surveillance detected both early and advanced cancers, and that the use of Lugol's iodine chromoendoscopy further increased the detection rate of early SCC and dysplasia.

To detect early AC in BE, a four-quadrant 1–2 cm blind biopsy has been used to detect dysplasia during endoscopic surveillance; another technique is to spray a contrast dye such as indigo carmine to enhance mucosal surface irregularities. Retrospective data suggest a survival benefit in patients with BE who undergo endoscopic surveillance due to detection of earlier stage AC, and a higher resectability rate, but such benefits have not been conclusively shown in prospective studies.

There are now optical 'virtual' chromoendoscopy techniques such as narrow band imaging (Olympus, Tokyo, Japan), i-scan (Pentax, Tokyo, Japan) and FICE (Fujinon, Tokyo, Japan) which can provide a less laborious alternative to traditional chromoendoscopy. In light of uncertain data on cost-effectiveness, but recognising the need for early detection of oesophageal cancer, the American Society of Gastrointestinal Endoscopy (ASGE) published recommendations in 2006 concerning the role of surveillance in individuals at risk of oesophageal cancer.[5]

◗ Management

In the presence of dysphagia, oesophageal dilatation can be performed with either through-the-scope balloon or wire-guided polyvinyl bougies for the temporary relief of dysphagia while awaiting definitive treatment. The definitive treatment of oesophageal cancer depends on the results of cancer staging. Definitive, potentially curative treatments include surgery with or without neoadjuvant chemoradiotherapy or adjuvant chemoradiotherapy, or definitive chemoradiotherapy alone. Unfortunately 50–60 per cent of patients with oesophageal cancer present with incurable, locally advanced or metastatic disease, so that palliation is the treatment goal for most patients.

Most reported studies on treatment have not distinguished between SCC and AC; the data on chemoradiotherapy are based mainly on SCC patients.

Management of premalignant lesions

In the East, foci of dysplasia in squamous mucosa detected during screening may be resected endoscopically. In the West, the main premalignant lesion is BE and, in this context, foci of dysplasia can also be resected endoscopically. Due to concern for occult synchronous lesions and the potential for disease progression in non-dysplastic BE, ablative strategies have been adopted.

Photodynamic therapy (PDT) has been used, but it is associated with very high complication rates. Radiofrequency ablation using the HALO[360] and HALO[90] systems (BÂRRX Medical Inc., USA) was introduced recently and has been shown to have a high rate of complete eradication of both dysplasia and intestinal metaplasia and a reduced risk of disease progression. Unlike PDT, adverse events were less common.[6]

Management of superficial oesophageal cancer (Stages 0–I: Tis–T1, N0, M0)

Superficial oesophageal cancer refers to cancer limited to the oesophageal mucosa (Tis and T1a) or submucosa (T1b). Intramucosal cancers are subdivided into m1 (limited to epithelial layer), m2 (invades lamina

propria) and m3 (invades into but not through the muscularis propria), while submucosal involvement is subdivided into sm1 (penetrates the shallowest one-third of the submucosa), sm2 (penetrates into the intermediate one-third of the submucosa) and sm3 (penetrates the deepest one-third of the submucosa). Surgery has traditionally been the treatment of choice for these superficial cancers. In the case of m1 and m2 tumours, there is no risk of nodal metastasis. In the case of m3 tumours with no lymphatic invasion, the risk of nodal metastasis is minimal. Hence these lesions are well suited to endoscopic resection.

In recent years, endoscopic mucosal resection and endoscopic submucosal dissection techniques have been shown to be viable alternative treatments for early intramucosal cancers with no lymphovascular invasion, and are standard alternative treatments to surgery when the technical expertise is available—this is especially so in Japan, Korea and some European centres.[7] Submucosal tumours entail a substantial risk of nodal metastases, and hence oesophagectomy with lymphadenectomy is required.

Management of localised oesophageal cancer (Stages I–III: T1–T3, N0–N1, M0)[8]

The optimal treatment for patients with localised oesophageal cancer is surgical resection. Surgical approaches include transhiatal oesophagectomy with anastomosis of the stomach to the cervical oesophagus, and abdominal mobilisation of the stomach and transthoracic excision of the oesophagus with anastomosis of the stomach to the upper thoracic oesophagus or the cervical oesophagus.

In stage I disease, surgery alone suffices. In cases of stages II or III disease, preoperative or neoadjuvant chemoradiotherapy is increasingly being used. In the context of completely resected node-positive oesophageal cancer patients who have not received neoadjuvant therapy, postoperative adjuvant therapy with chemotherapy alone or chemoradiotherapy are both options.

Chemoradiotherapy is recommended for inoperable or unresectable localised oesophageal cancer. Definitive chemoradiation therapy is an alternative to surgery in stages II and III oesophageal cancer.

Management of advanced and metastatic oesophageal cancer[6]

The management of advanced non-resectable oesophageal cancer is essentially palliative. Treatment options include:

- endoscopic insertion of self-expandable metallic stents for palliation of dysphagia and tracheo-oesophageal fistula
- radiation therapy with or without oesophageal dilation
- intraluminal brachytherapy to provide palliation of dysphagia

- endoscopic ablation of the cancer to palliate dysphagia or bleeding, using Nd:YAG laser or argon plasma coagulation
- palliative chemotherapy.

▷ Prognosis

The overall five-year survival rate is less than 20 per cent due to frequent late presentation.[1] After complete surgical resection, the five-year survival rate exceeds 95 per cent for stage 0 disease, from 50–80 per cent for stage I disease, 30–40 per cent for stage IIA disease, 10–30 per cent for stage IIB disease, and 10–15 percent for stage III disease.[9] The results of endoscopic resection of superficial oesophageal cancer are comparable to surgery.[6] The median survival of patients with stage IV disease treated with palliative chemotherapy is less than one year.[9]

Summary

There are considerable differences between countries in oesophageal cancer epidemiology, both in incidence rates and histological subtypes. SCC remains the most common subtype, but the incidence of AC has risen significantly in Western countries. When diagnosed at an early stage, the main treatment modality is surgery. In recent years, the technique of endoscopic resection, pioneered in Japan, has been shown to be a viable treatment alternative in the context of dysplasia and intramucosal cancers. In the West, where the prevalence of BE is high, radiofrequency ablation has shown promise for eradication of intestinal metaplasia, dysplasia and prevention of disease progression. Unfortunately most cases of oesophageal cancer are diagnosed at a late stage, and management is solely palliative. There is a need to better identify patients at risk of oesophageal cancer, and determine the appropriate cost-effective surveillance strategy, in order to improve the disease outcome.

References

1. Umar SB, Fleischer DE. Esophageal cancer: epidemiology, pathogenesis and prevention. *Nat Clin Pract Gastroenterol Hepatol.* 2008; 5:517–26.

2. Kamangar F, Chow WH, Abnet CC, Dawsey SM. Environmental causes of esophageal cancer. *Gastroenterol Clin North Am.* 2009; 38:27–57.

3. Seewald S, Ang TL, Groth S, Zhong Y, Bertschinger P, Altorfer J, Thonke F, Soehendra N. Detection and endoscopic therapy of early esophageal adenocarcinoma. *Curr Opin Gastroenterol.* 2008; 24:521–9.

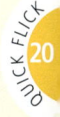
QUICK FLICK 20

4. Enzinger PC, Mayer RJ. Esophageal cancer. *N Engl J Med*. 2003; 349:2241–52.

5. Hirota WK, Zuckerman MJ, Adler DG, Davila RE, Egan J, Leighton JA, Qureshi WA, Rajan E, Fanelli R, Wheeler-Harbaugh J, Baron TH, Faigel DO. ASGE guideline: the role of endoscopy in the surveillance of premalignant conditions of the upper GI tract. *Gastrointest Endosc*. 2006; 63:570–80.

6. Shaheen NJ, Sharma P, Overholt BF, Wolfsen HC, Sampliner RE, Wang KK, Galanko JA, Bronner MP, Goldblum JR, Bennett AE, Jobe BA, Eisen GM, Fennerty MB, Hunter JG, Fleischer DE, Sharma VK, Hawes RH, Hoffman BJ, Rothstein RI, Gordon SR, Mashimo H, Chang KJ, Muthusamy VR, Edmundowicz SA, Spechler SJ, Siddiqui AA, Souza RF, Infantolino A, Falk GW, Kimmey MB, Madanick RD, Chak A, Lightdale CJ. Radiofrequency ablation in Barrett's esophagus with dysplasia. *N Engl J Med*. 2009; 360:2277–88.

7. Inoue H, Minami H, Kaga M, Sato Y, Kudo SE. Endoscopic mucosal resection and endoscopic submucosal dissection for esophageal dysplasia and carcinoma. *Gastrointest Endosc Clin N Am*. 2010; 20:25–34.

8. National Cancer Institute. General information about esophageal cancer. [Internet]. [Cited 2009 Dec 16]. Available from: www.cancer.gov/ cancertopics/pdq/treatment/esophageal/healthprofessional/allpages.

9. American Joint Committee on Cancer. AJCC cancer staging manual. 6th ed. New York: Springer; 2002. Esophagus; pp. 91–8.

Chapter 21: Global trends in gastric cancer: association with *Heliobacter pylori* and other factors

K.L. Goh (Malaysia)

Key points

- Gastric cancer incidence varies greatly throughout the world. High-incidence countries include countries in East Asia: Japan, China, Korea and Taiwan, and in South America: Colombia, Peru and Chile.
- A decline in the incidence of gastric cancer was first seen in the West and is now worldwide.
- The absolute number of cases of gastric cancer has increased because of the increase in population and ageing.
- *Helicobacter pylori* is the major factor in gastric cancer carcinogenesis.
- Cancer develops from the interaction of a virulent strain of *H. pylori* with a susceptible host in the presence of cancer-promoting environmental factors such as a high salt diet.

◊ Introduction

Gastric cancer (noncardia) (GCA) remains one of the most common cancers in the world. Its incidence varies greatly between different geographical regions of the world. The East Asian countries of China, Japan, Korea and Taiwan, and the South American countries of Colombia, Chile and Peru, for example, have a very high age-standardised incidence rate (ASR) of gastric cancer of 20–60 per 100 000 population per year, while developed countries in Europe and North America—especially the white population—and countries in Africa, have a relatively low incidence of GCA of less than 10 per 100 000 per year.

◊ Epidemiology

Time trends of GCA

In the West the incidence of GCA has been steadily declining since the 1940s, from more than 40 per 100 000 population to below 10 per 100 000. The reason for this decline may be that the introduction of refrigeration has led to a marked decrease in the consumption of salted and preserved foods.

A similar decline occurring some 40 years later has now been observed in the high GCA incidence countries of East Asia and appears to be correlated to the rising affluence and improved hygiene in these countries. Although the ASR has declined, the increase in the proportion of elderly population in, for example, Japan and Korea, has resulted in an increase in the absolute numbers of GCA cases. GCA continues to be a major health problem in these countries.

Pathogenesis

The role of *Helicobacter pylori* in GCA

The major aetiological factor in GCA is thought to be *H. pylori* infection. In 1993, the International Agency for Research on Cancer (IARC) classified *H. pylori* as a Class 1 carcinogen. Several bodies of evidence link *H. pylori* to the causation of GCA:

- A close association exists between *H. pylori* and GCA. Ecological comparison studies show a strong correlation between high GCA incidence and high *H. pylori* prevalence in various geographical regions of the world. Case-control studies show a strong link, with an odds ratio of up to 6.0 for GCA in the presence of *H. pylori* infection.
- *H. pylori* infection has been shown to precede the development of GCA.
- A plausible biological mechanism for the aetiological link exists. Correa hypothesised in 1992 that gastric carcinogenesis is a multifactorial, multistep cascade of events with *H. pylori* infection as the initiating step, progressing to chronic superficial gastritis, gastric atrophy, intestinal metaplasia, dysplasia and eventually gastric adenocarcinoma (see Figure 21.1).
- Animal studies in Mongolian gerbils infected with *H. pylori* demonstrated the development of chronic active gastritis, intestinal metaplasia and adenocarcinoma of the stomach. Further animal studies in gerbils have shown that exposure to the known carcinogen N-methyl-N-nitrosurea resulted in the development of gastric cancer only in the presence of *H. pylori*.
- Population-based observational longitudinal follow-up studies in Japan have shown that in *H. pylori*-positive compared to -negative subjects there is an increased risk of developing GCA by a large factor (in one study, a relative risk of 15–35 in patients with severe grades of gastritis).
- Interventional studies have been carried out in the population. Several studies are still ongoing. Patients with *H. pylori* infection without GCA were identified in the population and randomised to receive either *H. pylori* eradication therapy or no treatment, and were then followed up for many years with repeat gastroscopy to look for development

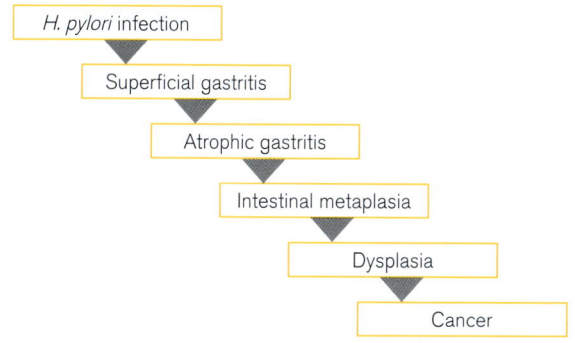

Figure 21.1 Correa's hypothesis on the development of gastric cancer
Source: Adapted from Correa (1992).

of cancer. In a study in China, Wong et al. (2004) showed that, in a
10-year follow-up of patients with no GCA precursor lesions, there was
significantly different occurrence of GCA in those who had been treated
for *H. pylori* and those who had not. For patients in whom GCA precursor
lesions were already present, however, no difference was observed
between those treated for *H. pylori* and those who had not been treated.
This indicated non-reversal of subclinical molecular changes that may
have taken place in the gastric mucosa.

Although, broadly, the distribution of high-prevalence areas of GCA and
H. pylori coincide, there are notable exceptions in India and Africa, where a
high *H. pylori* prevalence is not associated with a high GCA incidence.

Diet and gastric cancer

Dietary factors—in particular, salted, preserved and fermented foods—have
been implicated in gastric carcinogenesis. Several studies have shown a
positive correlation between high salt intake and increased cancer mortality.
Nitrates in the diet have also been associated with GCA causation, although
the epidemiological evidence is not as strong.

At the same time, fresh vegetables and fruits have been considered protective
against GCA. The allium vegetables garlic and onion, as well as antioxidant
vitamins C and E, beta-carotene, and micronutrients such as selenium, are also
thought to have a preventative effect on cancer. The protective effect of other
foods such as green tea and non-fermented soybean has also been reported,
particularly from Asia. There is a plethora of studies on cancer-causing and
cancer-protective factors related to gastric cancer, but dietary studies remain
difficult to perform and results often difficult to interpret.

Other factors

Tobacco smoking has been associated with GCA. The link with alcohol intake is weak. Other factors that have been studied include exposure to ionising radiation and asbestos, Epstein-Barr virus infection and pernicious anaemia. The risk of gastric cancer is about two to three times greater in first-degree relatives of patients with pernicious anaemia. This could be contributed to by familial clustering of *H. pylori* infection, or by a shared environment. Inherited GCA genetic syndromes are very rare.

Gastric cancer causation: interaction between *H. pylori*, host genetic factors and dietary factors

The biggest enigma with *H. pylori* infection is that only a small proportion of these patients ever develop gastric cancer. The reason for this lies in the interaction between different strains of *H. pylori* with host genetic factors and environmental factors, particularly diet (see Figure 21.2). Virulent *H. pylori* strains have been identified. For example, CagA-positive strains have been shown to be more carcinogenic than Cag-negative strains. Other bacterial virulence markers such as VacA and CagA submarkers have been identified: for example, the East Asian CagA-positive strains with stronger SHP-2 binding sequences that have been thought to be responsible for the higher incidence of GCA in the region. Studies on host genetic factors

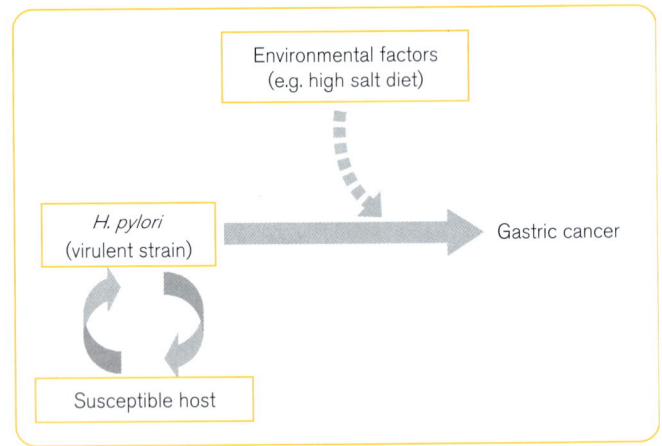

Figure 21.2 Interaction between *H. pylori*, host genetic factors and environmental factors

have pointed to GCA-susceptible hosts. The most studied host factor is interleukin-1beta (IL-1B) and its receptor antagonist (IL-1RN) gene polymorphisms. Subjects with these particular polymorphisms have been shown to have a proinflammatory phenotype, more severe gastritis and a predilection to gastric atrophy. Environmental factors, especially a high salt diet, can be considered cancer-promoting factors. GCA results from infection with a virulent *H. pylori* strain in a susceptible individual in the presence of a cancer-promoting diet.

Summary

Although the incidence of GCA has declined markedly, especially in the Western world, it remains an important cancer worldwide. The ASR in the East Asian countries and in South America is still high and, with an increase in the elderly population in these countries, the absolute numbers of GCA remain large. *H. pylori* is the predominant aetiological agent in GCA. Virulent or 'carcinogenic' strains have been identified. Infection in susceptible hosts with proinflammatory genotypes in the presence of cancer-promoting factors such as a high salt diet is likely to result in GCA.

Recommended reading

Camargo MC, Mera R, Correa P, Peek RM Jr, Fontham ET, Goodman KJ, Piazuelo MB, Sicinschi L, Zabaleta J, Schneider BG. Interleukin-1B and interleukin-1receptor antagonist gene polymorphisms and gastric cancer: a meta-analysis. *Cancer Epidemiol Biomarkers Prev*. 2006 Sep; 15(9):1674–87.

Correa P. Human gastric carcinogenesis: a multistep and multifactorial process: first American Cancer Society award lecture on cancer epidemiology and prevention. *Cancer Res*. 1992; 52:6735–40.

Huang JQ, Zheng GF, Sumanac K, Irvine EJ, Hunt RH. Meta-analysis of the relationship between cagA seropositivity and gastric cancer. *Gastroenterology*. 2003; 125:1636–44.

Sung JJ, Lin SR, Ching JY, Zhou LY, To KF, Wang RT, Leung WK, Ng EK, Lau JY, Lee YT, Yeung CK, Chao W, Chung SC. Atrophy and intestinal metaplasia one year after cure of *H. pylori* infection: a prospective, randomized study. *Gastroenterology*. 2000 Jul; 119(1):7–14.

Wong BC, Lam SK, Wong WM, Chen JS, Zheng TT, Feng RE, Lai KC, Hu WH, Yuen ST, Leung SY, Fong DY, Ho J, Ching CK, Chen JS, China

Gastric Cancer Study Group. *Helicobacter pylori* eradication to prevent gastric cancer in a high-risk region of China: a randomized controlled trial. *JAMA*. 2004 Jan 14; 291(2):244–5.

You WC, Brown LM, Zhang L, Li JY, Jin ML, Chang YS, Ma JL, Pan KF, Liu WD, Hu Y, Crystal-Mansour S, Pee D, Blot WJ, Fraumeni JF Jr, Xu GW, Gail MH. Randomized double-blind factorial trial of three treatments to reduce the prevalence of precancerous gastric lesions. *J Natl Cancer Inst*. 2006 Jul; 98(14):974–83.

Chapter 22: Clinical aspects of gastric cancer

I. Segal (Australia)

Key points

- ▶ Gastric cancer can be divided into intestinal and diffuse types, the latter having a worse prognosis.
- ▶ In Western countries proximal gastric cancer is more common than distal cancer and is usually of the diffuse type.
- ▶ Spread may be by blood, lymphatics, transcoelomic, or direct. Distant metastasis is uncommon if there is no lymph node involvement.
- ▶ Prognosis is generally poor due to advanced stage at presentation. Better results are obtained in Japan where screening programs and surgical treatment are of a high standard.
- ▶ Endoscopy, computed tomography (CT) scan and endoscopic ultrasound (EUS) are important in diagnosis and staging.
- ▶ Treatment of curable cases is by radical surgery, and the removal of the second tier of nodes may be advantageous.
- ▶ Endoscopic mucosal resection for early gastric cancer is considered a curative procedure.
- ▶ Chemotherapy improves survival in advanced disease.
- ▶ Presence of *H. pylori* infection.
- ▶ Risk factors: atrophic gastritis with or without intestinal metaplasia; pernicious anaemia, intestinal metaplasia, gastric adenomatous polyps >2 cm, postgastrectomy stumps, gastric epithelial dysplasia, Ménétrier's disease.

◖ Introduction

Approximately 90 to 95 per cent of gastric cancers are adenocarcinomas. Although the incidence of gastric adenocarcinoma localised to the distal stomach has decreased, the incidence of proximal gastric and gastro-oesophageal cancer has been steadily increasing in Western countries. Adenocarcinoma of the gastro-oesophageal junction presently accounts for 25 per cent of gastric cancers.

The usual age of presentation is between the ages of 50 and 70 years, and rates are higher each year in men than in women by 2 to 1 per cent. Survival is less than 20 per cent.

◯ Pathobiology

Most primary gastric cancers are adenocarcinomas. Histologically they can be subdivided into two categories: intestinal type and diffuse type. The intestinal type is a well-differentiated lesion that forms glandlike structures which ulcerate frequently. The diffuse type is characterised by infiltration and thickening of the gastric wall without the formation of a discrete mass.

There is believed to be a stepwise progression from chronic gastritis, atrophy and intestinal metaplasia to dysplasia and finally gastric cancer.

The decline of incidence in gastric cancer has been mainly in the distal stomach intestinal type, and there is a steady increase in the proximal stomach diffuse type.

◯ Clinical features

In the early stages, gastric cancer may be asymptomatic. In the later stages symptoms include dyspepsia, bloating, dysphagia, epigastric pain and early satiety. Dysphagia suggests a more proximal lesion near the gastro-oesophageal junction. Gastrointestinal haemorrhage and intestinal obstruction are rarely the initial manifestations.

Signs of gastric cancer include bleeding, iron deficiency anaemia, pain in the right upper quadrant, jaundice and metastases which can cause cough, hiccups and haemoptysis.

In the early stages of gastric cancer the physical examination may be unremarkable. In later stages, an epigastric mass may be palpated. If the tumour has invaded the liver, jaundice and ascites may be present. Splenic vein invasion may cause splenomegaly.

An enlarged Virchow's node indicates metastases to the left supraclavicular lymph node. A periumbilical lymph nodule (Sister Mary Joseph node) may indicate tumour spread along peritoneal surfaces.

◯ Staging

International Union Against Cancer (UICC) staging of gastric cancer is vital in treatment and prognosis. Initial staging of gastric cancer should include CT scanning of the abdomen to determine the presence or absence of metastatic disease. In the absence of metastases, EUS assists in deciding on surgical resectability (with 91 per cent accuracy) because it can accurately assess the depth of tumour penetration. Early gastric cancer (EGC) has been defined in Japan as gastric cancer confined to the mucosa or submucosa, with or without lymph node metastases. This group of patients has better than 90 per cent five-year survival. Other risk factors for lymph node metastases in EGC include lymphovascular invasion on histopathology, histologic ulceration, and tumour diameter more than 3 cm.

Upper gastrointestinal endoscopy and multiple biopsies are necessary to confirm the diagnosis. Due to sampling error, a repeat endoscopy and repeat biopsies, if necessary, are warranted 6–8 weeks after therapy for the ulcer.

▷ Management

Curative

This involves the complete removal or destruction of the lesion. Radical gastric surgery is the recommended option for cardia tumours and proximal gastric cancers with or without left thoraco-abdominal exposure. Although surgical resection remains the cornerstone of therapy for gastric cancer, the optimum extent of nodal resection is controversial: randomised studies have been unable to show that the more extensive D2 procedure improves survival compared with D1 dissection.

Endoscopic mucosal resection (EMR) for early gastric cancer

EMR is considered a curative procedure for EGC and, in Japan, it has increasingly replaced surgical resection for this indication, although it is not universally accepted in Western countries. EMR has also been used as a histologic staging technique to assess the depth of penetration in EGC to help determine the best definitive treatment.

Palliative

Chemotherapy (combination of epirubicin, cisplatin, fluorouracil) can improve the five-year survival rate by 23–36 per cent, both preoperatively and postoperatively, in patients with resectable gastro-oesophageal cancer. Similarly, combining chemotherapy with radiation therapy has been shown to improve median survival from 27 months to 36 months.

Radiotherapy alone is ineffective and is generally given only for palliative purposes where bleeding, obstruction and painful bone metastases occur.

Summary

There are two types of gastric cancer—intestinal and diffuse. Proximal gastric cancer of diffuse type is more common in Westen countries. Spread is usually by blood, lymphatics, transcoelomic or direct. Prognosis is generally poor. Endoscopy, CT scan and EUS are important in diagnosis and staging. Radical surgery is the best treatment. Chemotherapy is used in advanced cases.

Information for patients

When should I see a doctor?

It is important that you consult your doctor if you have symptoms such as epigastric pain, early satiety, bloating, nausea, vomiting or weight loss.

When should I have an endoscopy?

Discuss with your doctor the advisability of undergoing upper gastrointestinal endoscopy in order to find out if there are any abnormalities in the oesophagus, stomach or duodenum.

How can I decrease the risk of gastric cancer?

Social and dietary habits may require changes. Tobacco and alcohol consumption and the eating of 'junk foods' are risk factors for abdominal symptoms.

Recommended reading

Kelly S, Harris KM, Berry E, Hutton J, Roderick P, Cullingworth J, Gathercole L, Smith MA. A systematic review of the performance of endoscopic ultrasound in gastro-oesophageal carcinoma. *Gut*. 2001; 49:534–9.

Nomura AM, Hankin JH, Kolonel LN, Wilkens LR, Goodman MT, Stemmermann GN. Case-control study of diet and other risk factors for gastric cancer in Hawaii (United States). *Cancer Causes Control*. 2003; 14:547–58.

Rembacken BJ, Gotoda T, Fuji T, Axon ATR. Endoscopic mucosal resection. *Endoscopy*. 2001; 33:709–18.

Waxman I, Saitoh Y, Raju GS, Watari J, Yokota K, Reeves AL, Kohgo Y. High frequency probe EUS-assisted endoscopic mucosal resection: a therapeutic strategy for submucosal tumors of the GI tract. *Gastrointest Endosc*. 2002; 55:44–9.

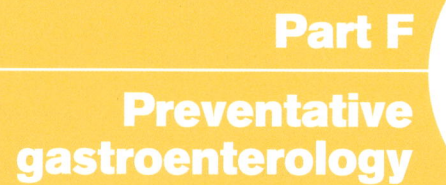

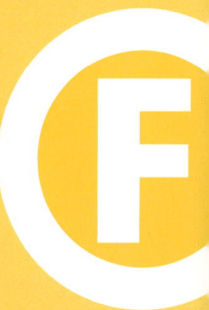

Part F

Preventative gastroenterology

Chapter 23: Preventative gastroenterology

S. Shah (India)

Key points

▶ The concept of preventive gastroenterology makes it possible to increase life expectancy and reduce the morbidity of digestive diseases.

▶ Preventive gastroenterology will have a major impact in controlling digestive disease in developing nations.

▶ Knowledge of molecular aspects of digestive disease, including cancer, has made the prevention and control of the spread of these diseases possible.

▷ Introduction

Preventative gastroenterology is not a major branch of clinical medicine, unlike preventative cardiology, even though in day-to-day practice there are more gastrointestinal (GI) problems than cardiological. An attempt has been made here to put forward the preventative aspect as a compendium of major digestive disorders.

▷ Impact of prevention

It is definitely possible to increase life expectancy and reduce morbidity with improved quality of life. This is despite a burgeoning human population, crumbling infrastructure, deteriorating sanitation and hygiene practices. Sedentary lifestyles, dependence on machinery, fatty foods and junk diets have made preventative gastroenterology essential.

There has been a major impact on some nations with regard to climate change, environmental pollution and the increasing incidence of natural disasters, global warming, decreasing agricultural land area, extinction of native food and food products and plants, and the introduction of genetically modified foods.

The knowledge of pathogenesis and molecular aspects of cancer has opened new possibilities for preventing cancer, including GI cancers, which may have an impact on screening algorithms, and preventative modalities.

A proven positive impact may lead to legislation to adopt these health reforms.

Gastro-oesophageal reflux disease (GERD)

Management of GERD requires small meals every two to three hours, raising the head of the bed, a gap of two to three hours between dinner and bed rest; in addition, avoiding tight clothes, reducing weight and eliminating factors that increase abdominal pressure. Other measures include avoiding smoking, avoiding excess of tea, coffee, alcohol, mint, citric juices, chocolates and carbonated drinks.

With regard to medications, minimise the use of calcium channel blockers or other smooth muscle relaxants, and alendronate.

Barrett's oesophagus

It is suggested that annual oesophagoscopy with biopsies after the age of 50 be carried out. Long-segment Barrett's requires endoscopic surveillance every two or three years. In addition, dysphagia may determine the frequency of endoscopy.

Peptic ulcer

Primary prevention

Avoid non-steroidal anti-inflammatory drugs (NSAIDs). (In theory, COX-2 inhibitors are superior; however, clinical use is not widely accepted.) Occasional sedative analgesics such as dextropropoxyphene may be worthwhile for short-term use.

Prevent *Helicobacter pylori* infection: a vaccine may be available.

Helicobacter pylori

H. pylori is the aetiological cause of gastritis. Trials using vaccination have shown encouraging results. Vaccination may be more important in South-East Asia because re-infection is fairly common.[1]

Vaccine is derived utilising different antigenic areas of *H. pylori*. Vaccines may also be effective for treating established infection. It is believed that the mucosal lining is not able to produce an effective immunoglobulin secretory IgA. Vaccination counteracts the ill effects on the mucosa.

On the horizon are newer types of vaccines using chimeric live virus vectors; interferon is an example of a chimeric drug in clinical use.

◗ Coeliac disease

Awareness and index cases have been recognised more frequently in South-East Asia. Treatment involves rigidly following a diet avoiding refined wheat products, barley, rye and oats.

◗ Short bowel syndrome

Much care is necessary immediately, and on a very long-term basis. Immediately there is a risk of massive upper GI bleed due to excess of gastrin. Patients require high doses of proton pump inhibitors (PPIs) to prevent massive bleeding.

On a very long-term basis, prevention will depend on the length of bowel resected: if it is more than 100 cm, steatorrhoea may occur and long-term total parenteral nutrition (TPN) may be necessary with concomitant complications, which should be prevented.

If the caecum is resected, the use of cholestyramine is necessary to prevent excess bile salts reaching the large bowel and causing diarrhoea.

◗ Inflammatory bowel disease (IBD)

Crohn's disease

There is evidence that there is an increase in the incidence of Crohn's disease in South-East Asia.

- Primary prevention—avoid smoking and avoid using NSAIDs.
- Secondary prevention—continued use of 5-aminosalicylic acid (5-ASA) or budesonide may prevent exacerbation.
- Post-operative prevention of relapse of Crohn's disease. As yet there is no conclusive evidence for this.[2]

◗ Viral hepatitis

Hepatitis is one of the major community health problems of South-East Asia. It is a waterborne disease, so that primary prevention involves the provision of potable, non-infective water.

Hepatitis A vaccine

- People visiting endemic areas should be vaccinated. Effective vaccine is available.
- Patients who are immunosuppressed or are partially immunocompromised should receive vaccine after confirming that they do not have IgG antibody titre above 10 IU. This includes individuals with cirrhosis of the liver, or who have long-lasting malignancy, or patients on immunosuppressive agents. It is rare that adults die from hepatitis A; based on this, it is a matter of public health policy whether or not to make hepatitis A vaccine compulsory for all adults in their region.
- Havrix vaccine (hepatitis A vaccine) is available in the South-East Asia area. It is given in two doses at six-month intervals. No booster is necessary. New vaccines of HAV and HBV will be available for both viruses to be given at initiation, one month and six months.

Toxic and drug-induced hepatitis

- Enquire about allergies to any drugs before beginning treatment.
- Avoid over-the-counter drugs.
- Regularly check levels of drugs with a low therapeutic window, such as carbamazepine or digoxin.
- Educate industrial staff and farmers regarding dangerous hepatotoxic substances such as pesticides, carbon tetrachloride and yellow phosphorus.
- Patients on anti-Koch's treatment (AKT) should have liver function tests at regular intervals and at the beginning of treatment to confirm tolerance of drugs. Similarly for patients on highly active antiretroviral therapy (HAART) treatment for AIDS.

NAFLD/NASH

For cases of non-alcoholic fatty liver disease/non-alcoholic steatohepatitis (NAFLD/NASH) it is most important to avoid obesity. If necessary, weight should be lost to improve body mass index (BMI). Regular exercise is recommended, as is diet modification (low-fat diet and promotion of healthy food), and unknown medications restricted or totally avoided.

Substance abuse[3–5]

- Complete abstinence from alcohol.
- Important to maintain nutrition—consumption of proteins of high biological value (that contain all nine essential aminoacids) including milk, casein and eggs.
- Avoid drugs excreted through liver.
- Preventative methods to be adopted for hepatitis B and C; screening of blood products.
- Avoid sharing of needles.

Prevent disabilities and complications

- First episode of variceal bleeding: prophylactic treatment with a non-selective beta-adrenergic antagonist (propranolol, nadolol) in patients with large, high-risk varices that have never bled, appears to decrease the incidence of bleeding by 40–50 per cent and prolong survival. Prophylactic banding of grade 3–4 varices, or varices with haemocystic and 'whiplash' marks.
- Recurrent bleeds: removal of varices by endoscopic band ligation reduces risk of recurrent haemorrhage by more than 50 per cent. Use beta blockers for prophylaxis.
- Ascites: restrict salt intake to 2 g/day; restrict fluid as determined by the extent of oedema, urine output and electrolytes.
- Spontaneous bacterial peritonitis: prophylactic antibiotics—unfortunately most of the quinolones are not effective, but bactrim can be used.
- Hepatic encephalopathy: avoid common precipitants of hepatic encephalopathy such as increased nitrogen load. Take care to prevent and treat gastrointestinal bleeding, excess dietary protein, azotaemia and constipation, and treat electrolyte and metabolic imbalance, hypokalaemia, alkalosis, hypoxia, hyponatraemia and hypovolaemia.
- Tolerated protein intake is at least 20–40 g per day or more (preferably vegetable proteins).
- Drugs that can precipitate hepatic encepahalopathy include narcotics, tranquillisers, sedatives and diuretics.
- Miscellaneous factors: infections, surgery, superimposed acute liver disease, progressive liver disease, portal systemic shunts.
- Hepatorenal syndrome: laxatives to avoid constipation, avoidance of all precipitating factors like alcohol, drugs excreted through kidneys, adjustment of drug dosage.
- Hepatocellular carcinoma: yearly ultrasonography, biennial alpha-fetoprotein level check.

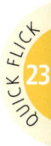

◗ Gall bladder

Prophylactic measures to avoid gallstones include weight loss to maintain BMI, avoidance of oral contraceptives, excessive fasting and high-calorie diet. Start enteral feeds as soon as possible if the patient is on total parenteral nutrition.

◗ Pancreas

Treat gallstones to prevent gallstone-induced pancreatitis. If the patient is alcoholic, provide advice on abstinence from alcohol and its correlation with hypertriglyceridaemia.

Treat with a low-fat diet, and advise on weight loss if appropriate.

Care should be taken with drug treatment, particularly azathioprine, 6-MP, sulfonamides, oestrogens, tetracyclines, valproic acid and anti-HIV medication. Patients with a history of acute pancreatitis attacks, or a family history of pancreatitis, should avoid drugs that are known to precipitate pancreatitis.

○ Cancer prevention

Public education is important, and awareness about the avoidance of risk factors, through school health courses, through print and electronic media, and through counselling adolescents and young adults.

Use the media to disseminate information about the hazards of smoking and alcohol, and the benefits of healthy diet and exercise (see Table 23.1), and:

- the use of screening methods and sun avoidance in order to prevent skin cancers
- chewing tobacco is a carcinogen linked to dental caries, gingivitis, oral leukoplakia and oral cancer
- dietary information—a diet that is high in fat increases the risk of cancers in the breast, colon, prostate and endometrium.

Table 23.1 Carcinogens in digestive diseases

Carcinogen	Associated cancer or neoplasm
Epstein-Barr virus	Burkitt's lymphoma, nasal T-cell lymphoma
Oestrogens	Cancer of the endometrium, liver, breast
Ethyl alcohol	Cancer of the liver, oesophagus, head and neck
Helicobacter pylori	Gastric cancer
Hepatitis B or C virus	Liver cancer
Human immunodeficiency virus (HIV)	Non-Hodgkin's lymphoma, Kaposi's sarcoma, squamous cell carcinomas (especially of the urogenital tract)
Human papilloma virus	Adult T-cell leukaemia/lymphoma type I Human T-cell lymphotropic virus type I (HTLV-I)

Carcinogen	Associated cancer or neoplasm
Immunosuppressive agents (azathioprine, cyclosporine, glucocorticoids)	Non-Hodgkin's lymphoma
Nitrogen mustard gas	Cancer of the lung, head and neck, nasal sinuses
Tobacco (including smokeless)	Cancer of the upper aerodigestive tract, bladder
Vinyl chloride	Liver cancer (angiosarcoma)

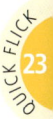

Diet

A low-fat diet provides some protection against cancer through anticarcinogens found in vegetables, fruits, legumes, nuts and grains. Protective substances found in these foods include phenols, flavones, fibre and sulfur-containing compounds. Dietary fibre may afford protection against colonic polyps and invasive cancer of the colon, and it absorbs inactivate dietary oestrogenic and androgenic cancer promoters.

Consuming at least five servings of fruits and vegetables a day decreases dietary fat and increases fibre. Such a diet may also lower the risk of cardiovascular disease.

A diet high in calcium lowers colon cancer risk. Calcium binds bile and fatty acids which cause hyperproliferation of colonic epithelial cells.

COX-2 inhibitors

COX-2 inhibiting drugs are effective in preventing colon cancer. Studies have shown that high-dose celecoxib reduces the number of colorectal polyps in patients with familial adenomatous polyposis (FAP), and it is currently being studied for prevention of sporadic colorectal cancer.

Cancer prevention by vaccination

- Hepatitis B vaccine to prevent hepatitis and hepatomas due to chronic hepatitis B infection
- Human papillomavirus (HPV) vaccine to prevent cervical cancer
- *Helicobacter pylori* eradication as part of cancer prevention strategy for gastric cancer.

Early detection does not in itself confer benefit. To be of value, screening must detect disease earlier and treatment of disease at this stage must yield a better outcome than treatment at the onset of symptoms. Reducing mortality, rather than survival after diagnosis, is the preferred end point.

Gastrointestinal cancer

The aetiology of squamous cell oesophageal carcinoma is correlated to the consumption of tobacco or cigarette smoking and excessive consumption of alcohol, ingestion of nitrites, smoked opiates and fungal toxins in pickled vegetables, as well as physical insults such as long-term exposure to extremely hot tea, the ingestion of lye, radiation-induced stricture and chronic achalasia (see Table 23.2).

Table 23.2 Aetiological factors associated with oesophageal cancer

- Excess alcohol consumption
- Cigarette smoking
- Other ingested carcinogens
- Nitrates (converted to nitrites)
- Smoked opiates
- Fungal toxins in pickled vegetables
- Mucosal damage from physical agents
- Hot tea
- Lye ingestion
- Radiation-induced strictures
- Chronic achalasia
- Host susceptibility
- Oesophageal web with glossitis and iron deficiency (Plummer-Vinson or Paterson-Kelly syndrome)
- Congenital hyperkeratosis and pitting of the palms and soles (tylosis palmaris et plantaris)
- Dietary deficiencies in molybdenum, zinc, vitamin A
- Coeliac sprue (gluten-sensitive enteropathy)
- Chronic gastric reflux (Barrett's oesophagus) for adenocarcinoma

▷ Gastric adenocarcinoma

Aetiology

Result of long-term ingestion of high concentrations of nitrates in dried, smoked and salted foods. One hypothesis suggests that dietary nitrates are converted to carcinogenic nitrites by bacteria (possibly *Helicobacter pylori*).

Exogenous sources of nitrate-converting bacteria include:

- bacterially contaminated food, which is common in less advantaged socioeconomic groups who record a higher incidence of the disease. This is diminished by improved food preservation and refrigeration
- *Helicobacter pylori* infection.

Endogenous factors favouring the growth of nitrate-converting bacteria in the stomach include:

- decreased gastric acidity
- prior gastric surgery (antrectomy) (latency period 15–20 years)
- atrophic gastritis and/or pernicious anaemia
- possibly, prolonged exposure to histamine H_2 receptor antagonists.

▷ Colorectal cancer

Aetiology

Colorectal cancer is associated with a diet high in animal fats. Risk factors include obesity, hereditary syndromes such as polyposis coli, inflammatory bowel disease, and possibly the use of tobacco.

Medical therapy with NSAIDs (COX-2 inhibitors celecoxib or aspirin) is protective by decreasing the number and size of polyps, but the effect is temporary only.

The children of patients with polyposis coli, who are often prepubertal when diagnosis is made in the parent, have a 50 per cent risk of developing the premalignant disorder and should be carefully screened by annual flexible sigmoidoscopy until age 35 years. Prophylactic colectomy is definitely recommended, along with explaining the risk of desmoids.

In patients with a history of inflammatory bowel disease (IBD) for more than 15 years, and who continue to experience exacerbation, the surgical removal of the colon can significantly reduce the risk of cancer and also eliminate the target organ for the underlying chronic gastrointestinal disorder.

Cigarette smoking is linked to the development of colorectal adenomas, particularly after 35 years of tobacco use.

The American Cancer Society suggests faecal screening annually, and flexible sigmoidoscopy every five years from the age of 50, for asymptomatic individuals having no colorectal cancer risk factors. They also propose a total colon examination (colonoscopy) every 10 years as an alternative to haemoccult testing, along with periodic flexible sigmoidoscopy.

▷ Tumours of the small intestine

Malignant tumours, while rare, occur in patients with longstanding regional enteritis and coeliac sprue as well as in individuals with AIDS.

▷ Cancer of the anus

Anal cancer is associated with infection by human papilloma virus (HPV). Vaccines may be preventative. The virus is sexually transmitted; homosexual males and both males and females suffering from AIDS are at greatest risk.

▷ Tumours of liver and biliary gut

The risk of liver adenomas is increased among those who take anabolic steroids and exogenous androgens. Oral contraceptives are also thought to contribute to this cancer.

Pregnancy should be avoided by women with large adenomas as it increases the risk of haemorrhage.

Hepatitis B and C viruses have a role in the aetiology. Prophylaxis includes hepatitis B vaccination and screening of blood products. Hepatocellular carcinoma may also occur following long-term androgenic steroid administration, with exposure to thorium oxide or vinyl chloride.

The risk factors for cholangiocarcinoma include occupations such as employment in rubber or automotive factories which may cause exposure to possible biliary tract carcinogens.

▷ Pancreatic cancer

Cigarette smoking is the most consistent risk factor. The disease is two to three times more common in heavy smokers than in non-smokers.

People with chronic pancreatitis or longstanding diabetes mellitus are at increased risk of pancreatic cancer. Obesity is also a risk factor for pancreatic cancer: risk is directly related to increased calorie intake.

Summary

The concept of preventive gastroenterology embraces the possibilities of increasing longevity, improving quality of life and reducing morbidity and mortality of digestive diseases.

The digestive diseases discussed include: GERD; Barrett's oesophagus; peptic ulcer, *H. pylori*; coeliac disease; short bowel syndrome; IBD; viral hepatitis, including hepatitis A and E; toxic and drug-induced hepatitis; NAFLD/NASH; hepatitis due to substance abuse; variceal bleeding; ascites; spontaneous bacterial peritonitis; hepatic encephalopathy; hepatorenal syndrome; gallbladder disease; and acute pancreatitis.

Cancer prevention is also discussed. Knowledge of the pathogenesis and molecular biology of cancer has made it possible prevent certain digestive disease cancers.

Information for patients

What are the symptoms of gastrointestinal illness if I am travelling?

Diarrhoea is the most common illness, especially in travellers. It is usually a short-lived, self-limited condition. It necessitates 40 per cent of affected individuals having to alter their scheduled activities, and another 20 per cent are confined to bed. The most important determinant of risk is your destination.

How often could this happen?

For a two-week stay in a given area, the incidence rates are as low as 8 per cent in developed countries, and up to 55 per cent in parts of Africa, Central and South America and South-East Asia.

What causes it?

Gastrointestinal sickness may be a bacterial or viral parasite infection. The main kinds of bacteria are *Escherichia coli* (the well-known *E. coli*), *Salmonella, Shigella* and *Campylobacter*; the main viruses are Norovirus (previously called Norwalk agent) and Rotavirus.

How can I take precautions when travelling?

Eat very hot food, avoid raw or poorly cooked foods or food sold by street vendors, and drink only boiled water or commercially bottled beverages, particularly those that are carbonated. Avoid ice cubes unless you know they are made from purified water.

Also, travellers should carry medication for self-treatment (see Table 23.3), loperamide, fluid replacements, and a three-day course of quinolone to be taken twice daily. A lactose-free diet for one week also helps.

In some areas, avoid walking barefoot because of the risk of infection by hookworm or threadworm (*Strongyloides*) and, of course, the risk of snakebite.

Is any extra information available for someone with HIV?

Yes. See Table 23.4 for information related to the HIV-infected traveller.

Table 23.3 Travel kit

- Analgesics

- Anti-diarrhoeals

- Anti-histaminics

- Laxatives

- Oral rehydration salts (ORS)

- Sunscreen with a skin protection factor of at least 30

- 2 insect repellents containing DEET for the skin (DEET is *N, N*-Diethyl-*meta*-toluamide)

- Insecticide for the clothing (e.g. permethrin)

- Antimalarial eye and skin ointment

Table 23.4 The HIV-infected traveller

- Abnormal levels of gastric acid may affect gastrointesinal mucosal immunity

- Other complications of HIV infection

- Medication taken for HIV infection

- Traveller's diarrhoea is likely to occur more frequently and be more severe and more difficult to treat, especially infections caused by Cryptosporidium or *Isospora belli*

- May benefit from prophylaxis, using bismuth salicyclate or a daily antibiotic, ideally a quinolone derivative

How can I treat the illness while travelling?

Table 23.5 has some information for patients regarding treatment while they are travelling.

Table 23.5 Treatment of diseases encountered when travelling

Disease/Disorder	Preventative measures
Primary bacterial peritonitis (recurrence)	Fluid restriction, salt restriction
Amoebic liver abscess Amoebiasis	Avoid eating improperly cooked food, cook food well. Wash vegetables with potassium permanganate solution Follow personnel hygiene and sanitation

Disease/Disorder	Preventative measures
Bacterial food poisoning: 1. Enterotoxigenic *E. coli* (Asia and Latin America) 2. *Shigella* 3. *Salmonella* 4. *Campylobacter* 5. *Vibrio cholerae* 6. Rotavirus 7. Norovirus 8. Botulism	Avoid excessive use of antacids and H_2 blockers Limit use of antimotility drugs Personal hygiene and sanitation Boil drinking water Avoid eating raw vegetables, salads and unpeeled fruit Wash vegetables before eating Avoid unpasteurised food products—milk, eggs Avoid milk and milk products (or other food containing lactose) during acute diarrhoea Eat hot, freshly cooked food Avoid canned food Drink plenty of fluids. Maintain adequate hydration Bismuth subsalicylate for indigestion etc. is inexpensive Prophylactic microbials
Travellers who are immunosuppressed or have other underlying illnesses that place them at high risk for morbidity from gastrointestinal infection	Prevent transmission by wearing gloves. Get rid of contaminated items
Clostridium difficile-associated disease (antibiotic-induced diarrhoea) For a parasitic infestation: 1. Deworming 2. Maintaining personal hygiene and sanitation 3. Eating only well-cooked food	Prevent outbreaks: Restrict use of clindamycin, 2nd and 3rd generation cephalosporins

References

1. Feldman M, Friedman LS, Brandt LJ, editors. Sleisenger and Fordtran's gastrointestinal and liver disease. 9th ed. Philadelphia: Saunders/Elsevier; 2010.

2. Keshava A, Bartolo DCC. Postoperative prevention of relapse in Crohn's disease. In: Delaini GG, editor. Inflammatory bowel disease and familial adenomatous polyposis: clinical management and patients' quality of life. Chapter 21. Milan: Springer; 2006.

3. Lashner BA, Silverstein MD, Hanauer SB. Hazard rates for dysplasia and cancer in ulcerative colitis. Results from a surveillance program. *Dig Dis Sci*. 1989 Oct; 34(10):1536–41.

4. Eaden J, Abrams K, Ekbom A, Jackson E, Mayberry J. Colorectal cancer prevention in ulcerative colitis: a case-control study. *Aliment Pharmacol Ther*. 2000 Feb; 14(2):145–53.

5. Loftus EV Jr. Epidemiology and risk factors for colorectal dysplasia and cancer in ulcerative colitis. *Gastroenterol Clin North Am*. 2006 Sep; 35(3):517–31.

Recommended reading

ASGE Standards of Practice Committee, Banerjee S, Shen B, Nelson DB, Lichtenstein DR, Baron TH, Anderson MA, Dominitz JA, Gan SI, Harrison ME, Ikenberry SO, Jagannath SB, Fanelli RD, Lee K, van Guilder T, Stewart LE. Infection control during GI endoscopy. *Gastrointest Endosc*. 2008 May; 67(6):781–90.

Buchman AL. The demise of modern medicine and gastroenterology. *J Clin Gastroenterol*. 1996 Sep; 23(2):91–3.

Cochrane Reviews database. [Internet]. Available from: www2.cochrane.org/reviews.

El-Omar EM, Oien K, Murry LS, El-Nujumi A, Wirz A, Gillen D, Williams C, Fullerton G, McColl KE. Increased prevalence of precancerous changes in relatives of gastric cancer patient: critical role of *H. pylori*. *Gastroenterology*. 2000 Jan; 118(1):22–30.

Health Protection Agency. [Internet]. Available from: www.hpa.org.uk.

U.S. Department of Health and Human Services. Agency for Healthcare Research and Quality. [Internet]. Available from: www.ahrq.gov.

U.S. Department of Health and Human Services. Agency for Healthcare Research and Quality. National Guideline Clearinghouse. [Internet]. Available from: www.guideline.gov.

World Health Organization publications and documents in multiple languages from WHO library database. [Internet]. Available from: www.who.int/publication/en.

Diagnostic features: The physical findings (emaciated appearance, diminished skinfold thickness and reduced arm muscle circumference) are due to extensive tissue and muscle wasting. Laboratory findings in marasmus are relatively within the normal range. Nutritional repletion should be done gradually over the first two weeks to allow re-adaptation of metabolic functions.

Kwashiorkor

'Kwashiorkor' in Ga (the Kwa language of coastal Ghana) is the effect on a child when a second child comes: the 'deposed child' who, after being weaned, then goes hungry. It is the oedematous PEM, occurring when the individual is not only starved, but also has acute severe illness (stress starvation). The body's response is hypermetabolic, and the adaptive responses of simple starvation, which conserve body protein, are overridden by the cytokine effects of injury. It is the protein deficiency which is the hallmark of kwashiorkor. In adults, this type of malnutrition is typically seen in intensive care units.

Diagnostic features: The clinical picture is characterised by painless pitting oedema in the lower extremities, skin changes, distended abdomen and, in severe cases, liver enlargement. The skin may be dry and hyperpigmented. Pressure ulcers, skin breakdown or poor wound healing are also common. The major criteria for diagnosis of kwashiorkor are severe reduction in the levels of visceral proteins such as albumin (<2.8 g/dL), transferrin (<150 mg/dL) or iron-binding capacity (<200 µg/dL). Differently from marasmus, patients with kwashiorkor require more aggressive nutritional support to meet protein and energy requirements.

Marasmic kwashiorkor

This combined form of PEM can develop when an acute stress—surgery, trauma or sepsis—is superimposed on an already marasmic patient. The clinical and biochemical features of both marasmus and kwashiorkor are evident. Severe protein deficiency is the predominant metabolic alteration. It is characterised by the combination of the oedema of kwashiorkor and the muscle wasting/decreased subcutaneous fat of marasmus (see Table 24.2).

Table 24.2 Marasmus and kwashiorkor diagnostic comparisons

Features	Marasmus	Kwashiorkor
Clinical setting	↓ Calorie intake	↓ Protein intake during stress state
Time to develop	Months or years	Weeks

Features	Marasmus	Kwashiorkor
Weight for age	<60% of expected	60–80% of expected
Basis for diagnosis	Triceps skinfold <3 mm Mid-arm muscle circumference <15 cm Growth retardation in children	Serum albumin <2.8 g/dL Poor wound healing, decubitus ulcers Oedema Stunted growth may occur in children
Appetite	Good	Poor
Appearance	Starved	May appear adequately nourished
Mood	Alert	Irritable
Laboratory findings	Creatinine–height index <60% standard	Serum albumin <2.8 g/dL Total iron-binding capacity <200 µg/dL Lymphocytes <1500/mm³

⟲ Management

Nutritional screening

Malnutrition is associated with negative health outcomes. Functional and organ alterations that occur in both over- and undernutrition can result in a risk of complications 10 to 20 times greater than in the well-nourished. Unfortunately, most cases are not recognised either in outpatient or inpatient settings; this is mainly due to a lack of awareness and inadequate screening. Nutritional screening should utilise simple and easy-to-use clinical tools which can help identify those at risk, who can then undergo a complete nutritional assessment.

Today, we have numerous nutritional screening tools designed for different target populations: Subjective Global Assessment (SGA) for adult hospitalised patients; Body Mass Index (BMI) for both hospitalised and non-hospitalised people; and Mini Nutritional Assessment (MNA) for elderly patients 65 and over (see Tables 24.3, 24.4).

Table 24.3 Nutrition screening Subjective Global Assessment (SGA)

- Physical examination (normal, moderate or severe)
  - Loss of subcutaneous fat (triceps, chest)
  - Muscle wasting (quadriceps, deltoids)
  - Ankle or sacral oedema
  - Ascites

continued

Table 24.3 *continued*

- SGA rating

A = well-nourished
B = mild or moderate malnutrition
C = severe malnutrition

Table 24.4 Nutrition screening Mini Nutritional Assessment (MNA) in the elderly

- First part: Screening—food intake, weight loss, recent illness, BMI, neuropsychological problem. If screening score suggests malnutrition, second part is administered

- Second part: Environment, medications, dietary habits, mid-arm and calf circumferences, need for assistance with meals, fruit and vegetable intake and co-morbid conditions.

Nutrition assessment

There are many components to a thorough and complete nutrition assessment, and while no single parameter is sufficiently sensitive or specific, they are most effective when used in combination. Tables 24.5 to 24.11 contain descriptions of the most commonly used tools for nutrition assessment.

Table 24.5 Nutrition assessment

- History
  - Body weight
  - Diet assessment

- Physical examination
  General
  Anthropometrics
  - Body weight
  - Body mass index (BMI), waist circumference (WC), waist-to-hip ratio (WHR)
  - Triceps skin fold (TSF) thickness
  - Mid-arm circumference (MAC)

- Laboratory tests
  - Albumin
  - Prealbumin
  - Transferrin
  - Retinol binding protein
  - Total lymphocyte count (TLC)

- Body composition
  - Bioelectrical impedance (BI)
  - Dual X-ray absorptometry (DXA)
- Functional tests
  - Hand dynamometry
  - Direct muscle stimulation
  - Respiratory function

Table 24.6 Weight history important characteristics

- Recent weight loss
- Weight loss of more than 5% in 1 month or 10% in 6 months before hospitalisation
- Ideal body weight for men = 48 kg for the first 152 cm + 2.7 kg for each 2.54 cm over 152 cm
- Ideal body weight for women = 45 kg for the first 152 cm + 2.3 kg for each 2.54 cm over 152 cm

QUICK FLICK 24

Table 24.7 Diet assessment

- Ability to digest food including chewing, swallowing and absorption
- Food intolerances/eating disorders
- Food/drug interactions
- Skills and ability to comply with dietary lifestyle changes

Table 24.8 Bedside physical examination general

- Head, eyes, ears, nose and throat (HEENT): hair loss, temporal wasting, glossitis, angular stomatitis
- Extremities: oedema, muscle wasting
- Skin: pallor, ecchymoses, pressure ulcers

Table 24.9 Physical examination anthropometrics

- Measurements that help estimate body fat and protein stores using Lange calipers/tape measure.
- Significant drawback: reliance on age, sex, and race-matched reference values

continued

Table 24.9 *continued*

- Skin fold thickness: triceps skin fold (TSF): Indirect marker of body fat stores
  Normal: Men 11 mm, women 19 mm
    35–45% : mild malnutrition; 25–35% : moderate malnutrition; <25% : severe
    malnutrition

- Mid-arm circumference (MAC): indirect marker of body protein stores
  Normal: Men 270 mm, women 213 mm
    35–45% : mild malnutrition; 25–35% : moderate malnutrition; <25% : severe
    malnutrition

Table 24.10 Laboratory tests

- Serum albumin: normal value: 3.5–5.5 gm/dl, half-life 14–21 days

- Serum transferrin: normal value: 260–430 mg/dl, half-life 8–9 days

- Serum prealbumin: 0.2–0.4 gm/dl, half-life 2–3 days

- Retinol binding protein (RBP): 30–60 mg/L, half-life 0.5 days

- Total lymphocyte count (TLC): <1500 suggests PEM

- Creatinine-height index (CHI): excellent means of assessing total skeletal
  muscle mass.
    24-hour urinary creatinine excretion divided by normative value for height and sex:
    values: <80% indicates moderate to severe PEM

Table 24.11 Functional measures

- Three different techniques to exploit impaired skeletal muscle function in PEM:

  - Fist-grip dynamometry (FGD): measures hand-grip strength.
  - Adductor pollicis electrical stimulation: measures contraction and relaxation.
  - Respiratory muscle strength evaluation: measures changes in peak flow and
    forced expiratory volume in 1 second (FEV1)

Overnutrition

In contrast to undernutrition, this is a form of malnutrition in which
nutrients are oversupplied far beyond the requirements for normal
growth and development. Add to this the technological triumphs of
television, computers and cars, and the two most powerful ingredients

for overnutrition emerge—an abundance of food and a sedentary lifestyle.

Worldwide, from Brazil to Kenya to India to Indonesia, overweight and obesity affect both adults and children. The prevalence of these conditions has doubled, even trebled, in the past two decades for certain age groups, resulting in a manifold increase in the risk of developing chronic illnesses such as diabetes mellitus type 2, hypertension, cardiovascular disease and different types of cancer. Thus, early adoption of techniques for evaluating patients for overweight/obesity would help clinicians intervene early with proper lifestyle modifications and/or therapeutic options (see Tables 24.12 to 24.14).

Table 24.12 Obesity-related co-morbidities

- Greatly increased (relative risk >3)
  - Diabetes mellitus (DM)
  - Gallbladder disease
  - Dyslipidaemia
  - Sleep apnoea
- Moderately increased (relative risk ~2 to 3)
  - Coronary heart disease
  - Hypertension
  - Osteoarthritis
- Slightly increased (relative risk ~1 to 2)
  - Cancer (breast cancer in postmenopausal women, endometrial cancer, colon cancer)
  - Polycystic ovary syndrome
  - Impaired fertility
  - Low back pain due to obesity

Overweight and obesity: assessment

Body mass index

Body mass index (BMI), established by the World Health Organization (WHO) in 1997, is the most practical and internationally accepted tool for evaluating the degree of overweight and its associated risks. In adults, it is calculated as the patient's weight in kilograms divided by the square of their height in metres (kg/m^2). In adults:

- optimal weight is defined by a BMI of 18.5 to 25 kg/m^2
- overweight is defined by a BMI between 25 and 29.9 kg/m^2
- obesity is defined by a BMI equal to or greater than 30 kg/m^2.

In children and adolescents, obesity is defined as a BMI greater than the 95th percentile.

The range for acceptable, normal or optimum BMI for Asian populations has been narrowed to 18.5–23 kg/m², because scientific data suggests that associations between BMI, percentage of body fat and health risks in Asian populations are different from those in European populations. A WHO expert committee has concluded that the proportion of Asian people at high risk of contracting type 2 diabetes and cardiovascular disease is substantial at BMIs lower than the currently recognised cut-off points for overweight (25 kg/m²). The BMI cut-off point for observed risk in different Asian populations varies from 22 to 25 kg/m²; for high risk, it varies from 26 to 31 kg/m².

Although the current WHO BMI points are being retained as the international classification, several Asian countries have modified the BMI cut-off points for overweight and obesity. Japanese and Indian health officials are finding high rates of diabetes at BMI values of 25 or more; both countries have redefined obesity as a BMI of 25 and above.

Table 24.13 BMI recommended classifications

Classification	BMI (kg/m²)
Severely undernourished	<16
Moderately undernourished	<16.9
Mildly undernourished	17–18.4
Underweight	<18.5
Normal weight	18.5–24.9
Overweight	25.0–29.9
Class I obesity	30.0–34.9
Class II obesity	35.0–39.9
Class III obesity	≥ 40.0

Since the BMI uses a standardised weight vs height formula, some controversy exists over its accuracy in setting obesity standards: for example, BMI does not distinguish between body fat and muscle mass, which is denser than fat and therefore weighs more. It also puts women and men in the same category as far as body weight is concerned, even though women are expected to have a higher percentage of body fat.

Table 24.14 BMI salient features

- Most practical tool for assessing weight-related health risks.
- Cut-off points are lower for Asians. India and Japan define obesity at BMI 25 or more.
- USA and EU countries recognise obesity at BMI 30 or more.
- Limitations exist. BMI does not account for frame size or whether weight is coming from fat or muscle.

Waist circumference (WC)

Determining waist circumference eliminates the inconsistencies of BMI. Increasing central adiposity is associated with an increased risk of morbidity and mortality. A waist circumference greater than 102 cm (40 in) for men and 88 cm (35 in) for women puts them at increased risk of heart disease, diabetes, hypertension and dyslipidaemia. In Asian females a waist circumference >80 cm and in Asian males a value >90 cm are considered abnormal.

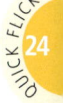

Waist-to-hip ratio (WHR)

Waist-to-hip ratio is another guideline for determining obesity. It determines how weight is distributed on the body. Weight distribution on the lower half of the body (pear-shape) generally does not pose the same serious consequences as weight that surrounds the abdominal area (apple-shape). Waist-to-hip ratio (WHR) is calculated by dividing the circumference of the waist (WC) by the circumference of the hips (WC). WC is measured at the midpoint between the lowest rib and the iliac crest, at the level of the umbilicus, or just above the iliac crest, with the patient standing, bare midriff, after exhaling, with feet together and arms hanging freely. Important features of WHR:

- A high WHR is defined as >0.9 in men and >0.85 in women.
- A high WHR is associated with an increased risk of cardiovascular disease and diabetes mellitus.
- It is a commonly recognised index of abdominal obesity.
- WHR is a more accurate tool than WC or BMI for diagnosing patients at increased cardiovascular risk.
- WHR is also considered a good predictor of cardiovascular morbidity and mortality.

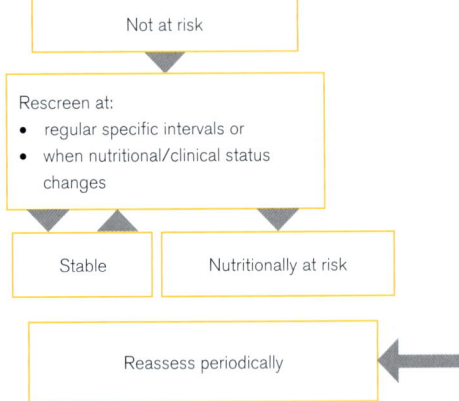

Figure 24.1 Algorithm for adult nutritional evaluation

Source: Adapted from Clinical pathways and algorithms for delivery of parenteral and enteral nutrition support in adults, Silver Spring, MD: American Society for Parenteral and Enteral Nutrition; 1998:4.

Summary

Having not completely escaped the ravages of undernutrition (still estimated at a billion globally), we now have to deal with the bigger and more challenging public health problem of obesity, for which there appear to be few good solutions.

Globally, there are more than 1.7 billion overweight adults, and at least 350 million of them are obese. The Centers for Disease Control and Prevention estimate that obesity-related diseases in the United States cost more than

> At risk

> Nutrition assessment, including:
> - review nutrition history/related information
> - evaluation of anthropometric and lab data
> - review of clinical status
> - nutritionally focused physical examination

> Develop nutrition care plan

$150 billion annually, and weight-related costs add $20 billion per year to the costs of employers nationwide in higher medical bills, decreased productivity, increased absenteeism, and higher health and disability insurance premiums.

What served us well during periods of prolonged starvation in our hunter-gatherer years has become a disadvantage in the modern world where food is abundant and lifestyles sedentary. For the first time in the history of humanity, we have more overnourished than undernourished people worldwide, a paradox of immense proportions that is straining healthcare systems globally. Clinicians have to be ever more vigilant to detect and assess the early signs of undernutrition, overweight or obesity to prevent potentially catastrophic outcomes.

Information for patients

How do I know if I am at my healthy weight?

The easiest and most practical way to identify weight problems is to calculate your body mass index (BMI), which is a measure of your weight in relation to your height. The equation is BMI = weight in kg ÷ (height in m)^2. BMI interpretation is as follows:

BMI (kg/m^2)	Classification
<18.5	Underweight
$\geq$ 18.5 and < 25	Healthy weight
$\geq$ 25 and <30	Overweight
> 30	Obesity

If you are in the 'obesity' category, the circumference of your waist should be measured. If it is more than 89 cm in women or more than 102 cm in men, it can increase your risk of obesity-related complications such as hypertension, heart disease and diabetes. People who are obese and also have a larger waist circumference may need more aggressive weight loss treatment. Talk to your doctor for advice.

BMI values are of even greater significance if they can be compared not only with the given ranges above but also with recent values in the same individual. If you are of Asian origin, the cut-off points are different. Talk with your health care provider for details.

When is weight loss considered abnormal?

Abnormal weight loss is a symptom of acute or chronic illness. There is a strong relationship between weight loss and mortality. Involuntary weight loss is nearly always a sign of serious medical or psychiatric disease, and requires evaluation. Weight loss more than 5 per cent of baseline weight over 6 to 12 months is considered clinically significant. Short-term weight changes—over days or weeks, for example—are more likely to reflect fluid balance rather than changes in tissue mass.

What is 'undernutrition'?

Undernutrition is the condition that occurs when you do not eat enough food. It may result from:

- inadequate or unbalanced diet
- maldigestion or malabsorption
- certain medical conditions.

Symptoms vary and depend on the cause, which needs to be investigated. Some general symptoms might be fatigue, dizziness and weight loss. Treatment usually consists of replacing missing nutrients, treating symptoms, and treating any underlying medical condition.

The prognosis depends on the cause of the undernutrition. Most nutritional deficiencies can be corrected. However, if undernutrition is caused by a medical condition, that illness has to be treated in order to reverse the nutritional deficiency.

If untreated, undernutrition can lead to mental or physical disability, illness and, possibly, death.

How is good nutrition maintained?

Eating a healthy, well-balanced diet helps to prevent most forms of malnutrition.

- Eat a variety of foods, including vegetables, fruits and whole-grains.
- Eat lean meats, poultry, fish, beans and low-fat dairy products.
- Limit the amount of red meat.
- Consume small amounts of salt and sugar.
- Avoid saturated fats and trans fats. Use monounsaturated and polyunsaturated fats such as olive oil and canola oil instead.
- Drink plenty of water—at least eight glasses a day.
- Avoid excessive alcohol intake.

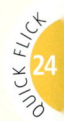

Recommended reading

Balko, R. The BMI problem. Risk: Regulation and Reality Conference, Toronto, Canada. Centers for Disease Control and Prevention. Defining Overweight and Obesity. 2004.

Bleich S, Cutler D, Murray C, Adams A. Why is the developed world obese? *Annu Rev Public Health*. 2008; 29:273–95.

Caballero B. The global epidemic of obesity: an overview. *Epidemiol Rev*. 2007; 29:1–5.

Capra S. Nutrition assessment or nutrition screening: how much information is enough to make a diagnosis of malnutrition in acute care? *Nutrition*. 2007; 23:356–7.

Centers for Disease Control and Prevention. Youth risk behavior surveillance: United States, 2007. Morbidity and Mortality Weekly Report. 2008; 57(SS-04):1–131. [Internet]. Available from: www.cdc.gov/mmwr/preview/mmwrhtml/ss5704a1.htm.

Chakravarthy MV, Booth FW. Eating, exercise, and 'thrifty' genotypes: connecting the dots toward an evolutionary understanding of modern chronic diseases. *J Appl Physiol.* 2004; 96(1):3–10.

Grover Z, Ee LC. Protein energy malnutrition. *Pediatr Clin North Am.* 2009 Oct; 56(5):1055–68.

Heimburger DC. Nutrition assessment. In: Heimburger DC, Ard JD, editors. Handbook of clinical nutrition. 4th ed. Mosby; 2006; 242–61.

Nutrition Assessment Online: 3 steps to better health. Evaluate BMI, energy needs, physical activity levels and risk for chronic illness. [Internet]. Available from: www.NutritionVista.com.

Ogden CL, Carroll MD, Flegal KM. High body mass index for age among U.S. children and adolescents, 2003–2006. *J Am Med Assoc.* 2008; 299:2401–5.

Russell MK, Mueller C. Nutrition screening and assessment. In: Gottschlich MM, editor. The A.S.P.E.N. nutrition support core curriculum: a case-based approach: the adult patient. Silver Spring, MD: American Society for Parenteral and Enteral Nutrition; 2007; 163–84.

WHO expert consultation. Appropriate body-mass index for Asian populations and its implications for policy and intervention strategies. *Lancet.* 2004; 363:157–63.

Chapter 25: Impact on children of global nutritional breakdown

R. Jackson (Australia)

Key points

- Malnutrition ranges from undernutrition to overnutrition.
- Increasing prevalence of malnutrition and obesity due to environmental factors.
- Spectrum of malnutrition depends on chronicity of energy or protein deficiencies.
- In developed countries, failure to thrive is important.
- Obesity complications are diverse and affect almost all systems.
- Detailed history and examination necessary. Inspect for all aspects of energy, vitamins and mineral deficiencies.
- Acanthosis nigricans in obese children.
- Tailored investigations depending on initial results.
- Look for risk and development of refeeding syndrome.
- Slow increase in caloric renourishment with electrolyte and vitamin B replacement.
- Multidisciplinary long-term strategic approach in obesity.

○ Introduction

Maintenance of good health and nutrition has been affected globally by increasing world population, which brings with it rising pollution and poor sustainability to maintain resources to feed communities nutritionally.

○ Epidemiology

Lead and mercury poisoning are examples of increasingly recognised extremely harmful environmental pollutants affecting health. They are of particular concern in poor countries where a significant percentage of children are in the workforce. Hazardous levels have been seen to result in severe risk factors affecting growth. There has also been increasing famine related to climate change and wars affecting the health of large populations. Over-population has been accompanied by an increased variety of infections and their rate of spread. All of these factors have contributed to an ever-increasing worldwide incidence of abnormal nutrition.

Diagnosis

The definition of *malnutrition* refers to abnormal nutrition ranging from undernutrition to overnutrition. At one extreme of the range it encompasses malnourished children or adults, and obesity is the other extreme. As a result, malnutrition is essentially a common phenomenon all over the world, from third-world countries to developed nations. Malnutrition from underfeeding or undernutrition affects more than one-third of all developing nations, but is rare in the Western world. The two ends of the spectrum are discussed here.

Balanced growth

To understand nutrition and normal growth, an appreciation of the concept of energy is needed. Total energy expenditure (TEE) is a helpful way of assessing a person's balanced growth. The resting metabolic rate (RMR) is by far the biggest contributor to our total daily energy expenditure: it is the level of energy required for healthy normal bodily functions and homeostasis. It can be measured to assist in managing chronic malnutrition; preferably it should be measured early in the day after fasting overnight, prior to any activity. The process is performed using indirect calorimetry with a ventilated-hood system. The metabolic rate is estimated from measurements of oxygen consumption and carbon dioxide production. RMR is influenced by nutritional state, thyroid function and sympathetic nervous system activity. Energy expenditure is also influenced by disease states such as fever, sepsis, neurological injuries, surgery, use of mechanical ventilation and chronic illness.

Exercise and physical activity play an important role in producing heat energy expenditure; they account for 15 to 30 per cent of TEE, and represent the energy cost of activity above basal levels. Digestion of food (thermic effect of food, TEF) accounts for approximately 10 per cent of TEE. This is the energy cost of ingestion of macronutrients (fat, protein and carbohydrate) and digesting, transporting, metabolising and storing the nutrients. Insulin resistance can affect TEF, and plays a part in obesity. Understanding the different components of TEE allows a better outcome in nutritional support when dealing with patients with medical causes of malnutrition (see Figure 25.1).

Clinical

Malnutrition can result in three main categories of clinical presentation: protein-energy malnutrition (PEM), stunting of growth impairing linear height and/or weight, and overweight with its large range of sequelae.

Figure 25.1 Components of energy expenditure

The spectrum of malnutrition of the undernutrition type can be subdivided on an organic and non-organic basis (see Table 25.1). Within this breakdown, the concepts of inadequate intake, inadequate digestion, inadequate absorption, increased losses and increased caloric expenditure are categorised. Poverty, leading to a lack of nutritional sources, is the most common cause in third world countries. The classic presentation often leads to severe PEM, which in turn depends on which of the three clinical findings is appropriate: kwashiorkor, marasmic kwashiorkor or marasmus.

Table 25.1 Causes of undernutrition

Organic
• Decreased caloric intake:
– poor oral intake (poverty)
– gastro-oesophageal reflux disease (GERD)
– vomiting (any cause)
– anorexia
– inability to suck
– iatrogenic (restricted diets)

continued

Table 25.1 *continued*

- Inadequate digestion (luminal)
  - bile salt deficiency
  - pancreatic insufficiency

- Inadequate absorption +/- increased losses
  - abnormal mucosa (coeliac disease, IBD, chronic giardiasis)
  - enzyme deficiency (disaccharidase deficiency—Type 1 and Type 2)
  - inadequate length (short bowel syndrome)

- Increased caloric expenditure +/- increased losses
  - thyrotoxicosis
  - chronic disease (cardiac, infections, burns, immunodeficiency, IBD, malignancy, diabetes mellitus, metabolic disorders)

Non-organic

- Münchausen syndrome

Kwashiorkor develops when a diet is persistently deficient in protein. It commonly occurs when babies in poor socioeconomic populations are given protein-poor formula or diluted formula. Hypoproteinaemia, oedema, fatty liver, lethargy and dry skin are common findings.

Marasmus occurs when the diet is persistently low in total energy. It is often a result of partial starvation in the first year of life. It is a physiological adaptation to starvation due to deficiency in energy, protein, vitamin and mineral intake, showing as stunted height and poor weight in the patient. Muscle wasting, loss of subcutaneous fat and dry skin are often evident. The enlarged fatty liver and oedema of kwashiorkor are not present.

Marasmic kwashiorkor refers to cases where there is a mixture of both types of deficiency. Table 25.2 outlines the common useful screens in patients with PEM. More specific testing can then follow, using the initial detailed history, an examination and the results of the screening laboratory testings.

Table 25.2 Screening tests in malnutrition

- Assessment of protein store
  - albumin

- Electrolytes
  - sodium, potassium, chloride, bicarbonate

- Mineral
  - calcium, phosphate, magnesium, zinc

- Renal function
  - urea, creatinine

- Liver function

- Other blood investigations
  - FBC
  - BSL
  - cholesterol
  - triglyceride
  - vitamins A, E and 25-OH D
  - coagulation

The most common presentation of poor nutrition in developed countries that leads to failure to thrive in infants is probably the common combination of GERD and cow's milk protein allergy. This combination can produce the opposite to the desired result of a thriving child if parents overfeed in response to the child's crying, interpreting it as hunger. When there is poor growth due to disruption of feeding from pain and losses in vomiting, there is often a complex interaction exacerbated by psychosocial factors. Ongoing poor intake and losses, and subsequent delayed progression to solid foods, contributes to poor weight gain. Failure to maintain adequate medical therapy can lead to extreme food aversion and poor oromotor skills (speech and swallowing), requiring intensive speech therapy later in life.

It is crucial to overcome poor weight gain in infancy: studies have shown an increased risk of cardiovascular disease in adulthood, developmental delay, and emotional and social problems associated with significant malnutrition. Long-term small stature and head circumference have been observed in children who continue to be malnourished between the ages of one and five years. The most common nutritional deficiency seen in these infants is persistent iron deficiency. Failure to correct long-term iron deficiency in children has also been shown to be associated with irreversible loss of IQ points.

Table 25.3 Common diseases causing undernutrition

- Eating disorder

- Burns

- Malignancies

- Cardiac

continued

Table 25.3 *continued*

- Neuromuscular

- Infections

- Gastrointestinal diseases
    - coeliac disease
    - pancreatic insufficiency (cystic fibrosis, Schwachmann's syndrome)
    - IBD
    - GERD
    - short bowel syndrome
    - cow's milk protein allergy

- Immunodeficiencies

- IUGR

- Liver disease

- Metabolic disease

- Lung disease

- Renal disease

- Psychological

In general, since each group of diseases in Table 25.3 is rare, screening laboratory tests are unhelpful for diagnosis. The yield rate from initial screening is said to be less than 2 per cent. More expanded and directed secondary investigations may need to follow, depending on the clues from the examination finding and observations of the child, and the psychosocial setting of the family. Table 25.4 lists some further potentially useful studies, but obviously the ability to carry out some tests may be limited depending on the local health resources.

Table 25.4 Further potential tests in malnutrition

- Immunoglobulins

- Coeliac screens (anti-gliadin, anti-endomycial and anti-tissue transglutaminase Ab)

- Growth hormones

- Urine metabolic screen

- Thyroid functions
- Stool for OCP and α_1-antitrypsin level
- Chromosome study
- Sweat test for chloride
- ECG
- CXR
- Bone age
- Skeletal survey
- Barium studies
- pH/impedance study of the oesophagus
- Upper and lower GI endoscopy
- Head CT or MRI.

QUICK FLICK
25

▶ Management

On renourishing a patient with medium- to long-term undernutrition, it is crucial to remember the frequently observed and potentially fatal entity of refeeding syndrome. It is a common complication when treating significant malnutrition with intravenous glucose, parenteral nutrition or enteral nutrition (orally or nasogastrically).

Refeeding syndrome

Refeeding syndrome comprises metabolic, cardiopulmonary and neurological complications. On refeeding, there is an insulin surge associated with restarting calories into the patient. The anabolic drive leads to increased phosphate, magnesium and thiamine usage, as well as driving potassium shifts, leading to hypophosphataemia, hypokalaemia, hypoglycaemia, hypomagnesaemia and hypocalcaemia (see Table 25.5 overleaf). Cardiopulmonary complications follow, due to fluid shifts, minute ventilation disturbance and arrhythmias from electrolyte changes. Management of refeeding includes slow increase of energy and protein intake, with concurrent regular monitoring and correction of electrolytes, early vitamin B-group replacement and cardiac monitoring until electrolyte shift ceases.

Table 25.5 Refeeding syndrome

• Hypoglycaemia
• Hypophosphataemia
• Hypokalaemia
• Hypomagnesaemia
• Hypocalcaemia
• Hyperlactic acidosis

Manifestations of deficiencies

Chronic malnutrition manifestations have been discussed with the various deficiencies of PEM. It is quite rare to have fat malnutrition alone. There are several isolated sugar-splitting enzyme deficiencies, but the manifestations of these are often associated with distension of the abdomen and chronic diarrhoea, without the major failure to thrive. When there is chronic malnutrition, there are often one or more vitamin and mineral deficiencies: Table 25.6 lists the common clinical manifestations of these. Despite the large number of clinical manifestations of nutritional deficiencies, in general iron deficiency is the most common.

Table 25.6 Manifestations of nutritional deficiencies

Nutrients		Manifestations of deficiencies
Carbohydrate		Hypoglycaemia, seizures, ketosis
Fat		Decreased subcutaneous fat (triceps, infrascapular, suprailiac), dry scaly skin associated with essential fatty acid deficiency
Protein		Muscle bulk loss, weakness, oedema, dry sparse hair
Vitamins	A	Night blindness, xerophthalmia, Bitot's spots (squamous metaplasia of conjunctival epithelia)
	C	4 H's of scurvy—haemorrhage (gum and skin), hyperkeratosis (follicle), hypochondriasis (with bony tenderness) and haematological abnormalities (anaemia). Pseudoparalysis.

	D	Rickets—craniotabes, widening of wrist and ankle, frontal bossing, delayed teeth eruptions, rickety rosaries and delayed motor milestones
	E	Loss of deep tendon reflexes, vibratory and position sense and balance, ophthalmoplegia and muscle weakness
	K	Bleeding tendency
Vitamin B$_1$ (thiamine)		Beriberi—cardiac failure, peripheral neuropathy, polyneuritis
Vitamin B$_6$ (pyridoxine)		Irritability, confusion, stomatitis, cheilosis, glossitis, peripheral neuropathy
Vitamin B$_{12}$ (cobalamin)		Megaloblastic anaemia, glossitis, ataxia, peripheral neuropathy and paresthaesia
Biotin		Thinning hair, dermatitis, paresthaesia
Folate		Anaemia and irritability
Niacin		Rash in sun-exposed areas, stomatitis, glossitis, loss of papillae
Riboflavin		Fatigue, cheilosis, angular stomatitis, corneal vascularisation, anaemia
Minerals		
Calcium		Abnormal bone and teeth mineralisation, tetany, rickets
Chromium		Abnormal glucose tolerance, peripheral neuropathy
Copper		Anaemia and leukopaenia
Fluorine		Dental caries
Iodine		Goitre, hypothyroidism
Iron		Anaemia, koilonychia, impaired psychomotor performance, behavioural changes
Magnesium		Tetany, positive Trousseau's and Chvostek's signs
Phosphorus		Rickets, muscle weakness
Selenium		Cardiomyopathy and muscle weakness
Zinc		Growth failure, acrodermatitis enteropathica, diarrhoea, alopecia, abnormal taste, circumoral and perianal rash.

QUICK FLICK 25

Monitoring of growth

Accurate measurement and serial plotting of weight, height and head circumference provides the best guide to the overall progress of normal children. The Centers for Disease Control and Prevention (CDC) provide excellent easy-to-download growth charts for different age and sex, including body mass index (BMI) vs age charts to allow clinicians to plot a child's progress; however, plotting of age-for-height, weight and head circumference are not always the best parameters, as different ethnicities possess different growth dynamics. It is increasingly challenging as the world becomes more accessible, leading to greater cultural and genetic mixing.

Reduction in percentage *ideal weight-for-height* ratio may signify malnutrition and is sometimes useful for distinguishing between acute and chronic malnutrition. The ratio is calculated by plotting the height on a standardised height chart. The subject's actual weight is then expressed as a percentage of the ideal weight-for-height by plotting the equivalent centile line as the height for the subject's age. This allows a percentage calculation ± two standard deviations, which is an easier target for battling obesity. The aim is to return to between 85 and 115 per cent of ideal weight for height.

Body mass index is defined as weight in kilograms divided by the square of height in metres. It is an indirect measure of body composition. It has flaws—a patient with heavy muscle or bone mass but little body fat can still fall into the category of being overweight or obese according to the BMI, something that is often seen in elite athletes.

Anthropometrics refers to a number of bedside body measurements used to assess nutritional status. Triceps skinfold can be measured using a caliper at the mid-upper arm (midway between the acromion and the olecranon process), giving an indirect representation of body fat mass. The mid-arm circumference is an indirect measure of lean body mass and is measured at the mid-upper arm point. Both can be plotted on standardised charts for age, which is then used to monitor progress in fighting weight issues (Table 25.7).

Table 25.7 Growth monitoring

- BMI
- Weight for age
- Height for age
- Ideal weight for height percentage
- Anthropometrics (skinfolds and mid-arm circumference)

Obesity

Overweight as a form of malnutrition is rapidly becoming the most common abnormality of nutrition, both in the developed and developing countries.

In countries where the population is being limited by the number of children allowed, boys are rapidly becoming extremely obese as a result of parental control and lack of physical activity. Long-established studies show that environmental factors also play a large part, for example in populations where there is high rainfall or snowfall. In seasons when outdoor physical activity is limited, there is a much higher level of BMI and associated complications.

The complications of obesity are widespread: the consequences range from intermediate to long-term complications involving physical and psychosocial damage (Table 25.8).

Table 25.8 Complications of obesity

- Cardiac
  - hypertension
  - dyslipidaemia
  - endothelial dysfunction
  - chronic inflammation

- Gastrointestinal
  - NAFLD
  - GERD
  - gallstones

- Endocrine
  - insulin resistance
  - impaired fasting glucose
  - type II diabetes mellitus
  - precocious puberty
  - polycystic ovary syndrome

- Respiratory
  - obstructive sleep apnoea
  - poor exercise tolerance

- Psychological
  - poor self-esteem
  - eating disorder thinking
  - depression
  - social stigmatisation

- Musculoskeletal
  - slipped femoral epiphysis
  - early osteoarthritis

QUICK FLICK 25

Non-alcoholic fatty liver disease (NAFLD) covers the range of liver abnormalities that affect children and adults as a consequence of obesity, despite being in the normal weight range.

Acanthosis nigricans may be found on the back of the neck or in the axillary region due to secondary hyperinsulinism from overeating. Most current treatments are based on improving the individual's quality of life in order to decrease morbidity and mortality. Lifestyle changes in the patient and in the family, dietary and exercise intervention are obviously the treatment of choice but, in general, long-term follow-up is the most crucial aspect, as failure is extremely high. Increasingly there is evidence to suggest that bariatric surgery is the most successful option in preventing long-term complications.

Physical impact of ageing and the impact on nutritional health

As we age, there is gradual thinning and loss of function of the secretory mucosa of the stomach. Over time this increases the micronutrient deficiency. As gastric acid production falls, absorption of iron, calcium, vitamins B_6, B_{12} and folic acid is reduced, and decrease in the intrinsic factor also affects B_{12} absorption.

As a result of the deficiency, common complaints are fatigue, weakness and impaired concentration. There is also an increased risk of anaemia, neurological damage and early dementia. Liver function also declines over time, and as a result many drugs have potentially adverse side effects, as well as their benefit being affected. Increasing immobility, dehydration and poor dietary habits then lead to increased faecal loading. It has been noted that subclinical malnutrition in the level of vitamins C and B_{12}, riboflavin and folic acid have been seen in many adults, along with impaired cognitive ability.

Summary

There is an increasing worldwide prevalence of malnutrition, including obesity. In developed countries it is characterised by failure to thrive. It is important to obtain the patient's history and carry out a detailed examination and routine screening blood and urine tests, followed by tailored investigations depending on initial results (see Figure 25.2). Care needs to be taken to avoid refeeding syndrome.

A multidisciplinary long-term strategy is vital to good management.

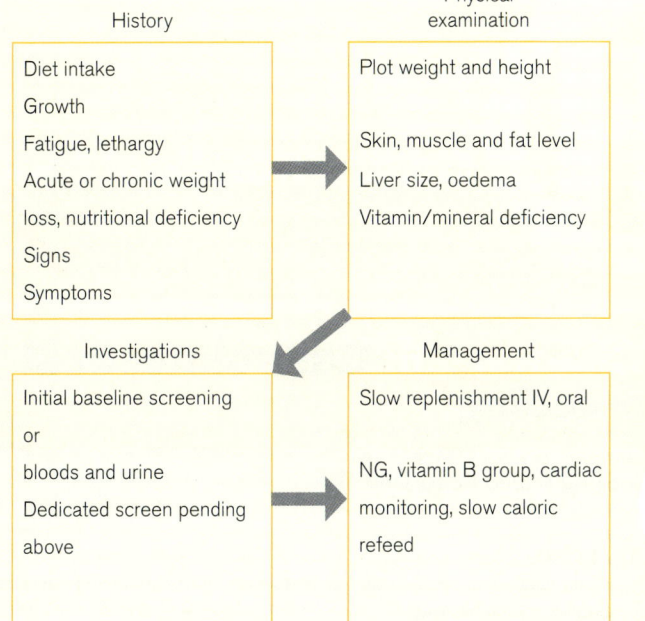

Figure 25.2 Algorithm of malnutrition

Recommended reading

Centers for Disease Control and Prevention: growth charts. [Internet]. Available from: www.cdc.gov/growthcharts.

James WP. The epidemiology of obesity: the size of the problem. *J Intern Med*. 2008 Apr; 263(4):336–52. Epub 2008 Feb 27.

Khoshoo V. Nutritional assessment in children and adolescents. *Curr Opin Pediatr*. 1997, Oct; 9(5):502–7.

Mager DR, Roberts EA. Nonalcoholic fatty liver disease in children. *Clin Liver Dis*. 2006 Feb; 10(1):109–31, vi–vii. Review.

Sheppard AA. Nutrition through the life-span. Part 2: children, adolescents and adults. *Br J Nurs*. 2008 Nov 27 – Dec 10; 17(21):1332–8.

QUICK FLICK 25

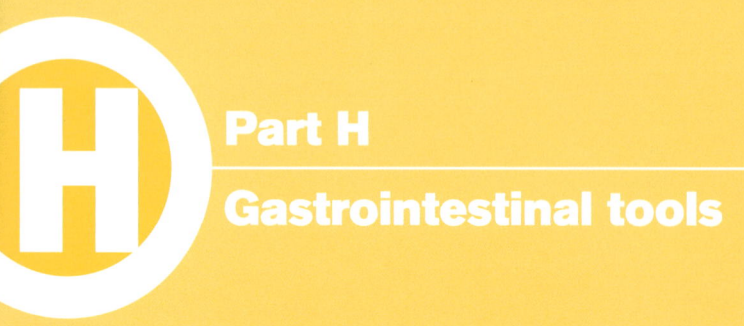

Part H
Gastrointestinal tools

Chapter 26: Gastrointestinal bleeding

J. Sung (Hong Kong, China)

Key points

- ▶ Resuscitation should be instituted irrespective of the underlying cause of gastrointestinal bleeding.
- ▶ A joint team of gastroenterologists, GI surgeons and intervention radiologists should manage a patient with gastrointestinal bleeding.
- ▶ Patients over 60 years old, and patients with co-morbid conditions, have a higher risk of mortality.
- ▶ Endoscopic examination should be made available to the patient within 24 hours or when the condition is stabilised.
- ▶ Proton pump inhibitors are recommended in high-risk peptic ulcer bleeding patients as an adjuvant to endoscopic therapy.
- ▶ Recurrent variceal bleeding is reduced by using octreotide as adjuvant therapy.
- ▶ Indications surgery include arterial bleeding that cannot be controlled by endoscopic haemostasis, and patients requiring massive transfusions.

▷ Introduction

Acute gastrointestinal bleeding is one of the most common emergency conditions associated with significant morbidity and mortality. Haematemesis (vomiting fresh blood) indicates that bleeding originates from a site proximal to the ligament of Treitz. A history of fresh haematemesis usually implies a significant bleed.

Coffee ground vomiting may arise from altered black blood, and often indicates that active bleeding may have ceased.

Melaena is the passage of black tarry stool, which occurs when haemoglobin is converted to haematin by bacterial degradation. Ingestion of as little as 200 mL of blood can produce melaenic stool. Although melaena generally connotes bleeding proximal to the ligament of Treitz, bleeding from the small bowel or proximal colon may also cause melaena, especially when colonic transit is slow.

Haematochezia—the passage of pure red blood or blood admixed with stool—usually occurs when bleeding comes from the lower gastrointestinal tract. It can also present in massive upper gastrointestinal bleeding.

◐ Aetiology

The most common cause of upper GI bleeding is peptic ulcer, followed by mucosal erosions, Mallory Weiss tear, oesophagitis and oesophageal/gastric varices. In the lower GI tract, the most common causes of bleeding are diverticular disease, vascular malformation, inflammatory bowel diseases and colorectal neoplasia (Table 26.1). In general, bleeding from the upper gastrointestinal tract is more common than from the lower gastrointestinal tract.

Table 26.1 Causes of acute upper and lower gastrointestinal bleeding

	Upper GI bleeding	Lower GI bleeding
Common	Gastric/duodenal ulcer Oesophageal/gastric varices	Diverticular disease Angiodysplasia Haemorrhoids
Less common	Gastroduodenal erosions Oesophagitis Mallory Weiss tear	Colonic neoplasms Inflammatory bowel diseases Ischaemic colitis Radiation colitis Upper GI bleeding Small bowel diseases
Rare	Upper GI malignancy Vascular malformation	Colonic ulcers Rectal varices

QUICK FLICK

26

High risk patient

Significant GI bleeding is indicated by syncope, haematemesis, systolic blood pressure below 100 mm Hg (13.3 k Pa), postural hypotension, and if more than four units of blood have to be transfused in 12 hours to maintain blood pressure. Patients over 60 years of age and with multiple underlying diseases are of higher risk of mortality. Those admitted for other medical problems (e.g. heart or respiratory failure, or cerebrovascular bleed) who develop GI bleeding during hospitalisation also have a higher mortality.

In about 80 per cent of patients, bleeding has stopped spontaneously upon presentation. In the other 20 per cent whose bleeding continues, or recurs during hospitalisation, mortality increases as much as eight times that

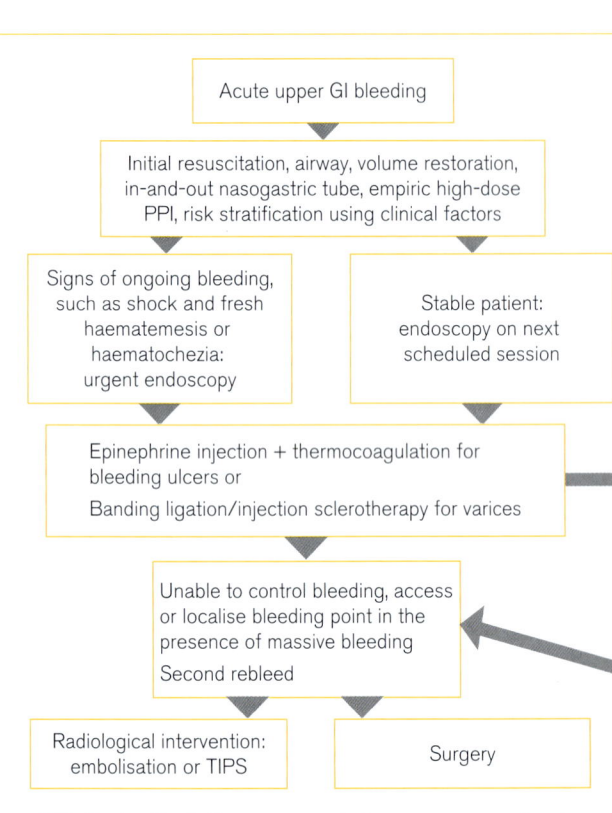

Figure 26.1 An algorithm in the management of common causes of acute upper GI bleeding

of patients without further bleeding. High-risk peptic ulcers that are actively bleeding, or have bled recently, may show stigmata of haemorrhage on endoscopy, including localised active bleeding (i.e. pulsatile, arterial spurting or simple oozing), an adherent blood clot, a protuberant vessel or a flat pigmented spot on the ulcer base. Stigmata of haemorrhage are important predictors of recurrent bleeding.

◗ **Management**

A multidisciplinary approach to the management of upper gastrointestinal bleeding is shown in Figure 26.1.

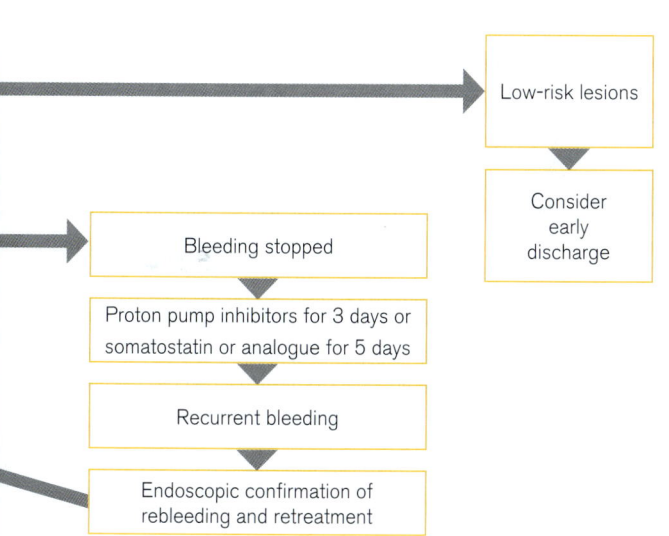

Resuscitation

Irrespective of the underlying cause of gastrointestinal bleeding, a patient should be resuscitated. The vital signs (blood pressure, pulse, oxygenation) should be carefully monitored. A large-bore peripheral drip should be inserted for fluid replacement and, if the patient is in shock, a central line would be useful. Blood transfusion should not be delayed if there is evidence of substantial volume loss. Patients with chronic liver disease might also benefit from fresh frozen plasma and platelet transfusion.

A patient with gastrointestinal bleeding is best taken care of jointly by a team comprising gastroenterologists, GI surgeons and intervention radiologists. Patients with severe acute bleeding require admission to a high-dependency or intensive care unit.

Endoscopy

Endoscopic examination offers three functions:

1. the most accurate diagnosis of the source of bleeding
2. risk assessment of the of recurrent bleeding (from an ulcer or varices)
3. endoscopic therapy, when a source of bleeding is found.

Endoscopic examination should be made available to the patient within 24 hours after index bleeding or when the patient is stabilised from his or her haemodynamic instability. It is the best tool for patient triage for hospital stay or home care. It has been shown that early endoscopy can reduce both mortality and the requirement for surgery. The following should be done during endoscopy:

- Removal of blood and blood clot. An effective suction system is mandatory, using either a large endoscope or a forceful suction device.
- Lavage of potential bleeding source (e.g. ulcer, varices, tumour) to assess the risk of recurrent bleeding. Some endoscopes are equipped with a washing device attached to the working channel. Targeted washing of the base of an ulcer to expose the underlying blood vessel is a prerequisite to effective treatment of the blood point to prevent recurrent bleeding. Sometimes, cold snaring of the blood clot using a polypectomy snare may help to expose the protuberant vessel underneath. In some cases when the stomach is filled with clots that cannot be evacuated, the use of intravenous erythromycin may hasten gastric emptying to give better vision in the stomach.
- Endoscopic haemostasis for peptic ulcers bleeding (either actively bleeding or showing protuberant vessel or fresh clot, i.e. Forrest I and IIa/b ulcers):
  - injection therapy using epinephrine or other sclerosants
  - thermocoagulation using heater probe or electrocoagulation
  - mechanical haemostasis using haemoclips or rubber band ligation.

It is generally accepted that a combination of injection and either thermal coagulation or mechanical haemostasis using haemoclips, for example, is effective in controlling acute bleeding and preventing recurrence. When injection alone is used, the effect is transient and there is therefore a high risk of rebleeding.

Thermal devices and mechanical devices are equally effective in the treatment of ulcer bleeding; they could be applied without added injection therapy.

After successful haemostasis, a routine second-look endoscopy on the following day is not necessarily conferring better protection for the patient, and therefore is not recommended.

- Endoscopic haemostasis for gastric or oesophageal varices:
  - injection of sclerosant such as ethanolamine or sodium tetradecyl sulphate (STD)
  - banding ligation using single- or multiple-band ligators
  - injection of cyanoacrylate for gastric varices.

  Banding ligation is now widely accepted as a better treatment than sclerotherapy for oesophageal varices. While their success is comparable in controlling acute variceal bleeding, banding ligation results in fewer complications such as perforation, mediastinitis and ulceration of the oesophagus and there is less risk of oesophageal stricture. There is some evidence, however, indicating that banding ligation of oesophageal varices is associated with earlier recurrence of the condition.

  Injection of cyanoacrylate ('tissue glue') should be used primarily to treat gastric varices or difficult cases of oesophageal varices when banding and sclerotherapy fail to stop the bleeding. It is associated with more serious complications such as systemic embolisation and ulceration.
- Endoscopic haemostasis for vascular malformation:
  - argon plasma coagulation
  - haemostatic clips.

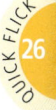

Pharmacological therapy

Acid-suppressing drugs

H_2-receptor antagonists and proton pump inhibitors (PPIs) are effective drugs for promoting ulcer healing; however, H_2-receptor antagonists cannot control acute bleeding. Since an acidic environment impairs platelet function and haemostasis, reducing the secretion of gastric acid should reduce bleeding. Potent acid suppression using intravenous PPIs (omeprazole, esomeprazole, pantoprazole and lansoprazole) reduces recurrent bleeding after endoscopic therapy.

A high-dose regimen with bolus injection followed by continuous infusion for 72 hours is recommended as the best strategy for raising intragastric pH. PPI infusion is recommended for high-risk peptic ulcer bleeding patients as an adjuvant to endoscopic therapy. It is also used before endoscopy can be arranged, as studies have shown that it probably halts active bleeding temporarily, providing a stop-gap therapy before endoscopy.

Vasoactive agents

Vasopressin (0.2–0.4 U/min) in the past was the most widely used agent for reducing portal blood pressure and controlling variceal bleeding; however, its adverse effects—cardiac ischaemia (in about 10 per cent of patients) and worsening coagulopathy (by release of plasminogen activator)—have discouraged its use in recent years. Terlipressin, a triglycyl synthetic analogue of vasopressin, has a longer half-life and fewer cardiac side effects, and appears more effective and safer when used in combination with glyceryl trinitrate.

Infusion of somatostatin and its analogues (octreotide, vapreotide) reduces portal blood pressure and azygous blood flow. They are safe and effective vasoactive agents for use in acute variceal bleeding; their benefit is more prominent if they are given early—even before endoscopy. Octreotide has also been shown to be effective when used as an adjuvant therapy in combination with endoscopic therapy. Recurrent bleeding episodes and the requirement for transfusion are significantly reduced.

Antifibrinolytic agents

Antifibrinolytic agents such as tranexamic acid have not been found useful in reducing the operative rate and mortality of acute GI haemorrhage.

Recombinant activated factor VII (rFVIIa) may be useful in difficult cases of bleeding from oesophageal varices.

Antibiotics

Antibiotics have been recommended as part of the management of variceal bleeding. Bacteraemia commonly occurs after endoscopic therapy. Prophylactic antibiotics (e.g. cephalosporin or quinolone) can prevent the development of infected ascites.

In patients at high risk of recurrent bleeding, pharmacological control without endoscopic haemostasis is inadequate: a combination of endoscopic and pharmacological therapy offers the best treatment for ulcer bleeding patients.

Radiological therapy

Angiography is an important tool in the diagnosis of gastrointestinal bleeding when endoscopy fails to identify the source. The advantages of angiography include its ability to accurately pinpoint the location of rapidly bleeding lesions, and the potential for achieving immediate control using several treatment modalities:

1. highly selective coil embolisation for bleeding ulcer and vascular malformation using:
   a. gelatin sponge pledgets
   b. microcoils
   c. polyvinyl alcohol particles
2. transjugular intrahepatic portosystemic shunt (TIPS) for gastric or oesophageal varices.

Surgery

Surgery remains the most definitive method of stopping haemorrhage. However, there is little agreement on the exact indications and best timing for surgical intervention. These issues are even less clear now that endoscopic and radiological intervention are so effective. Accordingly, good cooperation among intensivists, gastroenterologists, intervention radiologists and surgeons is essential. Indications for surgery can be:

- arterial bleeding that cannot be controlled by endoscopic haemostasis
- massive transfusion (i.e. total of 6–8 units of blood) required to maintain blood pressure
- recurring clinical bleeding after initial success in endoscopic and/or angiographic haemostasis
- evidence of GI perforation.

Bleeding of obscure origin

The source of bleeding remains unidentified after gastroscopy and colonoscopy in about 5 per cent of patients. The most common causes include angiodysplasia, small bowel neoplasms, Meckel's diverticulum, ectopic varices and conditions causing haemobilia. These often present difficult management problems. In the past, red blood cell scintigraphy and angiography were the two commonly used diagnostic tool but the yields are very low. The American Gastroenterological Association (AGA) Institute Position Statement recommendation is shown in Figure 26.2 overleaf.

With the advent of capsule endoscopy and double-balloon enteroscopy, the diagnosis and treatment success of these conditions is much improved. While capsule endoscopy is much more comfortable for patients and therefore better tolerated, double-balloon enteroscopy offers an opportunity to control the bleeding when a source is found. A new algorithm for the management of gastrointestinal bleeding of unknown origin is shown in Figure 26.3 overleaf.

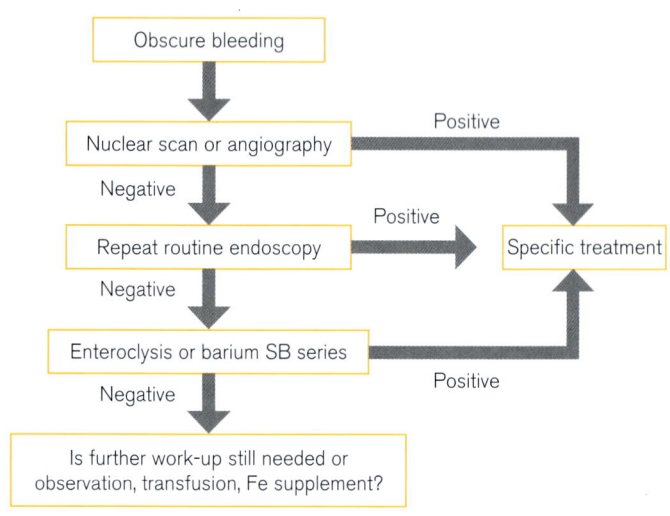

Figure 26.2 Bleeding of obscure origin

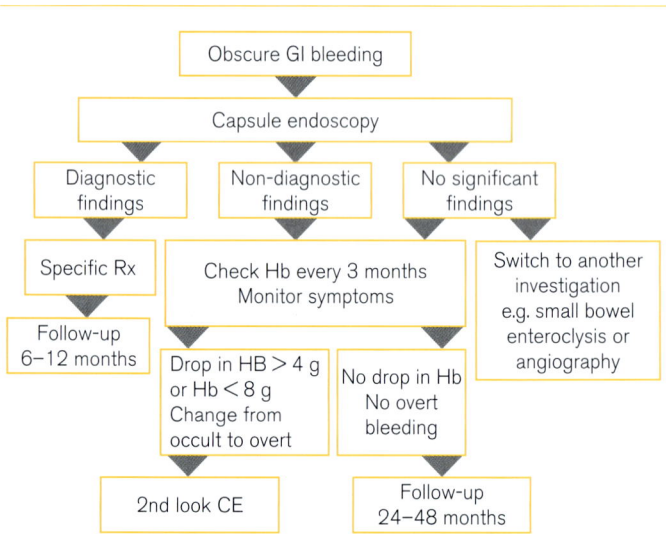

Figure 26.3 Management algorithm for gastrointestinal bleeding of obscure origin

Summary

Acute gastrointestinal bleeding is one of the most common emergency conditions associated with significant morbidity and mortality. The most common cause of upper GI bleeding is peptic ulcer. In the lower GI tract, the most common causes of bleeding are diverticular disease, vascular malformation, inflammatory bowel diseases and colorectal neoplasia. Patients over 60 who have multiple underlying diseases are at higher risk of mortality. Endoscopic examination should be made available to the patient within 24 hours or when the condition is stabilised.

Proton pump inhibitors are recommended in high-risk peptic ulcer bleeding patients as an adjuvant to endoscopic therapy. The most common causes include angiodysplasia, small bowel neoplasms, Meckel's diverticulum, ectopic varices and conditions causing haemobilia. Indications for surgery include arterial bleeding that cannot be controlled by endoscopic haemostasis, and patients requiring massive transfusions.

- the control section
- the insertion tube
- the connector section.

The insertion tube length, diameter and stiffness, the instrument channel size and the number and configuration of the distal end of the insertion tube characteristics vary according to the specific area to be examined and the purpose of the procedure. These features affect the ergonomics of an endoscope, the depth to which an endoscope can be inserted, and the type and size of accessories that can be used with an endoscope.

Control section

The control section is held in the operator's left hand. It has two knobs that direct up/down and left/right deflection of the endoscope tip. These control knobs can be locked in position. In some specialty endoscopes, such as the choledochoscope, there is only one knob with up/down deflection capability. The control section for the duodenoscope is modified for elevator control.

Valves on the upper front portion of the control section control air/water and suction, and remote switches for modifying or capturing the video image. The entry port to the instrument channel(s) is located on the lower front portion of the control section. A second instrument channel for special therapeutic procedures is available in some endoscopes.

Insertion tube

The insertion tube is attached to the control section and is the portion of the endoscope that is inserted into the patient. It contains the instrument channel, an air channel, a water channel, a CCD chip with wire connections, and angulation wires for deflecting the bending section of the insertion tube. The length, diameter and degree of stiffness of the insertion tube vary depending on the make and model of the instrument.

The endoscope tip contains the opening of the suction channel (also used for passage of the accessories), an air/water nozzle positioned to clear the lens of debris and permit air insufflations, an illumination system and an objective lens system. Different instrument models are designed with forward-, side- or oblique-viewing optics.

The connector

The connector section of the endoscope primarily comprises the processor/light source together with its electrical connections. This section also has side connectors for a water container and suction, including insertion tube venting.

◔ Types of endoscopes

Oesophagogastroduodenoscope (gastroscope)

The gastroscope is a forward-viewing instrument used primarily for evaluating the oesophagus, the stomach and the duodenum.

Enteroscope

The enteroscope is similar in design to the gastroscope except that the insertion tube is longer, allowing the evaluation of the duodenum and the proximal portion of the jejunum. An overtube may be used to avoid gastric looping, thus enhancing insertion depth.

Duodenoscope

The duodenoscope is a side-viewing instrument designed primarily for ERCP. The insertion tube length varies between 1000 mm and 1250 mm, and the diameter varies between 7.5 mm and 12 mm. Instruments with wider channels are used for the passage of the choledochoscope and choledochoscopy.

Choledochoscope

A choledochoscope is a fine-calibre endoscope that is passed through the instrument channel of a duodenoscope and inserted intraductally for the direct visualisation of the biliary and pancreatic ducts.

Echoendoscope

The echoendoscope is a hybrid instrument for high-resolution ultrasound imaging of the luminal digestive tract and adjacent organs.

◔ Indications

Upper gastrointestinal endoscopy

- Diagnostic and biopsy confirmation
- Unexplained anaemia (usually along with a colonoscopy)
- Upper gastrointestinal bleeding as evidenced by haematemesis or melaena
- Persistent dyspepsia in patients over the age of 40–45
- Heartburn and chronic acid reflux. This can lead to Barrett's oesophagus precancerous lesion
- Persistent vomiting
- Dysphagia: difficulty in swallowing
- Odynophagia: painful swallowing

Surveillance

- Surveillance of Barrett's oesophagus
- Surveillance of gastric ulcer or duodenal ulcer

Therapeutic

- Treatment of oesophageal varices (banding/sclerotherapy)
- For control of bleed: injection therapy (e.g. epinephrine for bleeding ulcers), argon plasma coagulation (APC) for vascular ectasias, endoclips for bleeding vessels
- Endoscopic snare resection, endoscopic mucosal resection, endoscopic submucosal dissection for premalignant and early malignant lesions, including polyps
- Removal of ingested foreign bodies
- Application of oesophageal/enteral stents for malignant obstruction
- Dilating and/or stenting of benign strictures
- Endoscopic balloon dilatation for achalasia cardia
- Percutaneous endoscopic gastrostomy (feeding tube placement)
- Endoscopic drainage of pancreatic pseudocyst

Newer interventions

- Endoscopic transgastric laparoscopy
- Placement of gastric balloons for obesity treatment

Colonoscopy and sigmoidoscopy

Diagnostic and biopsy confirmation

- Unexplained anaemia (usually along with an endoscopy)
- Lower gastrointestinal bleeding as evidenced by haematochezia or melaena
- Altered bowel habits (new onset) in patients over the age of 50
- Diagnosis of cause and site of acute bleed
- Diagnosis of type and extent of inflammatory bowel disease
- Diagnosis of large intestinal malignancy and histological confirmation
- Diagnosis of colorectal polyps and biopsy confirmation of the nature

Surveillance

- Surveillance of asymptomatic people over the age of 50 who are at average risk
- Personal history of prior adenomas or colon cancer
- Family history of cancer, familial adenomatous polyposis, hereditary non-polyposis colorectal cancer
- Surveillance for dysplasia in IBD

Therapeutic

- Endoscopic therapy of acute bleed: epinephrine injection, electrocautery, APC, application of bands and clips
- Colonic decompression of sigmoid volvulus

- Endoscopic polypectomy
- Stricture dilatation and stenting (obstructive malignant lesions)

◯ Small bowel enteroscopy

The small bowel had been one of the most endoscopically inaccessible areas of the gastrointestinal tract. Previously, most diagnosis and treatment of lesions within the small bowel required open surgery.

Enteroscopy now allows direct real-time visualisation of the small bowel. The newer double balloon/single balloon enteroscopy enables exploration of the entire small bowel. It also allows interventional therapy, including biopsies, haemostasis, polypectomy and tattooing. Sequential inflation and deflation of these balloons as the endoscope is advanced allows for pleating of the bowel over the scope and forward movement through the small intestine. It can be used from either an oral insertion (upper endoscopy) or an anal insertion (colonoscopy).

◯ Endoscopic retrograde cholangiopancreatography (ERCP)

ERCP has no role as a diagnostic procedure, particularly since magnetic resonance cholangiopancreatography (MRCP) has been available.

Therapeutic uses (see Tables 27.1–27.3)

- Removal of stones in choledocholithiasis (CBD) by endoscopic sphincterotomy, with or without mechanical lithotripsy or extracorporeal shock wave lithotripsy (ESWL)
- Biliary stenting and cytology in bile duct obstruction:
  – malignant obstruction: ampullary/pancreatic adenocarcinoma, cholangiocarcinoma
  – benign obstruction: chronic pancreatitis
- Endoscopic sphincterotomy for Sphincter of Oddi dysfunction (SOD)
- Pre-operative biliary decompression
- Cholangioscopy by ERCP scope for direct visualisation and targeted biopsies

Table 27.1 Therapeutic indications of ERCP

- Biliary disease
  – stones
  – biliary stenting/biliary cytology
  – sphincterotomy

continued

Table 27.1 *continued*

- Pancreatic disease
  - chronic pancreatitis (stenting/stone removal)
  - acute pancreatitis (duct damage/cyst drainage)

Table 27.2 Indications of endoscopic sphincterotomy

- Choledocholithiasis
- Acute obstructive cholangitis
- Malignant tumours
- Sphincter of Oddi dysfunction

Table 27.3 Complications of ERCP

- Acute pancreatitis
  - 0–39% post-diagnostic ERCP
  - significant pancreatitis ~2%
- Acute cholangitis
  - inadequate duct clearance
  - occurs in ~1% cases
  - unaffected by routine antibiotic administration
- Perforation in <1% of cases
- Bleeding

◔ **Complications of endoscopic procedures**

The diagnostic and therapeutic uses of endoscopic procedures of the GI tract are now well established for as a variety of complaints and disorders.

Complications related to diagnostic evaluations are rare. A survey conducted in 1974 by the American Society for Gastrointestinal Endoscopy estimated that the overall complication rate based on over 200 000 oesophagogastroduodenoscopy (EGD) examinations was only 0.13 per cent, with an associated mortality of 0.004 per cent.

Major complications related to diagnostic procedures can be classifed as:

- cardiopulmonary complications
- complications related to sedation
- infectious complications
- perforation
- bleeding.

Rates of complications are critically dependent on the method of data collection (prospective/retrospective), the definition of complication, and duration of follow-up. Early recognition of complication and prompt intervention may minimise patient morbidity.

Complications related to sedation

Complications related to sedation and analgesia are the most commonly seen complications with diagnostic endoscopy. Sedation-related complications are generally identified during the procedure and early resuscitation ensures recovery.

Cardiopulmonary complications

These range from minor changes in vital signs to myocardial infarctions, respiratory depression and shock/hypotension. Oxygen desaturation may occur in up to 70 per cent of patients undergoing various endoscopic examinations but is usually asymptomatic. Severe desaturation occurs rarely.

A difficult intubation, patient's age over 60, together with a history of cardiovascular/pulmonary disease, are common predisposing features.

Infectious complications

These result from the use of contaminated equipment. Transient bacteraemia may also occur during some therapeutic procedures. Retropharyngeal and retro-oesophageal abscesses have been reported rarely in patients who have had difficult intubations related to retropharyngeal trauma or non-clinically apparent perforations.

Perforation of the gastrointestinal tract

Related to diagnostic endoscopy, incidence is low and complications are rare.

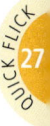

In the upper GI tract, perforation of the oesophagus is the most common and it is associated with a high mortality rate of about 25 per cent. Predisposing factors include the presence of anterior cervical osteophytes, Zenker's diverticulum, oesophageal strictures and malignancies. Pain is the most common and reproducible symptom. Fever, crepitance, chest pain, pleuritic chest pain, leukocytosis and pleural effusion may also be present.

The risk of perforation of the colon is 0.2–0.4 per cent after diagnostic colonoscopy. A higher rate is associated with polypectomy and hydrostatic balloon dilatation of colonic strictures. Perforation is more common in patients who are oversedated or under general anaesthesia, in the presence of poor bowel preparation, or with acute bleeding. Mechanical perforation by the tip of the instrument occurs at sites of weakness of the colon wall (e.g. diverticula, transmural inflammation) and proximal to obstructing points (e.g. neoplasms, strictures). Pneumatic perforation of the colon or ileum results from distension by insufflated air.

A small perforation that is recognised early may heal with conservative management. Surgical management is required for larger perforations and for failure to respond to medical management.

Significant bleeding

This is a rare complication of diagnostic endoscopy. Bleeding may be more likely in individuals with thrombocytopaenia and/or coagulopathy. Most cases resolve spontaneously.

Endoscopic procedures, including electrocoagulation, 1:10 000 epinephrine solution injection or application of endoscopic haemoclips may be required. In severe cases, transfusions, endoscopic therapy, angiography and even laparotomy may be required.

○ Novel endoscopic technologies

Wireless capsule endoscopy

Capsule endoscopy is now an accepted means for endoscopically visualising the small bowel. This involves ingesting a small capsule that contains a colour camera, battery, light source and transmitter.

Gastrointestinal peristalsis propels the capsule through the GI tract while the camera takes two pictures every second for eight hours, recording luminal detail in a 140-degree angle of view. Image data is transmittted to a data recorder worn by the patient at their waist. The images are later downloaded and processed into a video for viewing. The capsule is excreted with natural bowel movement; a rare retained capsule may require endoscopic/surgical removal.

The most common indications for capsule endoscopy is to evaluate GI bleeding, and to aid in the diagnosis of small bowel tumours and Crohn's disease. It also assists in the evaluation of malabsorption, chronic abdominal pain and chronic diarrhoea.

The primary advantage of capsule endoscopy is its non-invasive nature, avoiding the risks associated with sedation and radiation. The only shortcoming of capsule endoscopy is that it does not permit therapeutic procedures such as biopsy, ablation or control of bleed.

GI obstruction is an absolute contraindication for capsule endoscopy to prevent capsule retention. Other relative contraindications are pregnancy, GI motility disorders or large diverticuli within the small intestine.

A colon capsule endoscope for patients unable or unwilling to undergo conventional or virtual colonoscopy is under evaluation and has shown promising results.

Peroral direct cholangiopancreatoscopy

The first optical choledochoscope to assist with the intraoperative localisation of stones during bile duct exploration was described in 1941. The peroral approach was subsequently introduced in the early 1970s. Over the following 20 years the instrument was refined in scope diameter, up/down angulations and optics, permitting cholangiopancreatoscopy through the working channel of a standard therapeutic duodenoscope.

The technology was not widely adopted, however, mainly due to its limitations, including often-incompatible accessories and the requirement of a mother–daughter scope system requiring two operators.

Recently introduced peroral cholangioscopes enable direct cholangiopancreatoscopy without the need for duodenoscope or guidewire assistance, and require only one operator. The SpyGlass Direct Visualization System (Boston Scientific) and the high definition NBI capable scope (Olympus GIF-H180, Olympus America) have simplified cholangiopancreatoscopy.

These systems have been used to evaluate equivocal fluoroscopy findings during ERCP, treat difficult biliary and pancreatic duct stones, and investigate indeterminate biliary and pancreatic strictures with directed tissue sampling.

Newer imaging technology

Narrow band imaging

Narrow band imaging (NBI) technology involves narrow band filtering of the conventional white light source in an endoscope. The tissue is illuminated at selected narrow-wavelength bands, providing optical image enhancement in real time when required. The enhanced visualisation of the vascular network and surface texture of the mucosa assists in tissue characterisation, differentiation and diagnosis.

The NBI system components are identical to those in conventional red/green/blue (RGB) sequential or colour CCD endoscopes. The primary modifications are the narrow-bandwidth optical filter at the light source. NBI systems can also be coupled with electronic or optical zoom facilities for more detailed visualisation of mucosal details. Commercially available NBI systems include a two-band NBI RGB sequential endoscope (Evis Lucera 260 Spectrum) and a colour CCD endoscope (Evis Exera II 180, Olympus Medical Systems, Tokyo, Japan).

The foremost narrow band imaging application has been in analysing the surface architecture of the epithelium (pit pattern), and analysis of the vascular network. NBI can demonstrate and distinguish the alteration in the pit pattern and vasculature of the gastrointestinal mucosa in inflammatory and neoplastic (premalignant and malignant) lesions of the oesophagus, stomach and large bowel.

I-scan/FICE

I-scan from Pentax (Montvale, NJ) and Fuji intelligent chromoendoscopy (FICE) (Fujinon, Wayne, NJ) are based on post-imaging processing involving spectral estimation technology, where an endoscopic video image is reproduced at particular dedicated wavelengths using arithmetical estimation. Unlike narrow band imaging, no optical filter is used, with the result that the FICE simulated images are as bright as conventional white light images in large-diameter luminal regions of the gastrointestinal tract where NBI images are darker; this property could be more useful for screening purposes.

In vivo histologic assessment: confocal endomicroscopy, endocytoscopy

Recent advances in endoscopic imaging technology have now made microscopic observation possible at the cellular level, assisting in tissue characterisation of a variety of neoplastic and non-neoplastic lesions of the gastrointestinal tract.

Confocal endomicroscopy (CEM) provides images from layers of tissue using the principle of optical sectioning at the cellular and subcellular structures. CEM incorporates a confocal laser microscope into the tip of a flexible endoscope, giving 1000× magnification with high-resolution and real-time in vivo histology of the gastrointestinal tract mucosa.

Preliminary results have been encouraging in detecting intraepithelial neoplasias in Barrett's oesophagus, ulcerative colitis surveillance, characterisation of CBD strictures and differentiation of the nature of polyps.

The endocytoscope (E-C) system is based on the principle of light contact microscopy and enables on-the-spot assessment for cellular atypia: whereas normal cells are arranged homogenously with a normal nuclear cytoplasmic ratio, mitotic cells have heterogenous shape, altered nuclear cytoplasmic ratio and are arranged in irregular clusters. The E-C system has been used successfully in the detection of mitotic changes in vivo.

However, many challenges remain before these technologies are accepted into routine clinical practice. Personal skills and experience affect detection and diagnostic ability. Systematic additional training may be required before endoscopists can interpret cellular and subcellular images.

Summary

Gastrointestinal endoscopy has become the core of mainstream gastroenterology. The emergence of this imaging tool has transformed the perspective of the gastroenterologist and redefined gastroenterology in terms of disease processes, diagnoses, treatment and surveillance of many digestive diseases. Novel endoscopic technologies are emerging and the innovative potential continues to develop, allowing the expansion of endoscopic possibilities.

Recommended reading

Banerjee R, Reddy DN. A primer on narrow band imaging. Hyderabad: Paras Medical; 2009.

Baron TH, Kozarek R, Carr-Locke DL, editors. ERCP. Philadelphia: Saunders/Elsevier; 2008.

Cotton P, Leung J, editors. Advanced digestive endoscopy: ERCP. Boston: Blackwell; 2005.

Cotton PB, Williams CB, editors. Practical gastrointestinal endoscopy: the fundamentals. 6th ed. Oxford: Wiley-Blackwell; 2008.

Feldman M, Friedman LS, Brandt LJ, editors. Sleisenger and Fordtran's gastrointestinal and liver disease. 9th ed. Philadelphia: Saunders/Elsevier; 2010.

Wilcox CM, Munoz-Navas M, Sung JJY. Atlas of clinical gastrointestinal endoscopy. 2nd ed. Philadelphia: Saunders; 2007.

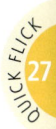

Chapter 28: Alimentary tract imaging

J. Chaganti (Australia)

Key points

- Multidetector CT scanning (MDCT) has replaced fluoroscopic contrast studies in the evaluation of suspected GI tract obstruction.
- In the evaluation of motility disorders, video fluoroscopic contrast studies precede capsule endoscopy and scintigraphy.
- While commenting on bowel gas pattern in plain radiographs, specific terminology has to be used to guide the next step in the management.
- In a suspected case of intestinal obstruction/inflammatory disease/tumours, neutral enteral contrast is preferred.
- CT enterography (CTE) is superior to fluoroscopic enteroclysis and has several advantages over conventional CT: better assessment of low-grade obstruction, enteric fistula and bowel wall thickening.
- CT colonography is as sensitive as optical colonoscopy for polyps measuring 10 mm or more.
- Magnetic resonance (MR) enterography is still evolving. Newer, faster and more robust sequences will make this procedure more attractive than CTE since it does not produce ionising radiation.

Introduction

Advances in imaging technology have changed the way the alimentary tract is interrogated. Historically, conventional imaging of the alimentary tract used plain film radiography to look for bowel gas pattern together with positive contrast (barium) to assess the motility of intestine, luminal filling defects and obstructive lesions. Double-contrast studies introduced a little later helped to visualise the mucosal pattern and also, to a limited extent, the bowel wall—useful in evaluating inflammatory disorders and neoplastic changes of both the small and large bowel.

Further developments in technique then saw the introduction of intubation of the intestine under fluoroscopy and infusing the barium under direct vision. This overcame the limitation of conventional non-intubation techniques—that is, poor distension of the intestine—enabling it to detect mild and subclinical mechanical obstruction. Clinical studies have shown that such intubation techniques correctly predict the presence of obstruction in all cases, the absence of obstruction in 88 per cent of cases, and the cause of obstruction in 86 per cent; however, intramural and extraluminal disease evaluation with these techniques was less than satisfactory.[1]

◗ Diagnostic studies

Multidetector computed tomography (MDCT)

In current medical practice, MDCT is more commonly performed than fluoroscopic studies for analysing the gastrointestinal tract. The new generation multidetector CT scanners can acquire up to 320 slices in one rotation. Dual-source scanners, that is, with two X-ray tubes mounted in the same gantry, usually acquire 520 slices in one rotation and can typically scan the entire abdomen in less than five seconds, producing isometric high-resolution images in multiple planes along with instantaneous three-dimensional data sets.

Intravenous contrast-enhanced scans can be tracked in multiple vascular phases, making it possible for the first time to assess the viability of intestine and/or tumour vascularity. Simultaneous visualisation of the arterial, capillary and venous anatomy has made catheter angiography largely redundant in the diagnosis of various vascular and related pathologies. Contrast enhancement is also helpful in accurately detecting extraintestinal findings.

MDCT is increasingly being used as the first investigation of choice for detecting free intra-abdominal air and intestinal obstruction, and is replacing plain film radiography for this purpose.

CT enterography (CTE)

Several developments in CT techniques have occurred in the past few years. Positive oral contrast, usually using diluted iodinated medium, has been routinely used in the past to assess the bowel. The current approach is to favour neutral contrast supplemented by intravenous contrast enhancement whenever inflammatory bowel disease, tumours or vascular malformations are suspected, using CT enterography. Enhancement of the bowel wall and mucosa are better appreciated against the backdrop of neutral contrast and there are fewer admixture artefacts than in positive-contrast techniques.[2]

The chief advantage of CTE is that intubation is obviated, and thus it has become more popular. While the distension of the small bowel may not be as consistent as with CT enteroclysis, the diagnostic yield still appears to be very high. CTE and CT enteroclysis appear to be equally sensitive in detecting mucosal and mural diseases and extraluminal abnormalities, although CTE is probably inferior to intubation techniques when there is subclinical obstruction.

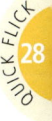

QUICK FLICK 28

CT enteroclysis

The use of CT enteroclysis was first reported in 1922; it was primarily intended to combine the advantages of contrast barium and CT scan. The procedure is the same as that of barium enteroclysis, with intubation of intestine under conscious sedation and infusing the contrast under pressure till the entire small bowel is filled. CT enteroclysis appears to be superior to conventional CT in the assessment of low-grade obstruction, enteric fistula and bowel wall thickening. The disadvantage is the relatively invasive nature of the procedure, including the insertion of a nasoenteric tube and the risks associated with conscious sedation.

CT colonography (virtual colonoscopy)

Historically, colonic polyps were diagnosed using colonoscopy examinations under direct vision; patients for whom colonoscopy was unsuccessful would then undergo a double-contrast barium enema. CT colonography is an attractive alternative for this group of patients. In this new and emerging technique, thin sections of colon are obtained from the patient in both supine and prone positions after the colon is adequately distended with room air or CO_2. The resulting multiplanar reformatted (MPR) images are studied using both minimum intensity projection algorithms and standard soft tissue window settings. The data set is also formatted into 'filet'-view and endoluminal fly-through view. The procedure requires colon preparation with laxatives on the day before the procedure, although recent studies have shown that limited prior bowel preparation together with tagging of the faeces using dilute contrast may have comparable accuracy.[3]

Current indications for CT colonography include unsuccessful colonoscopy cases, patients with increased risk for sedation, patients on anticoagulants, and evaluation of diffuse metastatic disease. It can also detect proximal synchronous polyps and cancers in patients with occlusive colorectal growths.

MR enterography

Magnetic resonance (MR) imaging has many unique properties that make it ideally suited for examining the gastrointestinal tract: the lack of ionising radiation, the ability to perform real-time and functional imaging, and the safety profile of gadolinium-based contrast agents, to name a few. In contrast, CT enteroclysis carries the risk of radiation exposure. Several diseases of the intestinal system such as polyposis, Crohn's disease and other inflammatory diseases occur in young patients and may require frequent imaging for surveillance, and CT can accumulate a possibly harmful radiation dose in such patients.

Because of its inherently superior contrast resolution, MR is ideally suited for evaluating perianal fistulas related to Crohn's disease. The enteroclysis procedure is same as for CT, with the study being performed using either positive, neutral or negative contrast. Water-based contrast using T2 weighted breath holds (HASTE, SSPE, etc) and post-contrast T1 fat-suppressed scan sequences are commonly used to interrogate the GIT. Administration of glucagon will help to reduce the artefacts caused by bowel movement. An intravenously administered contrast, gadolinium chelate, has become a critical MR imaging tool in the evaluation of GIT.

Unlike CT, where contrast enhancement depends upon volume, evaluation in MR is based on the signal change and is therefore more sensitive to subtle alterations in various disease processes. Therefore, areas of abnormal enhancement such as inflammation or infection or vascular tumours can be assessed with higher sensitivity. The common indications are Crohn's disease and the surveillance of tumours. The technique of MR colonography is still evolving; MRI is generally accepted as the 'gold standard' in the staging of rectal cancers and inflammatory bowel disease.[4]

Ultrasonography

The development of high-resolution real-time scanners and the graded compression technique has enabled sonography to evaluate the GIT very precisely. Transabdominal sonography is an elegant and safe procedure, and allows real-time evaluation of the GIT. Visualisation of the structures depends upon the luminal contents and the amount of gas present. The superior contrast resolution of ultrasonography allows visualisation of the intestinal wall, fluid-filled intestinal segments and the surrounding environment; this is particulary so in the paediatric age group, for which sonography is the investigation of choice for acute abdominal conditions.

Sonography can accurately describe changes associated with GI tract inflammation, such as wall thickening, surrounding oedema and associated lymphadenopathy. It can also localise and characterise the fluid collections and direct guided drainages. Similarly, Doppler techniques give insight into the vascularity, hyperaemia and perfusion of the given segment of the GIT. Application of intravenous ultrasound contrast agents has improved the detection of such findings.

Catheter angiography

Diagnostic catheter angiography for detecting the source of GI bleeding is becoming increasingly rare since the development of MDCT. One study has reported that detection of massive GI bleed by MDCT has 90.9 per cent sensitivity and 99 per cent specificity. Conventional angiography will continue to maintain its role in the diagnosis when other methods fail to identify the source of GI haemorrhage.[5]

Currently oesophagogastroduodenoscopy and colonoscopy are the main methods of diagnosing GI haemorrhage. Tagged red cell scans, capsule endoscopy and double-balloon endoscopy are all used with varying degrees of success. Increasingly, contrast-enhanced multiphase MDCT is being used to identify the source of haemorrhage.

Positron emission tomography with CT (PET CT)

Primarily used as research tool in the past, positron emission tomography (PET) has been developed as a powerful imaging tool in current medical practice, due largely to the fusion of CT technology with PET scanners—termed molecular imaging—which has radically changed the way imaging information is accessed. In the context of the gastrointestinal tract, PET CT is used mainly in oncological imaging for staging the malignancy.

Oesophagus

As it passes through the mediastinum, the wall of the oesophagus is impressed anteriorly and on the left side by the aortic arch. This anatomical relationship is important, as any indentation on the posterior wall and/or on the right side is pathological, often due to abnormal vascular rings, and may result in dysphagia lusoria. The complex anatomy of the cardio-oesophageal junction is beyond the scope of this chapter; however, in the present context it is sufficient to appreciate that this region is most commonly studied using endoscopy, replacing radiology as the main technique.

Imaging methods

Barium swallow remains the cornerstone of the initial assessment of the oesophagus for motility disorders. However, confirmation of the diagnosis is almost always done using manometry and/or radionuclide studies. Cross-sectional imaging methods are used to stage the cancers of pharynx and oesophagus.

Motility disorders

Pharyngo-oesophageal dysfunction is known to occur with advancing age, and in patients with neurological disorders, muscular dystrophies, structural disorders and GE reflux, and who are on medications, and for other, unknown, reasons. The characteristic feature in all of them is incoordination of the muscular contraction with weak propagation of the primary peristaltic wave. These features can be demonstrated by cinefluoroscopy while the patient is swallowing barium.

Oesophageal achalasia has a typical appearance on barium swallow and shows smooth tapering of the distal oesophagus, often expressed with the descriptive term 'bird beak'. Classically, the primary propulsive wave is also a lacking. Although considered pathognomonic, similar findings may also be observed in adenocarcinoma (pseudoachalasia) and therefore oesophagogastroduodenoscopy is essential for patients for whom the radiological diagnosis is achalasia.

Oesophageal carcinoma

Oesophageal carcinoma is a leading cause of cancer mortality worldwide. Complete resection of oesophageal cancer and adjacent malignant lymph nodes is the only potentially curative treatment, and accurate staging is crucial. On barium swallow the oesophageal cancers may present as polypoidal, infiltrative, varicoid or ulcerative lesions. While endoscopic ultrasonoscopy is considered ideal for assessing the depth of tumour invasion and the presence of regional lymph node involvement, MDCT is recommended for local resectability and in the assessment of distant metastasis. The classical CT findings include thickening of the wall, perioesophageal fat infiltration and vascular encasement. PET is useful for assessing distant metastases, but is not appropriate for detecting and staging primary tumours, and MRI provides little advantage over CT in staging oesophageal tumours.

Stomach and duodenum

The advent of endoscopy made radiological methods obsolete for evaluating the stomach and duodenum; however, the emergence of the MDCT technique has rekindled interest in the evaluation of gastric disorders. The same technology that is applied to CT colonography can be used to perform a detailed CT examination of the stomach. This technique, which uses water as contrast, is generally referred to as CT gastroscopy. The three-dimensional data set so generated can be used to reconstruct the endoluminal imaging of the stomach. Using virtual gastroscopy, one study has demonstrated the diagnosis of advanced carcinomas (with local invasion or metastatic disease) in 95 per cent of cases, in 93 per cent of cases for elevated early carcinomas (no local invasion or metastases), and 18 per cent for early depressed carcinomas.[6]

Simultaneous use of intravenous contrast enhancement and obtaining multiphase CT appears to increase the sensitivity. Virtual gastroscopy has also been used to study the various types of gastric lymphoma as well as gastrointestinal stromal tumour (GIST). These techniques are still evolving and at the time of writing had not been validated by multicentric controlled trials.

Small bowel

Small bowel obstruction: clinical considerations

Small bowel obstruction (SBO) remains difficult to accurately diagnose and treat. Radiological methods remain the main approach in the diagnosis and management of SBO. The commonest causes of SBO in Western countries are adhesions, Crohn's disease and malignancy; hernias predominate as the cause of SBO in some developing countries. The current mortality rate for patients with adhesive intestinal obstruction is in the 1–2 per cent range, indicating that the risks associated with conservative management may be acceptable.[1]

Recent literature has shown a substantial resolution rate, even in high-grade mechanical obstructions with conservative nasointestinal decompression, further supporting an even-handed approach for patients with SBO. It is important to realise, however, that preoperative diagnosis of strangulation is unreliable in 50–85 per cent of cases.

Abdominal radiography

The accuracy of abdominal radiography (AR) in SBO is 50–60 per cent.[7]

The following terminology has been suggested to describe the gas pattern in AR:

1. *Normal small bowel gas pattern*: up to four loops of small bowel less than 2.5 cm in diameter and with normal distribution of gas and faeces in non-distended colon.
2. *Abnormal but non-specific pattern*: three or more air fluid levels in the small bowel on horizontal beam films, with at least one loop distended to more than 3 cm, and the colon either of normal calibre or borderline distended. This appearance may represent low-grade SBO and may require further evaluation by barium enteroclysis or CT enteroclysis.
3. *Probable SBO pattern*: multiple gas- and fluid-filled loops of distended small bowel, with a moderate amount of colonic gas. It may be seen in early SBO, partial high-grade SBO or adynamic ileus. These patients should ideally have CT scanning; if this is inconclusive, CT enteroclysis should be considered.
4. *Definite SBO*: dilated fluid-filled small bowel loops with a gasless colon. This is diagnostic of SBO, and CT is required to assess for strangulation. In the absence of strangulation, barium enteroclysis or CT enteroclysis should be performed to determine the cause.

Barium radiography

Because barium does not inspissate in the adynamic gut, it can be safely administered orally to evaluate SBO. Ideally the small bowel should be examined with intubation and infusion using barium to help in unmasking an occult obstruction by challenging the distensibility of the bowel. Barium enteroclysis (EC) correctly predicts the site of obstruction in 86–100 per cent of cases. By EC criteria, the upper limit of the jejunum is 3 cm, and of the ileum is 2.5 cm.[1, 7]

CT

Similar to barium, the sensitivity of CT for low-grade obstructions is relatively low (63–66%) when compared to high-grade partial or complete obstructions (81%).[1, 7]

CT demonstrates the cause of obstruction and also any complications associated with it, such as closed loops and strangulation. Exclusion of these two complications is paramount for surgeons who believe in a trial of conservative non-operative management in simple mechanical SBO. Typical CT indications of closed loop obstruction include a whirl sign, which describes convergence of vessels to the twisted bowel, and also reversal of the normal relationship between artery and vein. Non-enhancement of the bowel wall is an indicator of ischaemia for which CT has a relatively low specificity (44%) but high sensitivity (95%).[7]

CT enterography (CTE) is clearly superior to conventional CT, with specificity reaching 100 per cent in diagnosing SBO, according to some reports. The classical CTE findings of obstruction are the identifiable transition zone. CTE combines the advantages of CT and EC and allows better recognition of bowel wall and mesentery. Adynamic ileus can be satisfactorily differentiated from SBO with 100 per cent specificity using CTE.[1, 7]

MRI

MDCT combines high sensitivity with high specificity in detecting acute SBO, and is the imaging method of choice. A few studies have reported that MRI imaging has a sensitivity of 95 per cent and specificity of 100 per cent in diagnosing SBO.[8]

MRI also characterises malignant and benign strictures with high sensitivity.

Crohn's disease

Crohn's disease can manifest with varied morphology—the presentation can be active inflammatory, fibrostenosing, chronic smouldering and fistulous types. MDCT is quite sensitive in identifying all of these subtypes. As discussed, the technique involves administering neutral enteral contrast along with intravenous dye enhancement. Classical findings include mucosal hyperenhancement, submucosal oedema, wall thickening and mesenteric hypervascularity (comb sign).[2]

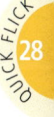

MR appears to be as sensitive as CT in moderate and marked disease. According to one study it appears to be more sensitive for milder disease forms, but this has not been well validated; further studies are required comparing these two techniques.

Small bowel tumours

Capsule endoscopy appears to be the first investigation of choice for detecting small bowel mucosal lesions. However, if mural or extramural disease is suspected, CT enteroclysis with neutral enteral and intravenous contrast is the preferred first investigation.

Large bowel—colon cancers

One of the seminal developments in CT has been virtual colonoscopy, which compares favourably with optical colonoscopy in the diagnosis of polyps greater than 10 mm in size.[2]

Currently this technology is used clinically in patients with incomplete or unsuccessful colonoscopy and for those with contraindications for sedation. MR imaging is the 'gold standard' for staging rectal cancers.

Summary

The practice of alimentary tract imaging will continue to evolve with technological advancements. The approach to the disease processes offered by the new technologies has resulted in a paradigm shift in management strategies, with better outcomes. Further advances in the diagnostic algorithms and advances in functional imaging are on the horizon.

Although one would like to think that we are in the modern imaging era of gastroenterology, this author believes we are still picking the pebbles.

References

1. Maglinte DDT, Heitkamp DE, Howard TJ, Kelvin FM, Lappas JC. Current concepts in imaging of small bowel obstruction. *Radiol Clin North Am*. 2003; 41(2):263–83, vi.

2. Maglinte DDT, Sandrasegaran K, Tann M. Advances in alimentary tract imaging. *World J Gastroenterol*. 2006; 12(20):3195–45.

3. Gryspeerdt S, Lefere P, Herman M, Deman R, Rutgeerts L, Ghillebert G, Baert F, Baekelandt M, Van Holsbeeck B. CT colonography with fecal tagging after incomplete colonoscopy. *Eur Radiol*. 2005; 15:1192–202.

4. Frøkjær JB, Drewes AM, Gregersen H. Imaging of the gastrointestinal tract: novel technologies. *World J Gastroenterol*. 2009; 15(2):160–8.

5. Woong Y, Yong YJ, Hyo SL, Sang GS, Nam GJ, Jae KK, Heoung KK. Acute massive gastrointestinal bleeding: detection and localization with arterial phase multi-detector row helical CT. *Radiology*. 2006 Apr; 239(1):160–7.

6. Horton KM, Fisherman EK. Current role of CT in imaging of the stomach. *Radiographics*. 2003; 23:75–87.

7. Sandrasegaran K, Maglinte DDT, Howard TJ, Kelvin FM, Lappas JC. The multifaceted role of radiology in small bowel obstruction. *Semin Ultrasound CT MR*. 2003; 29:319–35.

8. Fiddler J. MR imaging of the small bowel. *Radiol Clin North Am*. 2007; 45:317–31.

Recommended reading

Maglinte DDT, Howard TJ, Lillemoe KD, Sandrasegaran K, Rex DK. Small-bowel obstruction: state-of-the-art imaging and its role in clinical management. *Clin Gastroenterol Hepatol*. 2008; 6(2):130–9.

Schmidt S, Lepori D, Meuwly JY, Duvoisin B, Meuli R, Michetti P, Felley C, Schnyder P, van Melle G, Denys A. Prospective comparison of MR enteroclysis with multidetector spiral-CT enteroclysis: interobserver agreement and sensitivity by means of 'sign-by-sign' correlation. *Eur Radiol*. 2003; 13:1303–11.

Tae JK, Hyae YK, Kyung WL, Moon SK. Multimodality assessment of esophageal cancer: preoperative staging and monitoring of response to therapy. *Radiographics*. 2009 Mar; 29:403–21. doi:10.1148/rg.292085106.

Section 3

Pancreatic diseases

Chapter 29: Acute pancreatitis

C.S. Pitchumoni (USA)

Key points

▶ Acute pancreatitis most often results from gallstones (sludge/microlithiasis) and chronic alcoholism. There are many other aetiologic factors as well.

▶ The typical history of epigastric pain with elevation of serum levels of amylase/lipase to more than three times the upper limit of the normal range is diagnostic of acute pancreatitis. Only rarely is computed tomography (CT) abdomen scanning needed to confirm the diagnosis.

▶ An initial abdominal ultrasound helps to diagnose a biliary aetiology and to measure the common bile duct size, which is important in deciding the management options.

▶ Abdominal CT examination with contrast, although not needed in most cases initially, helps to assess the severity/necrosis/fluid collections when performed after 72 hours. Later in the clinical course, contrast-enhanced CT of the abdomen is needed if there is clinical suspicion of necrosis.

▶ Ranson's criteria, APACHE-II, Glasgow and various other single prognostic markers help to predict the severity and management options.

▶ Most patients with mild pancreatitis need only nil per os: nothing by mouth (NPO), intravenous fluids and pain medications in the management. Those with markers of severity need intensive care.

▶ Severe acute pancreatitis may cause multiple organ dysfunction—cardiac, respiratory, renal and metabolic.

▶ Patients with severe acute pancreatitis may need prolonged nutritional support; the preferred method is nasojejunal feeding rather than parenteral nutrition.

▶ Surgery in acute pancreatitis is needed in biliary pancreatitis, and in infected necrosis.

◐ Introduction

Acute pancreatitis is an acute inflammatory disease of the pancreas characterised clinically by sudden onset of upper abdominal pain, and biochemically by elevated levels of amylase and lipase in the serum. In mild acute pancreatitis the mortality is less than 1 per cent; in severe pancreatitis it is up to 20 per cent. Overall mortality is less than 5 per cent.

◗ Risk factors

A number of factors may cause acute pancreatitis (see Table 29.1), the most common of them being gallstone disease and chronic alcohol consumption. The incidence of acute pancreatitis is increasing worldwide. There are differences in the incidence and aetiology between, and within, countries.

Table 29.1 Common aetiologic factors in acute pancreatitis

Metabolic/toxic	Mechanical	Infectious	Vascular
Alcohol Hypertriglyceridaemia Hypercalcaemia Drugs Genetic Toxins – scorpion bite – organophosphorus	Gallstones Post-operative – biliary/gastric Pancreas divisum Trauma ERCP Tumours *Ascaris* Duodenal obstruction	Virus – Cytomegalovirus (CMV) – Epstein-Barr virus (EBV) – mumps – Coxsackie B Parasite – *Toxoplasma* – *Cryptosporidium* – *Ascaris* – *Clonorchis sinensis* – *Fasciola hepatica* Bacteria – *Legionella*	Ischaemia Vasculitis

Gallstone pancreatitis is more common in women, and alcoholic pancreatitis is more common in men. Gallstones (biliary sludge or microlithiasis) migrate from the gall bladder through the cystic duct via the common bile duct to the Ampulla of Vater and then into the duodenum. Acute pancreatitis results from transient obstruction of the ampulla, near the duodenal outlet of the pancreatic duct. Premature activation of intra-acinar trypsinogen to trypsin is the basis of acinar cell injury.

In alcoholic pancreatitis, the first episode that presents itself as acute pancreatitis usually occurs after 10–15 years of heavy drinking and at the mean age of 35–40 years. Cigarette smoking enhances alcohol-associated pancreatic injury.

Many medications are suspected to cause acute pancreatitis. They include oxycodone, azathioprine, aminosalicylates, didanosine, 6-mercaptopurine, valproic acid, furosemide and sulfonamides. Hypertriglyceridaemia with triglyceride levels usually above 1000/dL causes acute pancreatitis. Infection (bacterial, viral, parasitic), hypercalcaemia, trauma, abdominal surgery and endoscopic retrograde cholangiopancreatography (ERCP) are other causes.

A small number of patients may not have an identifiable aetiological factor.

The roles of pancreas divisum and Sphincter of Oddi dysfunction in causing pancreatitis remain controvertial. In pancreas divisum, the most

QUICK FLICK
29

common congenital anomaly of the pancreas, most of the pancreas is drained through minor papilla.

Clinical manifestations of acute pancreatitis

The terminologies of two different forms of acute pancreatitis and its complications are listed in Table 29.2.

Table 29.2 Acute pancreatitis (AP) terminologies

1. Mild AP—uneventful recovery in 3–5 days; no organ dysfunction
2. Severe AP—associated with sustained multi-organ failure (>48 hours and more than two systems) and/or local complications, extended necrosis (>50%).
3. Acute fluid collections—no defined wall seen on CT
4. Acute pseudocyst—collection of pancreatic juice enclosed by a wall of fibrous/ granulation tissue
5. Pancreatic necrosis: a. Sterile—a diffuse or focal area/areas of non-viable parenchyma b. Infected—diagnosed by fine needle aspiration
6. Pancreatic abscess—circumscribed intra-abdominal collection of pus in the pancreatic region

Source: Modified from: Atlanta system of classification. *Arch Surg*. 1993; 128:586–90.

Acute pancreatits presents itself morphologically in two distinguishable types, although there may be overlapping forms. Clinical manifestations depend on the type of pancreatitis: the mild oedematous (interstitial inflammations) form is a self-limiting disease; the necrotising form with a local necrotising inflammation and systemic local complications may be sterile or infected.

In over 95 per cent of cases the characteristic abdominal pain is the presenting feature. The typical pancreatic pain is epigastric radiating to the back, associated with nausea and vomiting, aggravated by food intake. The discomfort is lessened by sitting up and leaning forward and by fasting.

On physical examination there may be mild to severe tenderness in the epigastrium. Patients with more severe forms of pancreatitis look acutely ill. Low-grade fever, hypotension and tachycardia may be notable. Initial examination of the abdomen typically reveals distension and hypoactive or absent bowel sounds. Clinical evidence for pleural effusion, atelectasis, pneumonia or scleral icterus may be seen. Grey Turner sign (ecchymotic discolouration of the flanks) or Cullen's sign (periumbilical) are extremely rare and are not needed for diagnosis, but are among the list of single markers of severity.

Diagnosis

An algorithmic approach to the initial diagnosis of acute pancreatitis is shown in Figure 29.1. The differential diagnosis includes cholangitis, cholecystitis, peptic ulcer disease, perforated peptic ulcer and myocardial infarction.

Suspect AP based on history of sudden onset of upper abdominal pain

↓

Physical findings may only include epigastric tenderness/decreased or absent bowel sounds

↓

- Initial lab studies: blood count, haemoglobin, amylase/lipase, blood sugar
- Alkaline phosphatase, ALT, AST, total bilirubin, LDH, albumin
- Serum calcium, BUN, creatinine, serum electrolytes, serum triglycerides
- Arterial blood gas (only in selected cases if patient has dyspnea)
- CRP in 48 hours

↓

- Establish diagnosis of AP when serum amylase and/or lipase $>$ 3 times ULN
- Exception: hyperlipidaemic pancreatitis (amylase may be normal)

↓

Initial imaging studies:
- abdominal ultrasound to rule out a biliary aetiology
- CXR to rule out pleural effusion (a marker of severity)
- KUB to rule out other causes of sudden-onset abdominal pain

Figure 29.1 Acute pancreatitis (AP) diagnostic algorithm

Initial diagnostic tests

In acute pancreatitis the levels of serum amylase increase sharply after the onset of symptoms, and return to normal within four days. Modest elevation of serum amylase is seen in a number of conditions other than acute pancreatitis (see Table 29.3). Elevation of amylase level more than three times normal is a feature of acute pancreatitis. Amylase levels may *not* be elevated in hypertriglyceridaemic acute pancreatitis because high triglyceride levels interfere with amylase activity.

Table 29.3 Non-pancreatic causes of elevated serum amylase and lipase levels

Amylase elevation	Lipase elevation
Intestinal ischaemia, obstruction	Intestinal ischaemia, obstruction
Perforated peptic ulcer	Duodenal ulcer
Diabetic ketoacidosis	Diabetic ketoacidosis
Macroamylasaemia	Macrolipasaemia
Renal failure	Renal failure
After ERCP	After ERCP
Parotitis, mumps	Head trauma or intracranial mass
Coeliac disease	Coeliac disease
Ectopic pregnancy, salpingitis	
Alcoholism	
Anorexia nervosa	

Elevation of serum lipase levels is often considered to be more specific; however, it also occurs in other conditions. Lipase levels rise within eight hours of onset, peak in 24 hours and decrease within eight to 14 days.

Other laboratory studies (see Figure 29.2, page 310) are initially needed for predicting severity, and in identifying an aetiological factor.

The levels of elevation of serum amylase and lipase do not parallel the severity of pancreatitis. Serial amylase and lipase levels are not needed in the follow-up.

Once a diagnosis is established, the next step is to predict the severity (risk stratification). A number of well-known criteria based on multiple scoring—Ranson's (see Table 29.4), Imrie, Glasgow, APACHE-II scale—and other single markers of prognosis are available (see Table 29.5). The newer single markers of severity are easy to remember and use in clinical practice.

Table 29.4 Ranson's criteria

Parameter	1974 version (all aetiologies)
At admission	
Age (yr)	>55
White cell count (x 109/L)	>16
Blood glucose (mg/dL)	>200
LDH (U/L)	>350
AST (U/L)	>250
48 hours	
Haematocrit decrease (%)	>10
BUN rise (mg/dL)	>5
Uncorrected calcium (mg/dL)	<8
Arterial PO$_2$ (mm Hg)	<60
Arterial base deficit (mmol/L)	>4
Fluid sequestration	>6000

Table 29.5 Single markers of prognosis

1. Obesity: BMI > 30

2. Ecchymosis

3. Admission haemoconcentration > 44

4. Failure to correct haemoconcentration to < 44 in 24 hours

5. Serum creatinine >2 mg/dL on admission, failure to reduce to < 2 with fluid administration

6. Fasting blood sugar >125 mg/dL*

7. Urinary trypsinogen activation peptide <30 nmol/L (negative predictive value)**

8. Pleural effusion

9. C-reactive protein >150 mg/L at 48 hours

* Normal blood glucose on admission correlates with interstitial, not necrotising AP.
** 100% negative predictive value if UTAP is <30 nmol/L when tested within 12 hours.

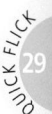
QUICK FLICK
29

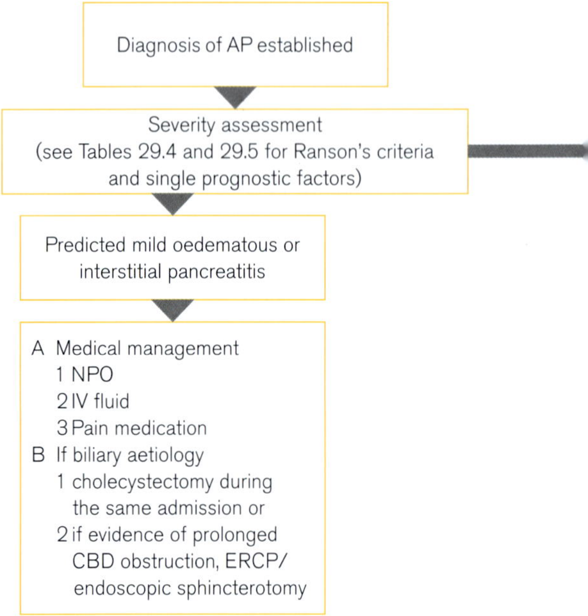

Figure 29.2 Management algorithm for acute pancreatitis

Imaging studies

An initial plain X-ray of the abdomen is more help in excluding the diagnosis of perforated ulcer or intestinal obstruction than in diagnosing pancreatitis. Dilated loops of small bowel ('sentinel loop') or transverse colon ('colon cut-off sign') are non-specific and infrequent. A chest X-ray helps to evaluate the lungs and to diagnose pleural effusion.

An initial abdominal ultrasound is essential in all cases except when an alcoholic aetiology is quite clear. The main purpose is to look for gallstones or sludge, and assess the common bile duct (CBD) size.

Computed tomography (CT) of the abdomen is not needed in all patients with suspected pancreatitis. Contrast-enhanced CT helps in assessing severity of acute pancreatitis.

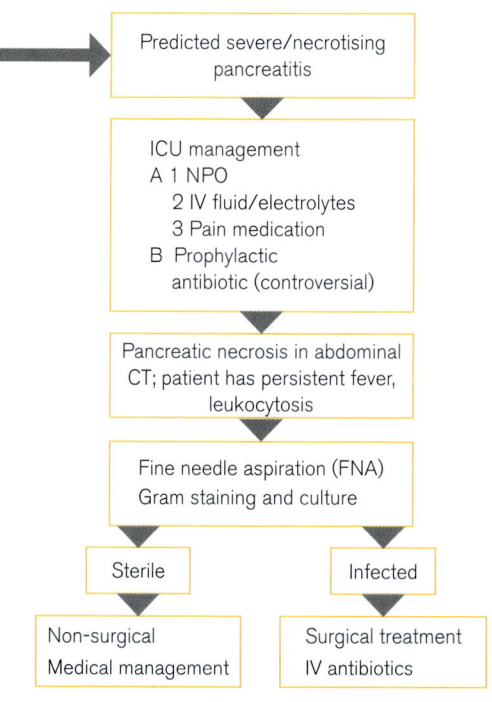

Specialised studies such as magnetic resonance imaging (MRI), magnetic resonance cholangiopancreatography (MRCP) and endoscopic ultrasound (EUS) have only limited value in routine management, but may be needed to exclude a CBD stone in the presence of a dilated duct or persistently abnormal liver enzymes. ERCP has no role in the diagnostic evaluation of acute pancreatitis. Its value is only in therapeutic endoscopy in reducing biliary obstruction.

Management

- 'Rest to the pancreas' is given by keeping the patient NPO. Routine use of nasogastric tube aspiration of the stomach is only needed in exceptional cases where the patient has protracted vomiting, or for a few patients with severe acute pancreatitis.

- Analgesic administration in pain management is crucial. Demerol, morphine or hydromorphone are frequently given.
- Aggressive fluid replacement, especially in the early phase, is crucial for maintaining haemodynamic stability.
- Early recognition of severity by appropriate prognostic evaluation, and transferring patients with predicted severe pancreatitis to intensive care (or to a tertiary care centre if needed).
- Those who do not respond promptly and are expected to be NPO for a long period need to be given nutritional support. Short-term peripheral parenteral nutrition may be helpful. Total parenteral nutrition (TPN) is to be discouraged—fungal sepsis is a severe clinical complication.
- The value of early enteral feeding is clearly proven. Intrajejunal tube feeding has many advantages over TPN, including reducing cost and reducing complications, and in providing a healthy bacterial flora that promotes gut immunity. Most importantly, jejunal feeding is not associated with a substantial stimulus to the pancreas.
- Surgical consultation is needed if a biliary aetiology is suspected. Cholecystectomy in the same hospitalisation is advocated. Complicated pancreatitis also requires surgical consultation.
- Prophylactic antibiotic therapy is not needed in most cases, although the topic is controversial. In patients with evidence of ascending cholangitis and in infected pancreatic necrosis, the indication for antibiotic therapy is quite clear. Sterile necrosis is not an indication for antibiotic therapy.

ERCP or endoscopicsphincterotomy (ES) are needed only in cases with demonstrated CBD obstruction and inpending ascending cholangitis. A patient with severe acute pancreatitis and multi-organ system dysfunction may also require ES as a temporising measure.

⊃ Prognosis

Mortality in acute pancreatitis occurs in two peaks. The first peak is usually in the first 72 hours (and, in a small number of cases, even before the patient reaches the hospital). The first peak of mortality cannot be assessed by imaging studies since it is not morphological, but by cytokine-activated and systemic inflammatory response, and multi-organ failure.

The second peak is associated with necrosis (irreversible death of tissues) and/or infection, and occurs two weeks later. Gross destruction of the pancreas (necrosis) is seen in about 20 per cent of patients. The pancreas fails to enhance after a rapid intravenous bolus injection of contrast followed by rapid CT imaging. Pancreatic necrosis is associated with local and systemic complications. Patients with sterile necrosis also display clinical signs resembling sepsis, characterised by fever, leukocytosis and abdominal pain.

Patients with severe pancreatic necrosis (>50%) are at high risk of infection. A CT-guided fine needle aspiration (FNA) and Gram staining of the aspirated material helps to diagnose infected necrosis. Infected necrosis is to be treated with antibiotics and by surgical debridement. Ciprofloxacin with metronidazole or imipenem (an intravenous beta-lactam antiobiotic) are among the choice of antibiotics.

⟡ Complications

Acute pancreatitis is a multi-system disease. The complications can be classified as intra-abdominal and systemic (see Table 29.6).

Table 29.6 Complications of acute pancreatitis

Systemic
Pulmonary: hypoxaemia, pleural effusion, acute respiratory distress syndrome (ARDS)
Cardiac: shock, pericardial effusion, electrocardiographic changes, arrhythmias
Haematologic: disseminated intravascular coagulation (DIC), thrombotic thrombocytopenic purpura (TTP)
Renal: azotaemia, oliguria, myoglobinuria
Metabolic: hypocalcaemia, hyperglycaemia, acidosis, hypoalbuminaemia
Central nervous system: psychosis, Purtscher's retinopathy
Peripheral: rhabdomyolysis, fat necrosis, bone necrosis, arthritis

Intra-abdominal
Pancreatic
Necrosis: sterile vs. infected; non-viable parenchyma
Fluid collections:
a. peripancreatic
b. pseudocyst (infection, rupture, haemorrhage)
c. abscess
Local extrapancreatic
Pancreatic ascites: high-protein, high-amylase ascites
Involvement of adjacent organs: splenic vein thrombosis, colonic infarction, lower GI bleeding
Obstructive jaundice

QUICK FLICK
29

A pseudocyst that usually forms after four weeks may be either asymptomatic or symptomatic. Asymptomatic pseudocysts need observation only. A pseudocyst that is painful, infected, pressing upon adjacent organs or growing under observation needs surgical, endoscopic or percutaneous drainage. Size alone does not determine the need for intervention. A pseudocyst may cause abdominal pain, may compress upon adjacent organs, rupture, bleed or become infected.

Pancreatic abscess needs surgery and antibiotic therapy. An open surgical debridement with continuous short-term lavage of the lesser sac is needed. Repeated surgery may be needed. The prognosis is better than for infected necrosis.

○ When to refer the patient

Most patients have mild (oedematous) pancreatitis. Patients with markers of severity, prolonged biliary obstruction, signs and symptoms of sepsis, or imaging evidence of necrosis, need to be referred to a gastroenterologist, a surgeon and an intensive care specialist. Severe acute pancreatitis is to be managed by a team of physicians comprising a gastroenterologist, surgeon, internist, an infectious disease specialist and an interventional radiologist. Patients with severe acute pancreatitis need intensive care management.

Summary

The commonest causes of acute pancreatitis are gallstones (sludge/microlithiasis) and chronic alcoholism. The typical history is of epigastric pain, often radiating to the back, and elevation of serum amylase and lipase to three times above the normal level. Imaging procedures include abdominal ultrasound (always) and abdominal contrast-enhanced CT scan, usually after 72 hours. Severity is predicted by various scoring systems, including Ranson's criteria, APACHE-II and Glasgow score. In mild cases management focuses on NPO, IV fluids and analgesia. Severe cases require ICU care as multiple organ dysfunction can occur. The latter complication can also occur after the second week following the onset. In those patients requiring prolonged nutritional support, nasojejunal feeding is the preferred method. Surgery is required for biliary pancreatitis and infected necrosis.

Information for patients

What is the pancreas? What is its function?

The pancreas is a gland that is about 17 cm long, located right at the back of the abdomen, across the vertebrae. The gland secretes many hormones, the two most important being insulin and glucagon that regulate the blood sugar, and it also secretes enzymes that digest food.

What is acute pancreatitis?

Inflammation of the pancreas, characterised by sudden upper abdominal pain that goes to the upper back, associated with nausea and vomiting. Children as well as adults can develop acute pancreatitis.

What causes acute pancreatitis?

There are many causes, but the two most frequent are stones in the gall bladder and alcoholism. Rarely, excessive fat in the blood (triglyceride), certain medications, physical injury to the gland and infections may cause acute pancreatitis.

How is acute pancreatitis diagnosed?

By the history of sudden onset of upper abdominal pain, together with increased levels of one or two pancreatic enzymes (amylase and lipase) in the patient's blood. Rarely, an abdominal ultrasound or a CT scan is necessary to diagnose the disease.

How serious is acute pancreatitis?

The disease can be mild in 80 per cent of cases, and the overall mortality is around five per cent. In serous acute pancreatitis, however, which occurs in almost 20 per cent of all cases, the disease can be very severe and the pancreatic enzymes that enter the blood can cause injury to the lungs, heart and kidneys. In rare cases the pancreas may be damaged, with dead areas which may become infected and may be associated with serious complications and even the death of the patient.

How is acute pancreatitis managed?

The patient is given intravenous fluids, and 'rest' to the pancreas is given by not taking food by mouth. If gallstones are found, surgical removal of the gall bladder is necessary.

Recommended reading

Banks PA, Freeman ML. Practice guidelines in acute pancreatitis. *Am J Gastroenterol*. 2006; 101:2379–400.

Beger HG, Rau BM. Severe acute pancreatitis: clinical course and management. *World J Gastroenterol*. 2007; 13:5043–51.

Bradley EL III. A clinically based classification system for acute pancreatitis. Summary of the International Symposium on Acute Pancreatitis; Atlanta 1992. *Arch Surg*. 1993; 128:586–90.

Yadav D, Agarwal N, Pitchumoni CS. A clinical evaluation of laboratory tests in acute pancreatitis. *Am J Gastroenterol*. 2002; 97:1309–18.

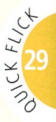
QUICK FLICK 29

Chapter 30: Chronic pancreatitis

C.S. Pitchumoni (USA)

Key points

▶ The most important cause of chronic pancreatitis (CP) is excessive consumption of alcohol for 10 or more years.

▶ Other causes or types of CP include tropical, hereditary, idiopathic, obstructive, hyperlipidaemic and hypercalcaemic chronic pancreatitis.

▶ The recent discovery of genetic mutations in hereditary pancreatitis explains predisposition to CP of other aetiologic factors.

▶ Recurrent abdominal pain, fat malabsorption and diabetes are the cardinal manifestations of CP.

▶ Autoimmune pancreatitis is a newly discovered type with distinctive clinical features that mimic pancreatic cancer. Other autoimmune disorders may coexist. Response to steroid therapy is characteristic.

▶ Plain X-ray of abdomen, ultrasound, computed tomography (CT) scan, magnetic resonance imaging (MRI) scan, endoscopic ultrasound and endoscopic retrograde cholangiopancreatography (ERCP) help in the diagnosis of CP. Secretin stimulation test is very sensitive, but time consuming.

▶ Abstinence from alcohol/cigarette smoking are important steps in the management.

▶ Pancreatic pain is multifactorial and medical management includes use of analgesics, pancreatic enzymes and antioxidants. Surgery may succeed in appropriate cases. Endoscopic therapy helps in a few cases.

▶ Patients with steatorrhoea need oral pancreatic enzyme therapy.

▶ Chronic pancreatitis has a number of complications including pseudocyst, pancreatic ascites and pancreatic cancer.

○ Introduction

Chronic pancreatitis is a chronic disease of the pancreas, characterised clinically by recurrent upper abdominal pain, associated with malabsorption of fat (steatorrhoea) and diabetes mellitus.

Pathological characteristics include varying degrees of irreversible fibrosis of the pancreas, loss of exocrine parenchyma, atrophic changes of acinar cells, and intraductal calculi (see Table 30.1). Tropical pancreatitis, hereditary pancreatitis, and two types of idiopathic pancreatitis (early onset and late onset), are also described.

Table 30.1 Chronic pancreatitis types, clinical features and pathogenesis

Types	Clinical features	Pathogenesis
Alcoholic	– Mean age of onset 30–35 yr – Alcoholism for > 15 yr, > 80 g/d – Painful episodes followed by calculi (9 yr), later steatorrhoea (13 yr), diabetes (20 yr)	1. Unfavourable secretory changes: viscous pancreatic juice–protein plugs 2. Early acinar cell injury
Tropical	– Prevalent in Afro-Asian countries – Affects young adults – Episodes of abdominal pain – Early onset of diabetes and calculi – High incidence of pancreatic cancer	– Non-alcoholic – No proven aetiologic factors – Genetic factors identified (SPINK1 mutation)
Hereditary	– Abdominal pain in childhood – Calculi later in life – Pancreatic cancer at a young age	– Autosomal dominant – Mutations in cationic trypsinogen genes (PRSS1)
Idiopathic	Two types: 1. Early onset: painful, calculi, steatorrhoea, diabetes 2. Late onset (senile): painless, pancreatic calculi are incidental	Idiopathic
Obstructive	– Calculi rare, marked dilated ducts – Relieved by surgery	– Post-traumatic ductal strictures – Periampullary tumours – Pancreas divisum
Autoimmune	More in men. Clinical features resemble those of pancreatic cancer.	Mutations in serine protease 1 gene most common genetic abnormality

Two other rare forms of the disease are obstructive chronic pancreatitis and the newly described autoimmune type with distinctive clinical and pathological findings.

○ Epidemiology and risk factors

The epidemiology of CP is closely associated with the extent of alcohol abuse in the community. Most available epidemiological data stems from Western countries and Japan. Annual incidence varies widely

(1.9 to 14.1 per 100 000). All over the world there has been an increase in alcoholism and alcoholic pancreatitis. In India, for example, the incidence and prevalence of alcohol-induced pancreatitis is on the rise. The epidemiology of CP in Western countries differs from that in Afro-Asian countries to some extent because of the prevalence of tropical pancreatitis in the latter countries.

The quantity and duration of alcohol consumption is linearly correlated with the risk of pancreatitis. Cigarette smoking, often associated with alcoholism, is an added risk factor.

◐ Alcoholic pancreatitis

Pathogenesis

The pathogenesis of alcoholic pancreatitis is not well understood; however, there are many theories, including the following.

Acinar cell injury (toxic-metabolite hypothesis)

A direct toxic effect of alcohol is suspected to cause acinar cell injury. Ongoing necrosis and fibrosis provides the basis for recurrent acute and ongoing chronic pancreatitis (Klöppel's theory). Pancreatic stellate cells (PSC) play a major role in cellular injury.

Small duct hypothesis (unfavourable secretory changes, protein plug theory) (Sarles' hypothesis)

Pathophysiological events begin with the formation of a protein plug inside the ducts and ductules. Sequential changes in the composition of pancreatic juice of alcoholic patients promote protein-plug formation. Highly viscous pancreatic secretion rich in proteins precipitate first, and calcium is then deposited to form stones. Acinar cells atrophy and fibrous tissue replaces the acinar cells.

Clinical

The profile of a patient with alcoholic pancreatitis is characteristic. In an alcoholic male with a history of consuming more than 80 g of alcohol per day for 10 to 15 years, usually the first attack of pancreatitis may occur around the age of 30.

The cardinal manifestations of clinical importance and prevalence are episodes of abdominal pain, steatorrhoea and diabetes mellitus.

Pancreatic pain is typically localised in the upper abdomen, radiating back to the vertebrae, partially alleviated by sitting up and leaning forward and by fasting. Associated nausea and vomiting may occur.

Tropical pancreatitis

Tropical pancreatitis is a form of CP characterised by recurrent abdominal pain, pancreatic calculi and diabetes mellitus, occurring mostly among children and young adults in many Afro-Asian nations such as Uganda, Nigeria, the Republic of Congo, Malawi, Zambia, Ghana, Ivory Coast and Madagascar; Sri Lanka, Indonesia, Malaysia, Thailand, India and Bangladesh; and also in Brazil.

Signs of malnutrition may be primary or secondary to chronic pancreatic insufficiency.

In advanced stages of the disease the pancreatic gland is small and the surface irregular and nodular because of fibrosis.

Microscopically, the characteristic feature is diffuse fibrosis of the pancreas. The main duct, the collecting ducts and small ductules show marked dilatation with periductular fibrosis.

With further advance of the disease, the islets of Langerhans (containig cells that produce hormones) become isolated and surrounded by dense fibrous tissue. In some instances, the islets appear hypertrophied and nesidioblastosis is seen.

There is a high incidence of pancreatic carcinoma in patients with tropical pancreatitis.

The exact aetiology of this disease has not been established. Protein malnutrition does not appear to be the initiating factor of this disease.

Chronic pancreatitis—alcoholic or tropical—has been hypothesised as one of the many diseases caused by unmitigated free radical (FR) injury. Reports of many recent studies describe searches for genetic abnormalities. In four such studies, three from India and the other from Bangladesh, tropical pancreatitis was noted to be associated with the SPINK1 N34S mutation.

Hereditary pancreatitis

Hereditary pancreatitis (HP) is a rare form of CP, transmitted by an autosomal dominant trait with a penetrance of 80 per cent. Mutations in the serine protease 1 gene (PRSS1) that encodes cationic trypsinogen are the most common genetic abnormalities associated with hereditary panceatitis. The mutations enhance premature activation of trypsinogen to trypsin in the acinar cell, initiating cell injury. Three genetic markers in relation to CP are currently recognised: cationic trypsinogen gene mutation, SPINK1 mutation and cystic fibrosis transmembrane regulator (CFTR) mutation. Of these, only cationic trypsinogen genetic mutation is aetiologically associated with hereditary pancreatitis. The main clinical significance of HP is the high predisposition for pancreatic cancer in patients with the disease.

�‣ Idiopathic pancreatitis

Idiopathic pancreatitis has two subsets. The juvenile form is characterised by male preponderance, age of onset before 25 years, and a long history of recurrent attacks of abdominal pain. The hallmarks of CP—calculi formation, pancreatic insufficiency and diabetes—develop 25 to 28 years after the onset of the disease. Prognosis is poor.

There is also a late-onset idiopathic CP (senile pancreatitis), which may occur after the age of 60. This type of pancreatitis, which is often painless, is diagnosed by the fortuitous discovery of pancreatic calculi in a routine abdominal radiograph or during the evaluation of a patient with steatorrhoea of uncertain aetiology.

◣ Obstructive pancreatitis

Obstructive pancreatitis is a very rare form of CP. It results from a blockage of flow in the large pancreatic ducts as a result of a scar or tumour. This may be a curable form of CP if the obstruction is relieved endoscopically or surgically.

◣ Clinical features of chronic pancreatitis (excluding autoimmune pancreatitis)

Abdominal pain

The mechanism of pain in CP is multifactorial. Intraductal hypertension is a major and probably a remediable cause. Intraductal stones, strictures and obstructions to the flow of stimulated pancreatic secretions may be responsible for postprandial pain.

Other pain mechanisms include ongoing pancreatic injury, pancreatic ischaemia (compartment syndrome), neuronal changes (neuronal hypertrophy, lack of nerve sheath with accumulation of perineural inflammatory cells), enhanced free radical injury (antioxidant deficiency), interleukin-mediated injury, extrapancreatic causes (biliary obstruction, duodenal obstruction, peptic ulcer) and pseudocysts.

Pancreatic pain in some patients may become less or disappear after many years ('burnt-out pancreas').

Malabsorption

Pancreatic insufficiency mainly affects fat absorption, and to a lesser degree absorption of protein and carbohydrate.

Steatorrhoea (fat malabsorption) does not occur until over 90 per cent of the exocrine tissue is destroyed. Steatorrhoea is characterised by the patient's noting fat or oil drops with the stool, which is often loose and foul smelling.

Weight loss becomes an added feature, with malabsorption of nutrients. Fat-soluble vitamins may also be malabsorbed. Stool fat determination is usually made on a collection of 72 hours of stool. Faecal fat excretion of <7 g/day with a 100 g/day fat diet excludes steatorrhoea.

Clinical vitamin B_{12} malabsorption is infrequent, but may occur.

Diabetes mellitus

Diabetes mellitus occurs approximately 10 years after the onset of CP.

Overt diabetic ketoacidosis is rare. Vascular complications and neuropathy may occur and are related to the duration of diabetes.

◑ Diagnosis of CP

Eliciting the typical history of pancreatic pain is the starting point in the diagnostic algorithm (see Figure 30.1 overleaf).

Radiological imaging studies are more popular, readily available and often performed instead of time-consuming pancreatic function studies. Imaging methods include:

- Plain film X-ray of the abdomen is the initial study. Pancreatic stones are diagnostic of CP, but occur late in the natural history of CP.
- Abdominal ultrasound suggests CP by demonstrating glandular atrophy, calculi, parenchymal heterogeneity, pancreatic pseudocysts, bile duct obstruction/dilatation, and other contiguous organ involvements. Splenomegaly will indicate portal hypertension as a result of splenic vein thrombosis.
- Contrast-enhanced CT scan of the abdomen provides a clear imaging of the pancreas in identifying most of the above findings. It has a sensitivity of 80 per cent and specificity of 85 per cent and currently it is the diagnostic procedure of choice.
- MRI with magnetic resonance cholangiopancreatography (MRCP) detects ductal morphology, dilatations and strictures, but it is expensive and not always available. Claustrophobic patients will not tolerate the procedure.
- ERCP findings include dilated main duct and side branches ('chain of lakes' appearance) which are highly sensitive (70–90%) and highly specific (90–100%). The limitations of ERCP include its high cost and the risk of ERCP-related complications (pancreatitis, perforation and sepsis).
- Endoscopic ultrasound (EUS) is emerging as a very sensitive diagnostic modality. EUS identifies parenchymal changes (hyperechoic foci), cystic abnormalities, stones or protein plugs in the ducts, and pseudocysts.
- The secretin stimulation test, in which duodenal pancreatic secretions are aspirated before and after IV secretin stimulation of the pancreas,

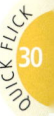
QUICK FLICK 30

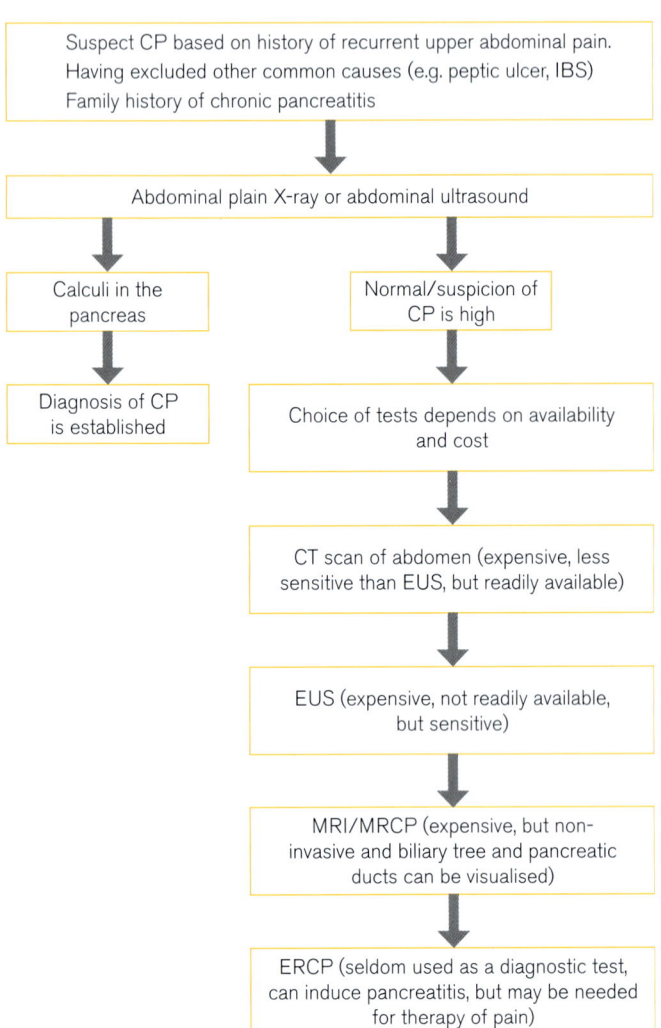

Figure 30.1 Algorithm of diagnosis of chronic pancreatitis (excluding autoimmune type)

is often considered to be the 'gold standard'. Only a few specialised centres perform this test. A decrease in the bicarbonate concentration (<80 mEq/L) is indicative of pancreatic insufficiency.

◐ Management

Management of pain

Management of chronic pancreatitis requires a team approach. A gastroenterologist, surgeon, radiologist and psychiatrist should work together to achieve success. It is difficult to assess the severity of pain in patients with CP since many of them are addicted to alcohol and/or narcotics.

Easily treated complications such as pseudocysts, bile duct obstruction and peptic ulcer disease should be ruled out first.

Abstinence from alcohol

The rate of pain relief is usually higher in abstinent patients and deterioration of pancreatic function is slower. Smoking cessation is also important.

Diet

The goal is to avoid excessive stimulation of the pancreas while maintaining adequate nutrition. The diet should be rich in calories and nutrients and low in fat. Frequent small meals should be helpful. The diet should also be modified if there is associated diabetes and/or steatorrhoea.

Supplementation with oral antioxidants

This is reported to reduce the intensity and frequency of pain, perhaps as a result of reduced free radical injury.

Analgesics

The first step is to try non-opioid analgesics such as acetaminophen, salicylates and nonsteroidal anti-inflammatory drugs (NSAIDs). Most patients, however, need opioid analgesics for symptomatic relief, and the initial doses should be low and administered infrequently.

Oral pancreatic enzyme therapy

Experimental evidence indicates that the presence of intraluminal proteases in the proximal small intestine inhibits the release of cholecystokinin and thereby inhibits stimulation of the exocrine parenchyma.

To affect feedback inhibition of pancreatic secretion, it is important to administer large doses of non-enteric coated pancreatic enzymes.

Endoscopic therapy

Techniques include endoscopic sphincterotomy, stenting and extracorporeal shock wave lithotripsy (ESWL).

QUICK FLICK 30

Endoscopic therapies are based on the premise that the most important mechanism of pain in CP is impairment of the outflow of pancreatic secretion by strictures or calculi in the main pancreatic duct. The attractive feature of an endoscopic drainage procedure is that it offers an alternative to surgical drainage.

Surgery

Surgical therapy for pancreatic pain is an option in selected cases. The type of surgery is based on the nature of the ductal disease (big duct vs small duct) as determined by ERCP or MRCP.

Longitudinal pancreaticojejunostomy or lateral pancreaticojejunostomy (modified Puestow procedure) is helpful only for patients with strictures and dilatations of the main pancreatic duct. Long-term pain relief is achieved in more than two-thirds of patients. Some 60–75 per cent of patients are pain-free for five or six years.

Pancreatic resective procedures are of choice when ducts are not dilated (small duct disease), or when a previous drainage procedure has failed, or if pathological changes predominantly involve a particular area of the pancreas.

Neurolytic therapies such as coeliac ganglion block offer only temporary relief.

Management of steatorrhoea

Dietary manipulation

A low-fat diet is generally recommended. In general a 20 g fat diet is prescribed.

The usual dietary fat, long-chain triglyceride (LCT), needs lipolysis by pancreatic lipase and micelle formation with bile acids for absorption through healthy villi.

Medium-chain triglycerides (MTC) with 6–12 carbon atoms undergo better intragastric lipolysis than LCTs; they also require less pancreatic lipolysis, and are effectively absorbed and delivered into the portal vein and not lymphatics. MCT supplementation offers excellent nutritional support.

Supplementary oral pancreatic enzyme therapy is important. Microencapsulated pancreatic enzyme preparations with high lipase concentrations are effective.

○ Autoimmune pancreatitis

Most cases of autoimmune pancreatitis (AIP) have been reported in the USA, Korea and Japan. AIP has been increasingly recognised only recently as a systemic fibroinflammatory disease that affects not only the pancreas but also other organs including the bile duct, salivary glands, the retroperitoneum and lymph nodes. The affected organs characteristically have lymphoplasmacytic infiltrate rich in IgG4-positive cells. AIP is associated with a number of other autoimmune disorders such as primary sclerosing cholangitis, Sjögren's syndrome and retroperitoneal fibrosis.

There is a male preponderance, with mean age of presentation 63 ± 18 years (range 14–85 years). The initial presentation is often obstructive jaundice with a pancreatic mass and mild or no abdominal pain. Many patients are mistakenly diagnosed initially as having pancreatic cancer and might even have undergone surgery.

Radiological findings include diffuse or focal pancreatic enlargement. A 'sausage-shaped' pancreas is reported, along with homogeneous attenuation, moderate enhancement and a peripheral rim, or 'halo', of hypoattenuation. The finding of pancreatic ductal narrowing on ERCP or MRCP is highly diagnostic.

Many diagnostic criteria (Japanese, Korean, Mayo Clinic) have been proposed. A CT scan shows diffuse or local gland enlargement; ERCP reveals long, attenuated segments of pancreatic duct. An elevated serum IgG4 level is seen in a large number of patients. Pathological confirmation is often difficult. Response to steroid therapy with prednisone 40 mg for four weeks is also a feature of AIP.

▷ When to refer the patient

Alcoholic patients require education by an internist, and referral to an alcohol rehabilitation program. Consultation with a pancreatic surgeon is needed if medical measures fail to relieve pain and when the patient's ductal morphology suggests the possibility of pain relief by surgery. The presence of pseudocysts or duodenal/biliary obstruction also needs surgical and/or therapeutic endoscopy consultation.

Difficult issues with managing diabetes may require endocrinology consultation. Consultation with a psychiatrist is helpful if the patient has drug addiction. Management of CP often requires a multidisciplinary approach.

Summary

Excessive alcohol consumption is the single most important cause of CP. Other causes or types of chronic pancreatitis include:

- idiopathic
- tropical
- hereditary
- obstructive

QUICK FLICK

30

- hyperlipidaemic
- hypercalcaemic.

The recent discovery of genetic mutations in hereditary pancreatitis explains how other aetiologic factors predispose the patient to CP. Recurrent abdominal pain, fat malabsorption and diabetes are the cardinal manifestations.

Imaging procedures greatly assist in diagnosis and management. Abstinence from alcohol and cigarette smoking are essential to management. Analgesics, pancreatic enzymes and antioxidants are used in the medical management. Selected patients may need to undergo surgery.

The complications of CP include pseudocysts, pancreatic ascites and pancreatic cancer.

Information for patients

What is chronic pancreatitis?

As a result of repeated injury to the pancreas, often due to prolonged alcoholism, the gland is permanently damaged, and scar tissue is formed in the place of healthy pancreatic cells. The tube or duct that transports enzymes to the intestine is involved in the scarring process, and stones may develop in the duct and obstruct the flow of pancreatic secretions.

What causes it?

In more than two-thirds of the cases, the disease is due to excessive consumption of alcohol for 10 or more years. In rare situations, chronic pancreatitis is hereditary. In some Afro-Asian countries, a form of tropical pancreatitis occurs. Rarely, chronic pancreatitis may have no identifiable cause.

How would I know if I had chronic pancreatitis?

You may experience frequent upper abdominal and upper back pain—more so on eating food—occasionally associated with nausea and vomiting. As the disease advances, diarrhoea and weight loss may occur. In advanced cases, digestion of fat suffers most, and you may notice droplets of fat in the stool (fat malabsorption, or steatorrhoea).

How is chronic pancreatitis diagnosed?

Generally by the history of repeated attacks of upper abdominal pain associated with a history of chronic alcoholism. Additional abdomen X-rays, CT scan, magnetic resonance imaging (MRI) scan and endoscopic ultrasound studies may be needed to confirm the diagnosis.

Is there treatment for chronic pancreatitis?

The most important step is to discontinue alcohol consumption. Medical treatment consists of managing abdominal pain with pain medications; in a few selected cases, surgery may be needed. When there is a defect in fat absorption, or diarrhoea, or weight loss, pancreatic enzymes are given by mouth. Treatment of diabetes is an important part of management.

Recommended reading

Garg PK, Tandon RK. Surgery in chronic pancreatitis in the Asia-Pacific region. *Gastroenterology*. 2004; 19:998–1004.

Otsuki M. Chronic pancreatitis in Japan: epidemiology, prognosis, diagnostic criteria and future problems. *Gastroenterology*. 2003; 38:315-26.

Park DH, Kim MH, Chari ST. Recent advances in autoimmune pancreatitis. *Gastroenterology*. 2009; 58:1680–9.

Pitchumoni CS. Pathogenesis and management of pain in chronic pancreatitis. *World J Gastroenterol*. 2000; 6:490–6.

Ryu JK, Lee JK, Kim YT. Clinical features of chronic pancreatitis in Korea: a multicenter national study. *Digestion*. 2005; 72:207–11.

Whitcomb DC. Mechanisms of disease: advances in understanding the mechanisms leading to chronic pancreatitis. *Nat Clin Pract Gastroenterol Hepatol*. 2004; 1:46–52.

Chapter 31: Pancreatic cancer

C.S. Pitchumoni (USA)

Key points

▶ Unexplained jaundice in a patient older than 50, weight loss, upper abdominal or back pain and anorexia should raise suspicion of pancreatic cancer.

▶ Pancreatic cancer has a dismal prognosis and is the fourth or fifth most common cause of cancer mortality in Western countries. The incidence is variable in Asian countries.

▶ Most cancers are adenocarcinomas that arise from the ductal epithelium.

▶ Among the aetiological associations, cigarette smoking is an important one. Use of other tobacco products also increases the risk.

▶ Chronic pancreatitis increases the risk of pancreatic cancer. In particular, hereditary pancreatitis and tropical pancreatitis are associated with high risk.

▶ Symptoms depend on the location of the tumour. The disease is nearly always diagnosed at a relatively late stage because of delayed onset of symptoms and signs. Classic presentation is painless jaundice, weight loss and back pain.

▶ The diagnosis is suggested by clinical history, supported by imaging studies including computed tomography (CT) scan, magnetic resonance imaging /magnetic resonance cholangiopancreatography (MRI/MRCP) and endoscopic ultrasound (EUS).

▶ Treatment consists of combination of pancreatioduodenectomy with post-operative adjuvant fluroracil and external beam radiation therapy. Gemcitabine therapy improves quality of life.

▶ Cystic lesions of the pancreas are frequently detected as incidental findings. Most of them are benign. Mucinous cystic neoplasms and intraductal papillary mucinous neoplasms (IPMN) are considered to be premalignant.

▶ Malignant cystic lesions need to be differentiated from benign lesions to decide the appropriate management procedure. Many imaging studies, fine needle aspiration of the cysts and analysis of cyst fluid are helpful.

◯ Epidemiology

The incidence of pancreatic cancer has wide geographical variations. The incidence is three to four times higher in Iceland, Finland and the USA than in countries closer to the equator such as Egypt, Tunisia and

Zimbabwe. In the US the incidence of pancreatic cancer is higher in blacks than in whites.

The peak incidence of pancreatic cancer is in the age group 65–75 years, and is more frequent in men than in women.

In India and China, where pancreatic cancer was once infrequent, the increased life expectancy in the general population combined with the resulting increase in the number of elderly has seen the incidence of pancreatic cancer also increasing. Another reason for the change is the increased prevalence of cigarette smoking, which is a major risk factor for pancreatic cancer. Greater availability of pancreatic imaging studies, in particular the routine use of CT scan of abdomen, has also contributed to the apparent increase.

Approximately 10 per cent of pancreatic cancers are associated with a hereditary predisposition. Peutz-Jeghers syndrome, hereditary pancreatitis, Von Hippel-Lindau disease, ataxia-telangiectasia, cystic fibrosis, familial adenomatous polyposis (FAP), hereditary non-polyposis colon cancer (HNPCC), and familial breast and ovarian cancer syndromes (BRCA2 mutations) are all associated with pancreatic cancer.

Diabetics are at increased risk, but no causative relationship is evident. A significantly increased risk is observed in those working in the chemical industry and in metals industries.

Pathology

Most exocrine pancreatic cancers (>85%) are ductal or acinar cell in origin, consistent with adenocarcinoma. Endocrine neoplasms account for 1–2 per cent of pancreatic tumours. Autopsy studies have shown that 60–70 per cent of tumours are localised in the head, 5–10 per cent in the body and 10–15 per cent in the tail of the pancreas. Metastasis from the pancreas can occur to regional lymph nodes, liver, lung and pleura, intestine and peritoneum. Symptoms vary depending on the location of metastasis.

Clinical features

Presenting features depend upon the location and extent of lesion. The major symptoms of pancreatic cancer are:

- abdominal pain of pancreatic type—postprandial epigastric and back pain, associated with nausea and vomiting
- weight loss
- jaundice
- loss of appetite
- clay-coloured stools

- diarrhoea
- depression
- new-onset diabetes mellitus.

Tumours of the head of the pancreas produce jaundice and abdominal pain symptoms earlier than tumours of the distal gland ('silent tumours'). Pancreatic cancer located in the body and tail of the pancreas causes splenic vein thrombosis and left-sided portal hypertension, as well as oesophageal and gastric varices.

Physical findings may include jaundice, epigastric tenderness and, in rare cases, a palpable gall bladder (Courvoisier sign), supraclavicular lymph node enlargement (Virchow's node), periumbilical mass (Sister Mary Joseph's nodule) and a palpable rectovaginal or rectovesical nodularity (Blumer's shelf). The 'Trousseau sign' is the migrating thrombophlebitis, and is not specific for pancreatic cancer.

◯ Diagnosis

Serum markers

CA19-9, a tumour marker, is not specific in tumours 2 cm in size. It may be immeasurable. False elevations occur in chronic pancreatitis and in benign cases of obstructive jaundice.

Imaging studies

Spiral CT (pancreatic protocol) is helpful in determining the extent of the disease in most cases. CT criteria for unresectability include tumours that have spread to the liver or peritoneum, contiguous invasion of adjacent organs other than duodenum or bile duct, arterial involvement or venous occlusion. MRI, positron emission tomography (PET) and EUS are helpful in selected cases. EUS is a minimally invasive but sensitive test that needs technical expertise, but offers the opportunity to do fine needle aspiration biopsies. ERCP may show a 'double-duct' sign, or enlargement of the biliary and pancreatic ducts; the sign is not specific. In advanced centres, tumour cytology can be performed. Tumour size, lymph node involvement, involvement of adjacent structures and distant metastasis are all factors to be included in the TNM tumour staging system.

◯ Management

Factors that influence the mode of therapy include the stage of the tumours, location, presence or absence of vascular involvement, nutrition of the patient, local availability of experienced surgeons, oncologists and radiotherapists. The approach to therapy is multimodal.

The Whipple procedure (pancreaticoduodenectomy) is a standard surgical operation that involves resection of the distal stomach, gall bladder, proximal jejunum and regional lymph nodes. The new pylorus-preserving procedure avoids post-gastrectomy symptoms.

Post-operative adjuvant chemotherapy with 5-fluororacil (5-FU) and external beam radiation therapy improves survival. Chemotherapy with gemcitabine improves quality of life, since gemcitabine inhibits DNA replication.

Palliation therapy for pain is possible by coeliac ganglion block (percutaneous or EUS approach).

Pancreaticobiliary stenting can be performed endoscopically, and improves jaundice and promotes drainage.

Pancreatic cystic neoplasms

Pancreatic cystic neoplasms (PCN) are being detected increasingly as incidental findings in CT abdomen imaging. Most patients are asymptomatic. Distinguishing features and differential diagnosis are listed in Table 31.1.

Serous cystadenomas (SCNs) represent 30 per cent of PCN, mainly occurring in women (65%) of fifth decade. The tumours are often located in the head of the pancreas. SCNs have low malignant potential.

Mucinous cystic neoplasms (MCNs) are much more prevalent in women than men (>95%), and are potentially malignant.

Intrapapillary mucinous neoplasms (IPMN) affect men and women equally. Most of these patients have a history of recurrent acute pancreatitis.

Table 31.1 Differential diagnosis of pancreatic neoplastic cysts

	SCA (30%)	MCN (45–50%)	IPMN (7.5%)
Gender	F > M	Mainly F (>95%)	F = M
Usual age	Middle age (35–84 yr)	Middle age	Elderly
History of pancreatitis	No	No	Possible
Morphology (imaging studies)	Microcystic and polycystic (>6 cysts) Honeycomb appearance Sunburst calcification (20%) <2 cm cysts	Unilocular cyst, septations, and wall calcifications Solid component indicates malignancy	Main duct dilatation or limited to side branches

continued

Table 31.1 *continued*

	SCA (30%)	**MCN (45–50%)**	**IPMN (7.5%)**
Location	Diffuse, head	Body and tail (>75%)	Head
Fluid	Thin	Viscous	Thick
Cytology	Cuboidal cells Stains for glycogen	Positive for mucin Columnar cells with variable atypia Ovarian-like stroma present	Positive for mucin Columnar cells with variable atypia
Malignant potential	Rare	Yes	Yes

SCA: serous cystadenoma; MCN: mucinous cystic neoplasm (cystadenoma); IPMN: intraductal papillary mucinous neoplasm.

Source: Adapted from Pitchumoni CS. Netter's gastroenterology. 2nd ed; 2009.

Summary

Upper abdominal pain, unexplained jaundice and weight loss in a patient older than 50 are key indications of pancreatic cancer. The prognosis is poor. Most cancers are adenocarcinomas arising from the distal epithelium. Aetiological associations include cigarette smoking and use of other tobacco products, chronic pancreatitis, hereditary pancreatitis and tropical pancreatitis. The classic presentation is painless jaundice, back pain and weight loss. History and imaging procedures aid in diagnosis.

Treatment consists of a combination of pancreaticoduodenectomy and post-operative adjuvant fluoracil and external beam radiation therapy. Most cystic lesions of the pancreas are benign. Mucinous cystic neoplasms and intraductal papillary mucinous neoplasms are premalignant.

Information for patients

What is pancreatic cancer?

Pancreatic cancer is a disease in which cancer cells grow in the pancreatic gland. There are three parts in the pancreas: head, body and tail. A growth may develop in any part, and symptoms vary depending on the location of the growth.

What causes pancreatic cancer?

There are many causes. The most important and preventable one is cigarette smoking. Chronic pancreatitis, which is due to alcoholism, or other factors such as heredity also cause pancreatic cancer.

What would make me suspect I have pancreatic cancer?

Pancreatic cancer usually occurs in the older adult (age over 60). When the tumour grows, there will be upper abdominal and/or back pain, progressive weight loss, loss of appetite and development of yellowish discolouration of skin and eyes (jaundice). Recent-onset diabetes is another feature.

Why is it that there is usually a delay in diagnosing pancreatic cancer?

In the early stages, pancreatic cancer mimics other, more common, causes of abdominal pain, such as a stomach ulcer. The organ cannot be easily examined without sophisticated X-ray studies, and biopsy of the gland is not easy. Chemical tests of the blood are not very sensitive in the diagnosis. Another reason is that the disease often has no symptoms until it spreads to the liver.

How is pancreatic cancer diagnosed?

A number of imaging studies help us to suspect and confirm a diagnosis of pancreatic cancer. A CT scan, where a number of pictures of the abdomen are taken after injecting a dye (IV contrast), is the initial test. Magnetic resonance imaging (MRI) is a technique that uses a magnet, radiowaves and a computer. These tests are expensive and not always definitive.

A new device is endoscopic ultrasound, in which an endoscope with an ultrasound probe is inserted into the upper small intestine (duodenum), and sound waves are recorded. A biopsy of the pancreas is taken for later microscopic examination.

Another diagnostic procedure known as endoscopic retrograde cholangiopancreatography (ERCP) utilises an endoscope which is passed through the mouth into the upper small intestine (duodenum). A dye is injected into the pancreatic duct and X-rays of the pancreas are obtained.

What is the outcome of pancreatic cancer?

Early diagnosis, before the cancer has spread to other organs, is vital for early surgical treatment. Overall, pancreatic cancer is associated with a poor outcome.

How is pancreatic cancer treated?

The treatment depends on the staging of the cancer, the condition of the patient and the local availability of experts in the field (surgeons, oncologists and radiotherapists). Surgery is the mainstay. A part of the pancreas or the whole organ is surgically removed. Radiation therapy uses high-energy X-rays to kill cancer cells.

Chemotherapy uses drugs to kill and stop the growth of cancer cells.

Symptomatic treatment with painkillers and nutritional support is important.

The patient is best treated in a tertiary care centre that is equipped with all the necessary facilities and where the services of an experienced pancreatic surgeon are available.

Are there different types of pancreatic cancer?

Although the above-mentioned are referred to as the common type of pancreatic cancer—which are solid growths—occasionally there are tumours of the pancreas that show on a CT scan image like small, fluid-filled cavities. This type of tumour has a better outcome with surgery.

Recommended reading

Brugge WR, Lauwers GY, Sahani D, Fernandez-del Castillo C, Warshaw AL. Cystic neoplasms of the pancreas. *N Engl J Med*. 2004; 351:1218–26.

Li D, Xie K, Wolff R, Abbruzzese JL. Pancreatic cancer. *Lancet*. 2004; 363:1049–57.

Lowenfels AB, Maissonneuve P. Environmental factors and risks of pancreatic cancer. *Pancreatology*. 2003; 3:1–8.

Rebours V, Boutron-Ruault M, Schnee M, Férec C, Maire F, Hammel P, Ruszniewski P, Lévy P. Risk of pancreatic adenocarcinoma in patients with hereditary pancreatitis: a national exhaustive series. *Am J Gastroenterol*. 2008; 103:111–9.

J. Chaganti (Australia)

Key points

▶ The pathophysiology in pancreatitis is autodigestion. Normal pancreatic parenchyma enhances intensely due to its rich vascular supply.

▶ One characteristic of acute pancreatitis is a swollen, non-enhancing gland.

▶ Computed tomography (CT) imaging of acute pancreatitis is used to confirm the diagnosis of inflammation both within and outside the pancreas.

▶ CT severity index (CTSI) is a powerful tool for prognosis.

▶ Pseudocysts (50%) resolve on their own. If not, they need to be drained by percutaneous methods or endoscopy.

▶ Radiological hallmarks of chronic pancreatitis are duct dilatation, fibrosis of the parenchyma and ultimately atrophy.

▶ Magnetic resonance imaging (MRI) and magnetic resonance cholangiopancreatography (MRCP) are powerful tools for early diagnosis of fibrosis and ductal morphology.

▶ Autoimmune pancreatitis has characteristic radiology, and findings are reversible if steroid treatment is started early.

▶ Positron emission tomography–computed tomography (PET CT) may replace other imaging modalities in the future in staging pancreatic cancer.

▶ Endoscopic ultrasound (EUS) is the imaging investigation of choice, both for diagnosis and characterisation of non-contour-deforming lesions of the pancreas.

▶ Intraductal pancreatic mucinous neoplastic lesions are potentially malignant; MRCP is the best method of assessing the risk.

◐ Introduction

As with other areas of gastrointestinal and biliary imaging, there have been exciting developments in pancreatic imaging. Multidetector CT (MDCT), MRI and EUS have all established their place in evaluating pancreatic disorders. PET CT is increasingly being used, both to diagnose and stage pancreatic tumours.

◯ Acute pancreatitis

Imaging strategies for acute pancreatitis involve establishing pancreatic inflammation, to identify the causes of pancreatitis and to exclude the mimics. The most common causes of pancreatitis are alcohol abuse and gallstones; others include hypertriglyceridaemia, hypercalcaemia, ductal obstruction caused by tumours and trauma, iatrogenic causes—endoscopic retrograde cholangiopancreatography (ERCP), for example—and developmental anomalies such as pancreas divisum and annular pancreas. Whatever the cause, the underlying pathophysiology of all pancreatitis is pancreatic autodigestion. All imaging strategies are tailored to identify this inflammation within the pancreas and outside it.

Mild acute pancreatitis is commonly an interstitial inflammation and self-limiting disease. Severe pancreatitis, also termed necrotising pancreatitis, is associated with organ necrosis and may lead to other complications such as pseudocyst, abscess and vascular complications. Contrast-enhanced CT is considered to be the 'criterion standard' for evaluating morphological changes, and has become an integral part of the new classification system.

Multidetector CT

The characteristic CT findings of acute necrotising pancreatitis are enlargement of the gland and necrosis.

Pancreatic necrosis

Pancreatic necrosis shows on dynamic arterial CT as areas of non-enhancing parenchyma. Although the initial CT scan establishes the diagnosis, it is useful to do a repeat scan 48 to 72 hours after onset in order to produce a more accurate assessment of pancreatic necrosis. Based on imaging findings, Balthazar et al. (1985) graded the severity of acute pancreatitis into five levels (A to E) (Table 32.1).[1]

Table 32.1 Grades of severity of acute pancreatitis based on imaging

A	Normal appearing pancreas
B	Focal/diffuse enlargement of pancreas
C	Gland abnormalities with mild peripancreatic inflammatory changes
D	Fluid collection in single location
E	Two or more fluid collections near or adjacent to pancreas

Source: Modified from: Balthazar et al. (1985).

Using this classification, the prognosis for patients with Grade D or E is poor, with a mortality rate of 14 per cent and a morbidity rate of 54 per cent. Severity grades A, B and C imply no mortality and a 4 per cent morbidity rate.

Patients showing less than 30 per cent necrosis on CT images, and who exhibited no increase in the mortality rate, in fact have a morbidity rate of 48 per cent. Balthazar later refined the original grading system to take into account the extent of pancreatic necrosis (CT severity index (CTSI): Balthazar 2002).[2]

The CTSI appears to have a very good correlation with prognosis. CT grades A to E are assigned 0–4 points plus 2 points for <30 per cent, 4 points for 30–50 per cent and 6 points for >50 per cent necrosis (Table 32.2). Patients with a CTSI rating of 0–3 have been shown to have a mortality rate of 3 per cent and morbidity of 8 per cent; those with a CTSI rating of 7–10 have morbidity of 17 per cent and mortality of 92 per cent.

Table 32.2 Modified CT severity index for acute pancreatitis

CT grade	Points	Necrosis (%)	Points	CTSI score
A	0	0	0	0
B	1	0	0	1
C	2	<30	2	4
D	3	30–50	4	7
E	4	>50	6	10

Source: From Balthazar (2002).

Necrosis of the parenchyma can become secondarily infected, since it is a good medium for the growth of the organisms. The demonstration of air in the necrosis is a sign of infection; however, caution should be exercised in interpreting such a finding, since partial volume averaging, fat necrosis and communication with the bowel by the inflamed necrotic tissue can give similar image morphology. Often such air locules mandate percutaneous aspiration and culture of the aspirate. When infected necrosis is diagnosed it is an indication for percutaneous intervention or necrosectomy.

Acute fluid collections

Acute fluid collections, consisting of enzyme-rich pancreatic juices, occur early in the course of the disease. Half of such cases resolve without intervention. Images of these collections differ from pseudocysts in that they do not have a wall of granulation or fibrous tissue.

Acute pseudocyst

If the fluid collection is enclosed by fibrous or granulation tissue it is referred to as pseudocyst. These take at least of four weeks to form.

Both pseudocyst and pancreatic fluid collections form in the vicinity of the pancreas and commonly dissect into lesser sacs. Since they are rich in digestive juices, they can dissect in any direction and may be located as far away as the mediastinum. They may dissect into solid viscera (liver, spleen, etc) or perforate into adjacent bowel (usually the transverse colon) and erode into arteries, producing pseudoaneurysms. Compression of adjacent vasculature may lead to thrombosis of the vessels (splenic or mesenteric thrombosis) and consequent complications.

Pancreatic abscess

When imaging is used with contrast, the walls of pancreatic abscesses show intense enhancement on both MRI and CT. With MRI, the fluid content can be characterised as proteinaceous and differentiated from pseudocysts.

Vascular complications

The most serious vascular complication is a pseudoaneurysm that can lead to life-threatening haemorrhaging. The two most common locations are the splenic artery and gastroduodenal artery. Venous thrombosis is not uncommon. Thrombosis of the mesenteric vein can lead to intestinal ischaemia, and splenic and portal venous thrombosis may lead to portal hypertension.

Extrapancreatic findings

The inflammatory process can extend locally into the peritoneal spaces and cause mesenteric panniculitis, or fat necrosis. On cross-sectional imaging, fat necrosis appears as 'dirty' fat, with linear stranding and patchy enhancement.

Extensive perirenal inflammation gives the characteristic renal halo sign—relatively well-preserved renal fat with inflammatory phlegmon enveloping both the anterior and posterior pararenal spaces and thickening their respective fascia.

Gastric wall thickening is frequently associated with acute pancreatitis.

Pleural effusions are often bilateral; however, when they are unilateral they tend to form on the left side.

MR imaging

Magnetic resonance imaging is comparable to CT in its ability to demonstrate morphological changes from acute pancreatitis and their complications.

Furthermore, MR cholangiopancreatography, or MRCP, can be performed at the same time to identify choledocholithiasis.

MRCP also demonstrates pancreatic ductal abnormalities such as dilatation, disruption and leakage. Demonstration of ductal communication with a pseudocyst would warrant surgical drainage rather than percutaneous intervention. Secretin-assisted MRCP is the preferred investigation in suspected cases of pancreatic fistula. Secretin gives functional information and is therefore a useful technique for diagnosing Sphincter of Oddi dysfunction (a cause of pancreatitis).

Most patients with pancreatitis are young, and therefore MR generally is a useful investigation method for follow-up, as it does not involve radiation and can be repeated as often as necessary. MRCP is also an excellent imaging tool for identifying the contributing causes of pancreatitis—tumours, anomalies and intraductal pancreatic mucinous neoplasia (IPMN), for example.

○ Chronic pancreatitis

The imaging spectrum of chronic pancreatitis depends on the type of the disease.

Phase of relapsing pancreatitis

In this stage of chronic pancreatitis, the glandular architecture does not show much change and the ductal structures may be normal. Diagnostic contribution is mainly to identify the cause of relapses. Causes include choledocholithiasis, Sphincter of Oddi dysfunction, ampullary tumours and congenital anomalies; the underlying mechanism in all causes is impairment of the flow of pancreatic juice and bile into the duodenum. MRCP, often combined with secretin, is the preferred investigation method for all these conditions.

Established chronic pancreatitis

Multiple attacks of pancreatitis cause irreversible changes in both the parenchyma and ducts; both CT and MRI are useful for diagnosing such changes. The primary role of these modalities is to differentiate obstructive chronic pancreatitis (OCP) from non-obstructive chronic pancreatitis (NOCP).

Obstructive chronic pancreatitis (OCP)

Parenchymal changes include fibrosis and atrophy. Imaging correlates of these findings are hypointense parenchyma on T-1 fat suppressed sequences, with poor enhancement in the arterial phases and hyperintensity of the parenchyma in the delayed phases (venous phase). Dynamic arterial CT shows similar findings, although the sensitivity of CT for identifying fibrosis is lower than the sensitivity of MRI. The delayed enhancement is often most striking in areas of focal fibrosis. This typical pattern of enhancement is possibly due to the slow uptake of contrast by the fibrous tissue.

Ductal changes of OCP are typically present even in the initial stages of the disease. They are characterised by uniform, regular dilatation of the main pancreatic duct (MPD) and relative preservation of the side branches. Over time, however, the side branches dilate and harbour calculi due to poor drainage. While the diagnosis of calcium is better by CT, MRI and MRCP are superior for identifying the location of stones as being either intraductal or parenchymal. The presence of stones in obstructive form is much less frequent than in other forms. MRCP with secretin is the preferred investigation method for demonstrating ductal abnormality. In patients with severe OCP, the duodenal filling is significantly less in post-secretin MRCP.

Secondary OCP

Adenocarcinoma of the papilla is the most common cause of tumour-producing OCP, and the mass can easily be identified by MDCT. Other, less common, causes of OCP include ductal adenocarcinoma and acinar cell carcinoma, and cystic pancreatic tumours; there are also other causes of OCP beyond the scope of this chapter.

Non-obstructive chronic pancreatitis (NOCP)

NOCP can be secondary to toxic agents such as alcohol and genetic mutations. In both these conditions the characteristic findings are initial enlargement of the gland and altered parenchymal enhancement, followed by fibrotic retraction of the parenchyma and atrophy. The collateral ducts show ectasia, and the main pancreatic duct shows stenotic tracts alternating with the focal areas of dilatation, producing a 'rosary crown' appearance. Calculi invariably accompany such dilated ducts.

MRI with diffusion-weighted imaging

Recent data indicates that diagnosis of chronic pancreatitis can be made with high sensitivity using diffusion-weighted imaging (DWI), which measures microscopic diffusion of water. In the liver, fibrosis and cirrhosis have both been shown to reduce diffusion. Similarly, in chronic pancreatitis both fibrosis and chronic inflammation are present, making DWI an attractive choice for interrogating parenchymal morphology. DW imaging of the pancreas in patients with chronic pancreatitis has shown significantly low apparent values of the diffusion coefficient (ADC) compared to healthy subjects. Further studies have shown that measured differences in the ADC values before and after the introduction of secretin enables the diagnosis of very early fibrosis.

Special forms of pancreatitis

Autoimmune pancreatitis

This distinct entity is a recognised cause of chronic pancreatitis and has characteristic imaging findings. These include:

- diffuse enlargement of the pancreas, with loss of lobularity, resulting in the characteristic featureless 'sausage-shaped' pancreas; although diffuse forms are the more common, focal forms do occur, and will ultimately progress to involve the whole pancreas if they are not treated
- moderate enhancement of the gland, with homogenous attenuation and sharp borders, and the absence of normal pancreatic clefts
- a rim of low attenuation that possibly represents inflammatory exudate
- a capsule-like rim of enhancement with CT/MR, which may represent periglandular inflammatory phlegmon/fibrosis
- characteristic ductal abnormality with ERCP/MRCP, demonstrating irregular narrowing of the main pancreatic duct and biliary ducts.

Inflammatory mass vs pancreatic adenocarcinoma

Although chronic pancreatitis is known to be associated with atrophy, it can at times cause focal enlargement of the gland and therefore poses a diagnostic difficulty. This is particularly concerning because patients with chronic pancreatitis are at increased risk of carcinoma.

One of the key imaging findings is the morphology of the pancreatic duct on MRCP, which may help to differentiate an inflammatory mass from pancreatic adenocarcinoma. If a non-dilated pancreatic duct courses through the pancreatic mass, then it is likely to be related to focal pancreatitis. A smooth stenosis is more often found in chronic pancreatitis.

Groove pancreatitis

This is a form of segmental chronic pancreatitis that is localised within the groove between the head of the pancreas, the duodenum and the common bile duct. The exact pathophysiology is unknown.

Characteristically, the pancreatic duct system is normal and there are no calcifications or other ductal anomalies. Contrast-enhanced CT demonstrates a poorly enhancing lesion extending between the pancreatic head and the duodenum. In the pancreaticoduodenal groove, on MRI is seen a sheet-like mass which is hypointense relative to the pancreatic parenchyma and slightly hyperintense on T2. Gadolinium contrast medium administration demonstrates delayed enhancement.

Pancreatic cancer

Both CT and EUS with fine needle aspiration are standard methods of diagnosing and staging pancreatic cancer; however, CT followed by surgical exploration is the most commonly used strategy for staging these cancers due to the limited availability of EUS.

Most pancreatic cancers arise in the head of the pancreas (60–65%), about 20 per cent in the body and 10 per cent in the tail. About 10 per cent involve the whole gland.

Pancreatic adenocarcinoma is a hypovascular tumour and appears as a relatively low attenuating mass compared to the rest of the gland in arterial phase CT. A helpful secondary finding is the presence of the double duct sign. Abrupt transition of the calibre of the pancreatic and bile ducts at the ampulla in the absence of a calculus favours malignancy. Dual-phase pancreatic CT (pancreatic phase 35–45 s delay; portal phase 65–75 s delay) after IV bolus injection, with thin re-formations, allows smaller pancreatic tumours to be detected and facilitates the detection of vascular encasement.

Vascular encasement is an important staging requirement. Both EUS and MDCT have equal sensitivity and specificity in this regard. It has been reported that cancers with definite vascular encasement have a higher incidence of liver metastasis and therefore imaging of this important finding may provide prognostic information. According to one study, MDCT has a positive predictive value (PPV) of 89–100 per cent for surgical resectability. However the negative predictive value (NPV) is low, with values of 45–79 per cent. Recent contrast-enhanced US has been used to image the vascular encasement, and has shown good correlation with digital subtraction angiography (DSA) in determining the vascular invasion.

The advent of CT fusion with the functional environment of PET has changed the way the cancers are managed. The hybrid PET CT combines all the benefits of CT and PET and therefore has the potential to become the imaging method of choice for staging pancreatic cancer. Table 32.3 lists general guidelines of resectability.

Cystic pancreatic neoplasms

The apparent incidence of cystic neoplasms has increased, attributable to increased resolution of the imaging techniques. The common cystic lesions of the pancreas include benign inflammatory cysts (pseudocysts), benign cystic neoplasms (serous cystadenomas) and premalignant cystic neoplasms (mucinous cystic and intraductal papillary mucinous neoplasms or IPMN). The imaging investigation of choice for most of these cystic neoplasms is EUS, which allows fine needle aspiration of the cysts. Only IPMN is discussed here, as it has created lot of interest and is being increasingly recognised.

Table 32.3 General guidelines for resectability in pancreatic cancer

Resectable	Unresectable
Involvement of peripancreatic lymph nodes	Ingrowth into stomach, colon, mesocolon
Ingrowth into duodenum	Presence of hepatic metastases, peritoneal metastases or para-aortic lymph node
Involvement of the gastroduodenal artery	Ingrowth into the coeliac axis, hepatic artery or superior mesenteric artery.
Vascular encasement <180°	

Intraductal papillary mucinous neoplasm (IPMN)

Excessive production of mucin by these neoplasms results in cystic dilatation of the pancreatic duct and possibly spillage of mucin from the Ampulla of Vater, a diagnostic finding on ERCP. Depending on their involvement, the pancreatic ducts are classified into main duct and branch duct, or mixed variants. Main duct IPMNs show higher malignant potential (60–70%) than branch duct IPMNs (22%).

MRCP is the preferred imaging technique, both for establishing the diagnosis and for characterising the morphology of IPMN. Main duct IPMN does not come under differential diagnosis of cystic pancreatic tumour, presenting either as diffuse or segmental main pancreatic duct dilatation. Chronic pancreatitis does come under differential diagnosis, but the associated signal changes of chronic pancreatitis are absent in IPMN.

Branch duct IPMN is commonly seen in the region of the pancreas head. It presents as a cystic lesion on CT and MR, and on occasions it may mimic mucinous cystadenoma; however, communication with the duct differentiates the IPMN from the others.

In one large study, Baba et al. (2004) compared the accuracy of imaging for predicting benign and malignant disease in 121 patients with pathologically confirmed IPMN. The techniques included EUS, CT, MRCP and radial EUS. The variables measured included maximum cyst diameter, maximum duct diameter, and height of protruding lesions (mural nodules). The results indicated that EUS was the most effective method for differentiating benign and malignant tumours by assessing the height of the nodule. MR imaging features that may favour associated adenocarcinoma detection include enhancing soft tissue nodularity, size more than 3.5 cm, and thick walls.[3]

Summary

Advancement of imaging techniques has pushed back the frontiers and established new boundaries. As a result of this altered dynamic, management of pancreatic diseases is rapidly changing. In this changing equilibrium, we would do well to remember that the patient comes first, and prudence in choosing the optimal technique must assume paramount importance: this depends not necessarily on a specific modality, but rather on utilising the best expertise in the imaging modalities available.

References

1. Balthazar EJ, Ranson JHC, Naidich DP, Megibow AJ, Caccavale R, Cooper MM. Acute pancreatitis: prognostic value of CT. *Radiology*. 1985; 156:767–72.

2. Balthazar EJ. Acute pancreatitis: assessment of severity with clinical and CT evaluation. *Radiology*. 2002 Jun; 223:603–13. doi:10.1148/radiol.2233010680.

3. Baba T, Yamaguchi T, Ishihara T, Kobayashi A, Oshima T, Sakaue N, Kato K, Ebara M, Saisho H. Distinguishing benign from malignant intraductal papillary mucinous tumors of the pancreas by imaging techniques. *Pancreas*. 2004 Oct; 29(3):212–7.

Recommended reading

Akisik MA, Aisen AM, Sandrasegaran K, Jennings SG, Lin C, Sherman S, Lin JA, Rydberg M. Assessment of chronic pancreatitis: utility of diffusion-weighted MR imaging with secretin enhancement. *Radiology*. 2009 Jan; 250(1):103–9.

Graziani R, Taparelli M, Malago R. The various imaging aspects of chronic pancreatitis. *JOP*. 2005; 6(1):73–88.

Kalb B, Sarmiento JM, Kooby DA, Adsay NV, Martin DR. MR imaging of cystic lesions of the pancreas. *Radiographics*. 2009 Oct; 29(6):1749–65.

Kwon SR, Brugge RW. New advances in pancreatic imaging. *Curr Opin Gastroenterol*. 2005; 21:561–7.

Manfredi R, Graziani R, Motton M, Mantovani W, Baltieri S, Tognolini A, Crippa S, Capelli P, Salvia R, Pozzi Mucelli R. Main pancreatic duct intraductal papillary mucinous neoplasms: accuracy of MR imaging in differentiation between benign and malignant tumors compared with histopathological analysis. *Radiology*. 2009 Oct; 253(1):106–15. doi:10.1148/radiol.2531080604/-/DC1.

Pereira SP, Gillams A, Sgouros SN, Webster GJ, Hatfield AR. Prospective comparison of secretin-stimulated magnetic resonance cholangiopancreatography with manometry in the diagnosis of sphincter of Oddi dysfunction types II and III. *Gut*. 2007; 56(6):809–13.

Sahani DV, Kalva SP, Farrell J, Maher MM, Saini S, Mueller PR, Lauwers GY, Fernandez CD, Warshaw AL, Simeone JF. Autoimmune pancreatitis: imaging features. *Radiology*. 2004 Nov; 233:345–52.

Saokar A, Rabinowitz BC, Sahani VD. Cross-sectional imaging in acute pancreatitis. *Radiol Clin North Am*. 2007; 45:447–60.

Zamboni GA, Kruskal JB, Vollmer CM, Baptista J, Callery MP, Raptopoulos VD. Pancreatic adenocarcinoma: value of multidetector CT angiography in preoperative evaluation. *Radiology*. 2007 Dec; 245(3):770–8.

Section

4

Hepatology

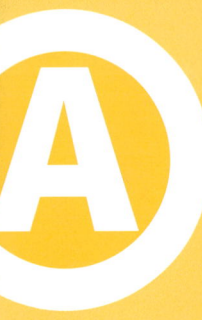

Part A

Diseases evoking a global impact

Chapter 33: Cirrhosis and complications

P. Sharma, S.K. Sarin (India)

Key points

▶ Cirrhosis is a response to chronic liver injury.

▶ It leads to portal hypertension and end-stage liver disease.

▶ Complications include variceal haemorrhage, ascites, spontaneous bacterial peritonitis, hepatic encephalopathy, hepatorenal syndrome, bacterial infections and iatrogenic causes.

▶ Alcohol remains the predominant cause of significant liver disease.

▶ In the Indian subcontinent, hepatitis B virus (HBV)-related liver disease predominates.

▶ In Japan and Pakistan, hepatitis C virus (HBC)-related liver disease predominates.

▶ Non-alcoholic fatty liver disease (NAFLD) has become significant in recent times.

▶ Cirrhosis is sometimes suggested by abnormalities in liver function tests.

▶ Thrombocytopaenia is the most common first haematologic abnormality.

▶ New diagnostic non-invasive tests have recently been evaluated.

▶ Transient elastography correlates with the elasticity of the underlying liver.

▶ Portal hypertension and ascites are common complications.

▶ Ascites is the most common complication.

▶ Recent advances include satavaptan, a V2 receptor antagonist.

◑ Introduction

Cirrhosis is … the histological development of regenerative nodules surrounded by fibrous bands in response to chronic liver injury, which leads to portal hypertension and end-stage liver disease.[1]

Advanced cirrhosis is regarded as irreversible, with liver transplantation as the only option, although reversal at earlier stages by treating the cause has been reported. Complications include variceal haemorrhage, ascites, spontaneous bacterial peritonitis (SBP), hepatic encephalopathy, hepatorenal syndrome (HRS), bacterial infections, and complications following medical procedures.

◑ Epidemiology

More than 27 000 deaths and 421 000 hospitalisations per year are recorded in the USA annually due to cirrhosis of the liver. Alcohol is the main cause of significant liver disease in most countries, including the Indian subcontinent (HBV-related liver disease), Japan and Pakistan (HCV-related liver disease).

Regular, moderate alcohol consumption, and being male and over 50, increase cirrhosis risk of chronic HCV infection; and older age, obesity, insulin resistance or type 2 diabetes, hypertension and hyperlipidaemia increase risk of non-alcoholic steatohepatitis.

Recent studies, including that of Das et al. (2010) have shown significant prevalence of NAFLD and cryptogenic cirrhosis in non-obese, non-affluent populations.[2]

◑ Clinical features

Physical examination

A number of physical findings are often described in patients with cirrhosis (see Table 33.1 overleaf).

Patients with cirrhosis may also present with a diverse range of features suggesting the underlying cause such as cryoglobulinaemia and diabetes from hepatitis C, diabetes mellitus and arthropathy in patients with haemochromatosis, and extrahepatic autoimmune diseases.

Table 33.1 Physical findings in patients with cirrhosis

	Descriptions	**Aetiology**
Jaundice	Yellow colouring of the skin and mucus membranes	When bilirubin is >2–3 mg/dL due to liver disease
Nail changes	Muehrcke's nails: paired horizontal white bands separated by normal colour Terry's nails: proximal two-thirds of the nail plate appears white whereas the distal one-third is red	Hypoalbuminaemia
Ascites	Fluid in the peritoneal cavity	Portal hypertension
Splenomegaly	Enlarged spleen	Portal hypertension
Palmar erythema	Erythema on thenar and hypothenar eminences while sparing the central portions of the palm	Altered sex hormone metabolism
Spider angiomata	Vascular lesions consisting of a central arteriole surrounded by many smaller vessels	Increase in the estradiol/free testosterone ratio
Clubbing and hypertrophic osteoarthropathy	Distal finger has a drumstick appearance and painful chronic proliferative periostitis of the long bones	Hypoxia due to right-to-left shunting and portopulmonary hypertension
Gynaecomastia	Benign proliferation of the glandular tissue of the male breast	Increased production of androstenedione, enhanced aromatisation of androstenedione to oestrone, and increased to oestradiol
Testicular atrophy	Manifested by impotence, infertility, loss of sexual drive seen predominantly in alcoholic cirrhosis and haemochromatosis	Direct toxic effect with increased serum FSH and LH concentrations
Nodular liver	Irregular hard surface on palpation	Fibrosis and regeneration
Dupuytren's contracture	Thickening and shortening of the palmar fascia	Oxidative metabolism of hypoxanthine
Caput medusa	Dilated veins resemble the head (caput) of the mythical Gorgon Medusa	Portal hypertension leading to opening of umbilical vein

	Descriptions	**Aetiology**
Fetor hepaticus	Pungent smell	Increased concentrations of dimethylsulphide
Asterixis	Flapping motion of dorsiflexed hands	Disinhibition of motor neurons

◇ Diagnosis

Laboratory findings

The presence of cirrhosis is sometimes suggested by laboratory abnormalities. Hyponatraemia is common in patients with cirrhosis with ascites and is related to an inability to excrete free water. This results primarily from high levels of antidiuretic hormone secretion.

Haematologic abnormalities include disorders of coagulation and varying degrees of cytopaenia. Thrombocytopaenia is the most common first haematologic abnormality; leukopaenia and anaemia develop later in the course of the disease.

New diagnostic non-invasive tests for liver fibrosis have recently been evaluated in a number of trials (Table 33.2).

Table 33.2 Examples of biomarker components and constituents of panel markers

Biomarker groups	**Examples of individual components**	**Examples of panel biomarkers using at least one component**
Direct		
Collagen and extracellular matrix components	HA MMP 1 MMP 8 PIII NP Laminin	ELF Fibrospect HA score Hepascore Leroy score
Hepatic stellate cell and fibrogenic cell mediators	TIMP 1 TGF b Angiotensin II YKL 40	ELF Fibrospect

continued

Table 33.2 *continued*

Biomarker groups	Examples of individual components	Examples of panel biomarkers using at least one component
Indirect		
Portal hypertension	Platelet count Spleen size	Fibrometer Fibroindex FIB 4 Pohl index
Synthetic parameters	Albumin Platelet count	PGAA index Fibrometer
Liver enzymes and bilirubin	AST ALT AST/ALT ratio GGT Bilirubin	APRI BAAT score Fibrometer Fibroindex Fibrotest Forns Hepascore HA score NAFLD simple index

Most of these biomarkers have a diagnostic accuracy approaching 80 per cent for the differentiation between mild fibrosis (Metavir F0–1) and moderate to severe fibrosis (F2–4). Transient elastography is a technique which correlates with the stiffness or elasticity of the underlying liver.

Radiographic findings

Radiography is mainly used to detect complications of cirrhosis such as ascites, hepatocellular carcinoma, and hepatic or portal vein thrombosis (see Table 33.3).

Table 33.3 Radiological modalities for diagnosis of cirrhosis

Modalities		Findings	Diagnostic tool
Ultrasonography (USG)	Non-invasive, well tolerated, widely available but low sensitivity and operator-dependent	Increased diameter of the portal vein with surface nodularity, increased echogenicity of liver parenchyma	Screening test for complications of portal hypertension, e.g. hepatocellular carcinoma, ascites, and hepatic and portal vein thrombosis

Modalities		Findings	Diagnostic tool
Computed tomography (CT)	Non-invasive, not operator-dependent Radiation and contrast exposure	Findings similar to those of USG	Used for confirming the findings on USG. Triple phase for HCC diagnosis
Magnetic resonance imaging (MRI)	Non-invasive, not operator-dependent No radiation exposure, limited availability and added cost	Substantiate the findings of CT and USG	Estimate hepatic iron concentration MR angiography is more sensitive in diagnosing portal vein thrombosis
Nuclear studies (99mTc sulfur colloid)	Limited studies and usefulness in presence of other modalities	Heterogeneity in uptake by the liver and increased uptake by the spleen and bone marrow	Rarely used now

Testing for specific diseases

A liver biopsy remains the standard for establishing the presence of cirrhosis and can also help uncover its cause in a few cases (see Table 33.4).

Table 33.4 Laboratory investigations for cirrhosis

Disease	Serological tests	Indication of liver biopsy
Hepatitis B-related cirrhosis	HBsAg, HBeAg, HBc-antibodies, HBV DNA	+ (especially in patients with age >40 yrs and normal ALT)
Hepatitis C	HCV antibodies, HBV RNA and genotype	+ (severity of disease and evaluating for contributing causes)
Alcohol	History + AST:ALT ratio ≥ 2, increased and γ-GT	+ (Mallory bodies, infiltration by neutrophils in perivenular distribution)
Autoimmune	Autoantibodies (ANA, ASMA, LKM antibodies, SLA antibodies), increased γ-globulins	+ (bridging necrosis, plasma cells)

continued

Table 33.4 *continued*

Disease	Serological tests	Indication of liver biopsy
Wilson	Decreased serum ceruloplasmin with increased copper in 24 h urine; Kayser-Fleischer ring and penicillamine challenge test	+ (for hepatic copper estimation)
Haemochromatosis	HFE mutation and increased transferrin saturation ($\geq$60% in men and $\geq$50% in women) and ferritin	+ (for hepatic iron load estimation)
$\alpha 1-$ antitrypsin	Reduced $\alpha 1$-antitrypsin and $\alpha 1$-antitrypsin subtyping	+ ($\alpha 1$ loaded hepatocytes)
NASH	Insulin resistance, triglyceride level, uric acid	+ (ballooning of hepatocytes with lobular inflammation)
PBC	Antimitochondrial antibodies (AMA-M2); increased ALP, and total cholesterol	+ (paucity of bile ducts)
PSC	pANCA antibodies (70%), increased ALP and γ-GT, imaging: MRI + MRCP/ERCP Beaded intrahepatic and extrahepatic bile ducts	+ (in small duct PSC)

⊙ Complications

Portal hypertension

The hallmark of portal hypertension is a pathological increase in the pressure gradient between the portal vein and the inferior vena cava, which is measured by the hepatic venous pressure gradient (HVPG). Briefly, the wedged hepatic vein pressure (WHVP), a marker of sinusoidal pressure, and the free hepatic vein pressure (FHVP) are measured with radiologic assistance. HVPG is calculated by the formula HVPG = WHVP – FHVP.

According to Garcia-Tsao (2008): 'HVPG >10 mm Hg is the best predictor of variceal development and decompensation and should be used to stratify patients with compensated cirrhosis in clinical trials'.[3]

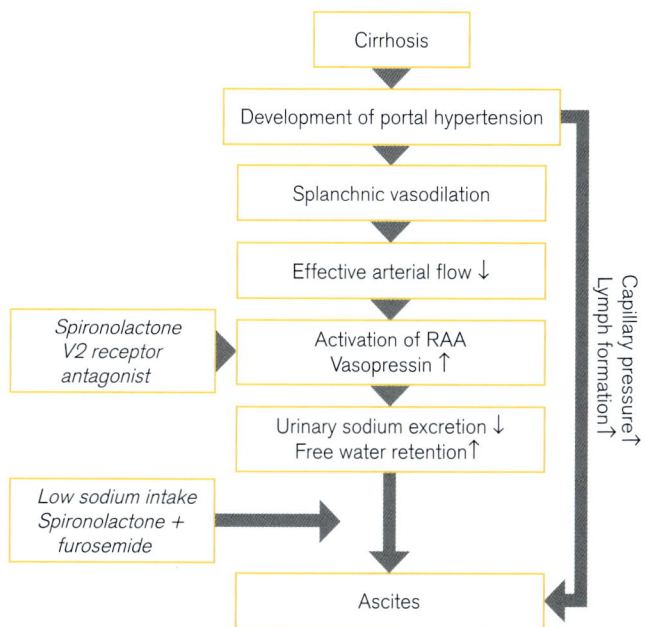

Figure 33.1 Pathogenesis of ascites formation

In cirrhosis, the principal site of increased resistance to outflow of portal venous blood is within the liver itself, due to: (1) mechanical obstruction to flow because of fibrotic disruption of architecture, and (2) a dynamic component produced by contraction of vascular smooth muscle cells and activated stellate cells. The high morbidity and mortality of cirrhosis is secondary to devastating complications.[4]

Ascites

Ascites is the accumulation of fluid within the peritoneal cavity. It is the most common complication of cirrhosis. The first step leading to fluid retention and ultimately ascites is the development of portal hypertension. Patients without portal hypertension do not develop ascites or edema. Those with ascites have several circulatory, vascular, functional, and biochemical abnormalities that contribute to the pathogenesis of fluid retention.[5]

Nearly 60 per cent of all patients with compensated cirrhosis will develop ascites in 10 years. The two-year survival of patients with ascites is approximately 50 per cent.[6]

Management of ascites

The US National Guideline Clearinghouse, Agency for Healthcare Research and Quality, recommendations are as follows:[7]

1. Abdominal paracentesis should be performed and ascitic fluid should be obtained from inpatients and outpatients with clinically apparent new-onset ascites.
2. Because bleeding is sufficiently uncommon, the routine prophylactic use of fresh frozen plasma or platelets before paracentesis is not recommended.
3. The initial laboratory investigation of ascitic fluid should include an ascitic fluid cell count and differential, ascitic fluid total protein, and serum ascites albumin gradient (SAAG).
4. If ascitic fluid infection is suspected, ascitic fluid should be cultured at the bedside in blood culture bottles prior to initiation of antibiotics.

Depending on severity, management of ascites consists of diverse strategies (Table 33.5).

Table 33.5 Management of ascites

Grade	Characteristics	Management
Grade 1, mild	Detected only by examination (ultrasound/CT)	Advice to reduce sodium intake and regular follow-up
Grade 2, moderate	Can be detected through physical examination	Grade 1 + low sodium diet (70–90 mEq/d) + diuretics (aldactone and frusemide)
Grade 3, severe	Marked distension of the abdomen	Grade 2 + therapeutic paracentesis with synthetic plasma expanders or albumin (8 g/L of ascites removed)
Refractory ascites	Lack of response to intensive diuretics Early ascites recurrence Occurrence of diuretic-induced complications	Grade 3 ± TIPS (transjugular intrahepatic portosystemic shunt) or liver transplantation

Recently, advances in medical therapy have been made with satavaptan, a V2 receptor antagonist.[8]

Single-agent furosemide has been shown in a randomised controlled trial to be less efficacious than spironolactone. The doses of both oral diuretics can be increased simultaneously every 3–5 days (spironolactone : furosemide, 100 mg : 40 mg ratio) if weight loss and natriuresis are inadequate. Usual maximum doses are 400 mg/day of spironolactone and 160 mg/day of furosemide. Once the oedema has resolved, 0.5 kg weight loss is probably a reasonable daily maximum. Uncontrolled or recurrent encephalopathy, serum sodium 120 mmol/L despite fluid restriction, or serum creatinine >1.5 mg/dL, should lead to cessation of diuretics, reassessment of the situation, and consideration of second-line options.[7]

Spontaneous bacterial peritonitis

Spontaneous bacterial peritonitis (SBP) is a bacterial infection of ascites without definite evidence of a surgically treatable, intra-abdominal infection.[8]

According to Lee et al. (2009):

The translocation of bacteria from the intestine into the mesenteric lymph nodes is considered an important step in the development of SBP. Translocation of intestinal bacteria is somewhat organism-specific; Gram-negative bacteria translocate more efficiently than Gram-positive bacteria or anaerobes. Translocation is facilitated by the increased intestinal permeability that occurs with bowel edema and portal hypertension. When the bacteria outgrow the capacity of lymph nodes, they spill over into the blood stream.[8]

The AASLD Practice Guidelines state:

The characteristic analysis in the setting of free perforation is polymorphs (PMN) count 250 cells/mm³ (usually many thousands), multiple organisms (frequently including fungi and enterococcus) on Gram stain and culture, and at least two of the following criteria: total protein >1 g/dL, lactate dehydrogenase greater than the upper limit of normal for serum, and glucose <50 mg/dL.[7]

Furthermore, as Murra-Saca points out:

SBP is almost always seen in the setting of end-stage liver disease. Manifestations of SBP include fever, abdominal pain, abdominal tenderness, and altered mental status.[6]

The diagnosis of SBP is made when there is a positive ascitic fluid bacterial culture and/or an elevated ascitic fluid absolute PMN count (i.e. >250 cells/mm³) without an evident intra-abdominal, surgically treatable source of infection. Without early treatment, mortality is high. Patients with ascitic fluid PMN counts >250 cells/mm³ in a clinical setting compatible with ascitic fluid infection should receive empiric antibiotic therapy.

Relatively broad-spectrum therapy is warranted in patients with suspected ascitic fluid infection until the results of susceptibility testing are available (see Table 33.6 overleaf).[9]

Table 33.6 Prevention of SBP

Group	Duration of antibiotic therapy	Degree of benefit	Drugs used
Prior episodes of SBP (secondary prophylaxis)	Lifelong	Definite	Norflox/ trimethoprim/ sulfamethoxazole
Upper gastrointestinal bleeding (primary prophylaxis)	7 days	Definite	Norflox/ceftriaxone
Ascitic fluid protein <1.5 g/dL and at least one of the following is present: serum creatinine >1.2 mg/dL, blood urea nitrogen >25 mg/dL, serum sodium <130 mEq/L or Child-Pugh >9 points with bilirubin >3 mg/dL (primary prophylaxis).	Lifelong	Definite	Norflox/ trimethoprim/ sulfamethasoxazole

The notes for the Internal Medicine Residency Program at Abbott Northwestern Hospital, Minneapolis MN, include the following relevant information:

> *Cefotaxime, a third-generation cephalosporin, has been shown to be superior to ampicillin plus tobramycin in a controlled trial. Cefotaxime or a similar third-generation cephalosporin appears to be the treatment of choice for suspected SBP; it covers 95 per cent of the flora including the three most common isolates:* Escherichia coli, Klebsiella pneumoniae, *and pneumococci.*[10, 11]

The role of albumin

A recent study has shown that albumin should be given when the serum creatinine is >1 mg/dL, blood urea nitrogen >30 mg/dL, or total bilirubin >4 mg/dL, but is not necessary in patients who do not meet these criteria. Albumin has been shown to be superior to hydroxyethyl starch in treatment of SBP.[12]

Hepatorenal syndrome (HRS)(see Figure 33.2)

Severe hepatic decompensation leads to marked splanchnic and systemic vasodilation, a reduction in cardiac function, and a marked decrease in effective arterial blood volume. These result in severe renal vasoconstriction, low renal perfusion, and a decrease in glomerular filtration rate, although the histology of the kidney remains preserved. The incidence of HRS in patients who have advanced cirrhosis and ascites is 8–10 per cent.

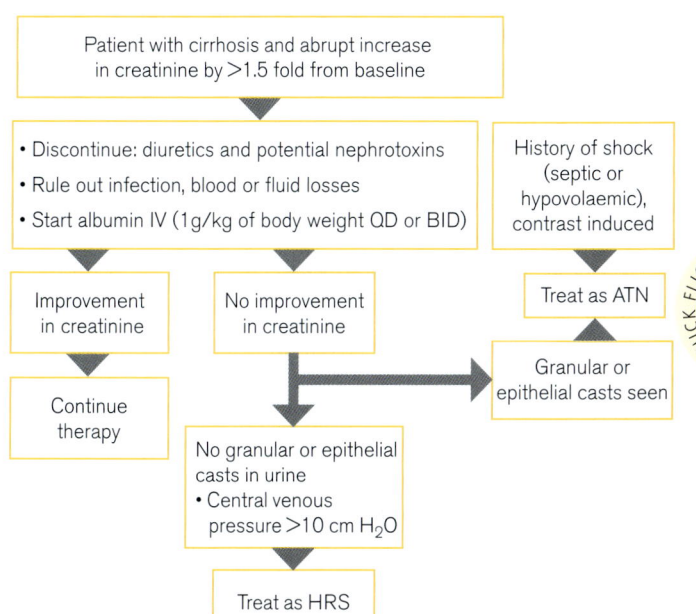

Figure 33.2 Approach to patients with suspected hepatorenal syndrome

There are two types of hepatorenal syndrome. Type I is characterised by rapidly progressive reduction in renal function as defined by a doubling of the initial serum creatinine to a level >2.5 mg/dL in less than two weeks. Type II does not have a rapidly progressive course and is a common cause of death in patients who not die of other complications of cirrhosis. Once the diagnosis of HRS is suspected, specific treatment with vasoconstrictors plus albumin should be initiated.

Best evidence supports the use of terlipressin, which should be started at a dose of 0.5 mg intravenously every six hours. If there is no early response (25% decrease in creatinine levels) after two days of therapy, the dose can be doubled every two days up to a maximum of 12 mg/day (in other words, 2 mg intravenously every 4 hours). Treatment can be stopped if serum creatinine (SCr) does not decrease by at least 50 per cent after seven days at the highest dose, or if there is no reduction in creatinine after the first three days.

In patients with early response, treatment should be extended until reversal of HRS (decrease in creatinine below 1.5 mg/dL) or for a maximum of 14 days. Vasoconstrictor therapy should be restarted if HRS recurs after discontinuation of therapy. Once creatinine normalises, TIPS should be considered, particularly if transplantation is not foreseeable in the near future and the patient has refractory ascites. Patients with cirrhosis, ascites and type I hepatorenal syndrome should have an expedited referral for liver transplantation.

Diagnostic criteria for HRS

- Cirrhosis with ascites
- Serum creatinine >1.5 mg/dL (133 mmol/L)
- HRS-1 doubling of the initial serum creatinine concentrations to a level >2.5 mg/dL (>226 mmol/L) in less than two weeks
- No improvement in serum creatinine (decrease to 1.5 mg/dL or less) after at least two days of diuretic withdrawal and expansion of plasma volume with albumin (1 g/kg body weight/day up to a maximum of 100 g/day)
- Absence of shock
- No current or recent treatment with nephrotoxic drugs or vasodilators
- Absence of parenchymal kidney disease as indicated by proteinuria >500 mg/day, microhaematuria (>50 red blood cells per high power field), or abnormal renal ultrasonography.

Variceal haemorrhage

'Variceal haemorrhage is a devastating complication that occurs in 25 to 40 per cent of patients with cirrhosis. … Although survival has improved with modern techniques for controlling variceal haemorrhage, mortality rates remain high.'[6]

Screening for varices

The frequency of surveillance endoscopies in patients with no or small/large varices depends on their natural history. Endoscopy should be performed once the diagnosis of cirrhosis is established.[12]

Oesophageal varices develop in most patients with advanced cirrhosis, and progress over time. New varices arise in 5–8 per cent of cirrhotic patients within a year, and in 28 per cent of patients within three years. The overall risk for bleeding from all varices is 15 to 20 per cent and 30 per cent in larger varices over a two-year period. The risk for rebleeding in the absence of intervention is approximately 70 per cent over the following two years. A low platelet count (80 000–100 000) and splenomegaly predict a higher likelihood of finding varices but cannot replace an initial screening endoscopy.[14]

Patients without varices develop them at a rate of 5–8 per cent per year, and the strongest predictor for development of varices in those with cirrhosis who have no varices at the time of initial endoscopic screening is an HVPG >10 mm Hg. Endoscopy should be repeated every two to three years for patients who do not have varices at the first endoscopy, because they have a less than 10 per cent risk of bleeding in the next three years. Because the expected progression of small varices to large varices is 10–15 per cent per year, endoscopy should be repeated every one or two years in patients who had small varices on initial endoscopy.

Patients with advanced cirrhosis, large varices or alcoholic liver disease are advised to have yearly endoscopy.

Preprimary prophylaxis

In patients with cirrhosis and small varices that have not bled but have criteria for increased risk of haemorrhage (Child-Pugh classification B/C, or presence of red wale marks on varices), non-selective beta-blockers should be used to prevent first variceal haemorrhage. For patients with cirrhosis and small varices that have not bled and have no criteria for increased risk of bleeding, beta-blockers can be used, although their long-term benefit has not been established.

Patients who receive beta-blockers for small varices do not need a follow-up EGD. For patients with medium/large varices that have not bled and are not at the highest risk of haemorrhage (Child-Pugh A patients, with no red signs), non-selective beta-blockers (propranolol, nadolol) are preferred and EVL (endoscopic variceal ligation) should be considered for patients with contraindications or intolerance to beta-blockers, or non-compliance. For patients with medium/large varices that have not bled but have a high risk of haemorrhage (Child-Pugh B/C or variceal red wale markings on endoscopy), non-selective beta-blockers (propranolol or nadolol) or EVL may be recommended for the prevention of first variceal haemorrhage. If a patient is placed on a non-selective beta-blocker, it should be adjusted to the maximal tolerated dose; follow-up surveillance EGD is unnecessary. If a patient is treated with EVL, it should be repeated every one to two weeks until obliteration, with the first surveillance EGD being performed one to two months after obliteration, and then every six to twelve months to check for variceal recurrence.

The addition of isosorbide mononitrate to beta-blocker therapy seems to lower the risk for initial bleed further in those who did not respond to beta-blockers alone. In clinical practice, 15 to 20 per cent of patients have a relative or absolute contraindication to beta-blockade; five per cent of these develop intolerance while on treatment. A recent study showed that in patients who have high-risk varices, defined as large varices or moderate-sized varices with red wale signs, those treated with propanolol had a higher rate of a first bout of bleeding and mortality than patients who underwent banding.[14]

Management of acute variceal bleed

The mortality from active haemorrhage has declined over the last decade to between 15 and 20 per cent. Only 40 to 50 per cent of all active bleeds stop bleeding spontaneously. Any bleeding that occurs more than 48 hours after the initial admission for variceal haemorrhage and is separated by at least a 24-hour bleed-free period is considered to represent rebleeding. Rebleeding that occurs within six weeks of onset of an acute bleed represents early rebleeding, and bleeding episodes that occur at later times are defined as late rebleeding episodes.

General measures

Packed red cells are transfused to keep the target haemoglobin after transfusion to about 7–8 gm/dL (haematocrit: 21–25%); overtransfusion increases the risk of rebleeding. Fresh frozen plasma and platelets, although frequently used, do not reliably correct coagulopathy and can induce volume overload. Recombinant factor VII has not been found to improve survival. Empiric use of a third-generation cephalosporin, given intravenously, improves the outcomes of active variceal haemorrhage (see Figure 33.3).

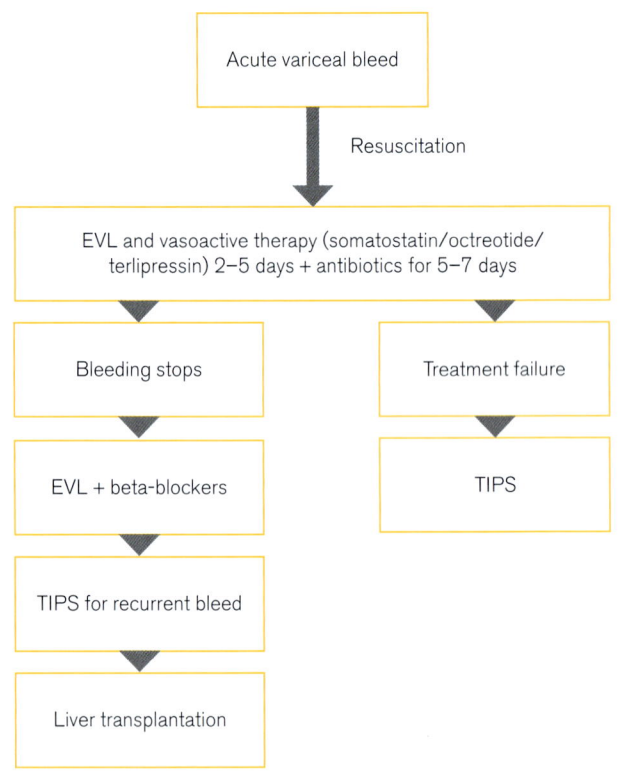

Figure 33.3 Flow diagram in case of acute variceal bleed

Control of bleeding

Terlipressin, somatostatin and octreotide are effective for controlling bleeding. A combination of endoscopic treatment (usually EVL) and pharmacologic treatment (octreotide in the United States) is the preferred first-line treatment to achieve haemostasis. Active bleeding at the time of endoscopy, hypotension, HVPG >20 mm Hg and advanced liver disease Child-Pugh C status are risk factors for failure to control bleeding and early rebleeding. EVL may be attempted once more for early rebleeding, but the decision to use this must be weighed against the risks of complications and the need to provide definitive therapy. Balloon tamponade can effectively produce temporary haemostasis in 80 to 90 per cent of cases. TIPS is the salvage procedure of choice in most subjects. TIPS produces haemostasis more than 90 per cent of the time, and is effective for both gastric and oesophageal variceal bleeding.

Secondary prophylaxis

After an index oesophageal variceal bleed, patients should be beta-blocked and undergo endoscopic band ligation on a bi-weekly basis until the varices are eradicated. Combined therapy is better than ligation alone and lowers the rate of variceal bleeding. The non-selective beta-blocker should be adjusted to the maximal tolerated dose. EVL should be repeated every one or two weeks until obliteration. The first surveillance EGD should then be performed between one and three months after obliteration, then every 6 to 12 months to check for variceal recurrence.

TIPS should be considered in patients who are Child-Pugh A or B and who experience recurrent variceal haemorrhage despite combination pharmacological and endoscopic therapy. In centres where the expertise is available, a surgical shunt can be considered in Child-Pugh A patients. Although TIPS reduces rebleeding, it offers no survival advantage over first-line medical and endoscopic therapy.

Gastric varices

Gastric varices are present in 5 to 33 per cent of patients with portal hypertension and a reported incidence of bleeding of about 25 per cent in two years, with higher bleeding incidence for fundal varices. Risk factors for gastric variceal haemorrhage include the size of fundal varices (>10 mm), Child class (C>B>A), and endoscopic presence of variceal red spots (defined as localised reddish mucosal area or spots on the mucosal surface of a varix). Gastric varices are commonly classified based on their relationship with oesophageal varices as well as their location in the stomach (see Figure 33.4 overleaf).

Patients who have gastric varices still may bleed despite lowering the hepatic venous pressure gradient (HVPG) to less than 12 mm Hg. Anatomically this may result from the preferential drainage of the

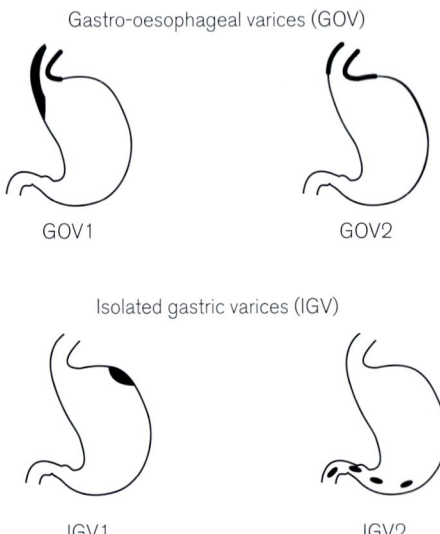

Figure 33.4 Classification of gastric varices

superior mesenteric vein via the short and posterior gastric veins, resulting in formation of gastric varices and a high likelihood of forming a spontaneous splenorenal shunt, which lowers the portal pressure. For patients who have bled from isolated gastric varices, type 1 (IGV1) or gastro-oesophageal varices or type 2 (GOV2), N-butyl-cyanoacrylate or TIPS are recommended. Patients who have bled from gastro-oesophageal varices, type 1 (GOV1) may be treated with N-butyl-cyanoacrylate or band ligation. In a recent study it has been shown that cyanoacrylate injection is more effective than beta-blocker for preventing gastric variceal rebleeding and improving survival.

Hepatopulmonary syndrome

Hepatopulmonary syndrome is defined by a widened alveolar–arterial oxygen gradient in room air more than 15 mm Hg, or more 20 mm Hg for patients older than 64. A pulse oximetry of less than 97 per cent on room air should prompt a blood gas analysis, and a PaO_2 less than 70 mm Hg is indicative of HPS in the absence of underlying cardiopulmonary disease— although they may coexist. Prevalence of HPS among patients with chronic liver disease ranges from 5 to 45 per cent, depending upon the diagnostic criteria and methods used.

The main clinical features are the insidious onset of dyspnoea, platypnoea (shortness of breath exacerbated in the upright posture), orthodexia (hypoxaemia in the upright posture), clubbing and cyanosis. The diagnosis of HPS can be confirmed by contrast echocardiography performed by injecting agitated saline. The study is positive in 40 per cent of patients who have cirrhosis, although only a subset has all the criteria for HPS.[14]

In patients who have intrinsic cardiopulmonary disease, a technetium-labelled macroaggregated albumin (MAA) scan is useful.[15]

Currently there are no effective medical therapies for HPS, with liver transplant being the only effective surgical treatment. Spontaneous resolution of HPS is rare. Liver transplantation leads to significant improvement in arterial hypoxaemia in 85 per cent of patients who have HPS, although it may take up to a year for the resolution of symptoms.

Other pulmonary syndromes

Hepatic hydrothorax and portopulmonary hypertension are two other pulmonary complications that may develop in patients with cirrhosis.

Hepatic hydrothorax

This is defined as the presence of a pleural effusion in a patient with cirrhosis but no evidence of underlying cardiopulmonary disease. It is initially managed by sodium restriction, diuretics and intermittent thoracentesis. TIPS have been used effectively in some patients with refractory hydrothorax.

Portopulmonary hypertension

POPH is defined as the development of pulmonary arterial hypertension associated with increased pulmonary vascular resistance (PVR), further complicated by portal hypertension with or without advanced hepatic disease. This means an increase in mean pulmonary arterial pressure (mPAP) to more than 25 mm Hg in the setting of portal hypertension. Transthoracic Doppler echocardiography (TTE) is a useful non-invasive screening method. Right-heart catheterisation is the 'gold standard' test for the diagnosis, quantification and characterisation of portopulmonary hypertension.

Epoprostenol, a prostacyclin analogue and potent pulmonary and systemic vasodilator, can significantly improve the pulmonary haemodynamics. Iloprost is an alternative to epoprostenol which, if combined with bosentan, an ET-1 receptor antagonist, may extend survival of patients with POPH with recurrent right-heart failure. Sildenafil, a lung tissue–selective phosphodiestrase-5 inhibitor, blocks the degradation of NO and may improve POPH. Liver transplantation is generally not done if mPAP is more than 50 mm Hg.[16]

Hepatic encephalopathy

Hepatic encephalopathy (HE) is defined as a metabolically induced, potentially reversible, functional disturbance of the brain.[17]

While HE may be a complication of acute or chronic liver disease, it is most commonly associated with cirrhosis. The diagnosis of HE requires the presence of liver disease or a portosystemic shunt. The two major mechanisms responsible for the development of HE are severe intrinsic hepatic dysfunction or the presence of portosystemic shunts leading to the diversion of portal blood to the systemic circulation before toxic intestinal substances are removed. HE is characterised by personality changes, impaired intellect, disturbed sleep pattern and depressed level of consciousness. In the presence of chronic liver disease, HE is a marker of decompensation and, as with other complications of liver disease, survival correlates better with the Child-Pugh score than the outcome of the complication itself. There are three types—acute, recurrent and persistent.[17]

According to Bass (2007):

Effective treatment options for hepatic encephalopathy are limited. Based on the principle that intestinal-derived ammonia contributes to the pathogenesis of hepatic encephalopathy, current therapeutic approaches are directed at reducing bacterial production of ammonia and enhancing its elimination. Non-absorbable disaccharides are first-line therapy for hepatic encephalopathy. Alternative therapies such as benzodiazepine receptor antagonists, branched-chain amino acids, and l-ornithine-l-aspartate also have limited clinical data supporting their use. ... Studies of antibiotics indicate that they are effective in the treatment of hepatic encephalopathy, but adverse effects and concerns about long-term safety have limited the widespread use of most. Rifaximin is a minimally absorbed antibiotic that concentrates in the gastrointestinal tract and is excreted mostly unchanged in faeces. It has been studied extensively in the treatment of hepatic encephalopathy and appears to confer therapeutic benefits greater than those of placebo and non-absorbable disaccharides and at least comparable with those of systemic antibiotics. Rifaximin was also well tolerated in patients with hepatic encephalopathy and is not associated with clinical drug interactions or clinically relevant bacterial antibiotic resistance ... and may help to improve patient outcomes.[18]

Summary

Cirrhosis is defined as the histological development of regenerative nodules surrounded by fibrous bands as a result of chronic liver injury, which leads to portal hypertension and end-stage liver disease. The complications of cirrhosis are variceal haemorrhage, ascites SBP, hepatic encephalopathy, hepatorenal syndrome and bacterial infections. The major causes are alcohol and, in the Indian subcontinent, HBV. In Japan and Pakisan HCV predominates. NAFLD has become a significant entity in many countries. New non-invasive diagnostic tests have recently been evaluated, including transient elastography which correlates with the stiffness or elasticity of the underlying liver. A recent advance in medical therapy is the use of satavaptan, a V2 receptor antagonist.

References

1. Schuppan D, Afdhal NH. Liver cirrhosis. *Lancet*. 2008 Mar 8; 371(9615):838–51. Abstract.

2. Das K(ausik), Das K(shaunish), Mukherjee PS, Partha S, Ghosh A, Ghosh S, Mridha AR, Dhibar T, Bhattacharya B, Bhattacharya D, Manna B, Dhali GK, Santra A, Chowdhury A. Nonobese population in a developing country has a high prevalence of nonalcoholic fatty liver and significant liver disease. *Hepatology*. 2010 May; 51(5):1593–602.

3. Garcia-Tsao G, Bosch J, Groszmann RJ. Portal hypertension and variceal bleeding—unresolved issues: summary of an American Association for the Study of Liver Diseases and European Association for the Study of the Liver single-topic conference. *Hepatology*. 2008 May; 47(5):1764-72. doi:10.1002/hep.22273.

4. Goldberg E, Chopra S. Overview of the complications, prognosis, and management of cirrhosis. *UpToDate*. [Internet]. Available from: www.uptodate.com/patients/content/topic.do?topicKey=~pTF_aGHk3QQGSd.

5. Such J, Runyon BA. Pathogenesis of ascites in patients with cirrhosis. *UpToDate*. [Internet]. Available from: www.uptodate.com/patients/content/topic.do?topicKey=~eisIcgz_MJJgCi&source=see_link.

6. Murra-Saca JA. Hepatic cirrosis [sic]. Complications. [Internet]. Available from: www.murrasaca.com/Hepaticirrosis.htm.

7. Runyon BA. AASLD Practice Guidelines Committee. Management of adult patients with ascites due to cirrhosis: an update. *Hepatology*. 2009 Jun; 49(6):2087–107.

8. Lee JM, Han K-H, Ahn SH. Ascites and spontaneous bacterial peritonitis: an Asian perspective. *J Gastroenterol Hepatol*. 2009; 24(9):1494–503.

9. Shalaby GGT. A comparative study between once daily oral levofloxacin 750 mg versus intravenous cefotaxime 2 gm three times daily in spontaneous bacterial peritonitis. Thesis: Master of Internal Medicine. Cairo: Ain Shams University; 2007.

QUICK FLICK
33

10. Abbott Northwestern Hospital. Internal Medicine Residency Program: Paracentesis. [Internet]. Available from: www.anwresidency.com/simulation/guide/para.html.

11. Felisart J, Rimola A, Arroyo V, Perez-Ayuso RM, Quintero E, Gines P, Rodes J. Randomized comparative study of efficacy and nephrotoxicity of ampicillin plus tobramycin versus cefotaxime in cirrhotics with severe infections. *Hepatology*. 1985 May/Jun; 5(3):457–62.

12. Rena NMRA, Wibawa IDN. Albumin infusion in liver cirrhotic patients. *Acta Med Indones*. 2010 Jul; 42(3):162–8.

13. Garcia-Tsao G, Sanyal AJ, Grace ND, Carey W. Practice Guidelines Committee of the American Association for the Study of Liver Diseases; Practice Parameters Committee of the American College of Gastroenterology. Prevention and management of gastroesophageal varices and variceal hemorrhage in cirrhosis. *Hepatology*. 2007 Sep; 46(3):922–38.

14. Grewal P, Martin P. Pretransplant management of the cirrhotic patient. *Clin Liver Dis*. 2009; 11(2):431–49.

15. De Franchis R editor. Portal Hypertension IV: Proceedings of the Fourth Baveno International Conference and Workshop on Methodology of Diagnosis and Treatment. Oxford: Blackwell; 2006.

16. Singh C, Sager JS. Pulmonary complications of cirrhosis. *Med Clin North Am*. 2009 Jul; 93(4):871–83. doi:10.1016/j.mcna.2009.03.006.

17. Cash WJ. Current concepts in the assessment and treatment of hepatic encephalopathy. *QJM*. 2010 Jan; 103(1):9–16. doi:10.1093/qjmed/hcp152.

18. Bass NM. Review article: the current pharmacological therapies for hepatic encephalopathy. *Aliment Pharmacol Ther*. 2007 Feb; 25 Suppl 1:23–31.

Recommended reading

Bosch J, Berzigotti A, Garcia-Pagan JC, Abraldes JG. The management of portal hypertension: rational basis, available treatments and future options. *J Hepatol*. 2008; 48 Suppl 1:S68–92.

Sanyal AJ, Bosch J, Blei A, Arroyo V. Portal hypertension and its complications. *Gastroenterology*. 2008 May; 134(6):1715–28.

Sarin SK, Lamba GS, Kumar M, Misra A, Murthy NS. Comparison of endoscopic ligation and propranolol for the primary prevention of variceal bleeding. *N Engl J Med*. 1999; 340(13):988–93.

Chapter 34: Acute liver failure

D. Amarapurkar (India)

Key points

▶ Acute liver failure (ALF) is characterised by rapid deterioration of liver function.

▶ In patients without pre-existing liver disease, ALF causes coagulopathy and hepatic encephalopathy.

▶ Paracetamol (acetaminophen) toxicity and idiosyncratic drug reaction is the main cause of ALF in Western countries.

▶ Hepatitis E, B and A viruses (HEV, HBV, HAV) are the main causes of ALF in Asian countries.

▶ In developing countries, infectious diseases such as malaria, leptospirosis, dengue fever and typhoid fever can mimic ALF.

▶ Aetiology is a strong predictor of outcome in ALF.

▶ ALF patients need the disease to be assessed and treated urgently.

▶ A multidisciplinary approach provides the best outcome.

◗ Introduction

Massive liver cell necrosis in ALF can threaten the patient's life; the mortality rate is high, even with liver transplantation.

Patients with ALF usually have jaundice, and may behave abnormally. In developing countries it is essential that ALF is differentiated from other potentially curable infectious diseases such as *Plasmodium falciparum* malaria, leptospirosis, dengue fever and enteric fever. Early recognition of ALF and transferring these patients to specialised units with liver transplant facilities is important for improved survival of patients. Viruses are the most common cause of ALF, but drug-induced ALF—especially anti-tubercular drugs—is also an important preventable cause.

◗ Definition

Acute liver failure is defined by evidence of coagulation abnormality (international normalised ratio, INR ≥ 1.5) and any degree of prior encephalopathy with an illness lasting less than 26 weeks in a patient who does not have pre-existing cirrhosis. The modified terminology, which is based on the interval from the onset of jaundice to the development of encephalopathy, was introduced in 1993 by O'Grady and colleagues (see Table 34.1 overleaf).

By dividing ALF into hyperacute (<7 days), acute (8–28 days) and subacute (between 29 days and 12 weeks), this classification distinguishes between patients with a distinct clinical course characterised by greater frequency of cerebral oedema, better prognosis in hyperacute fulminant hepatic failure (FHF), and worse prognosis in subacute liver failure.[1]

Table 34.1 Classification of acute liver failure

Type	Onset of Encephalopathy after jaundice (days)	Common aetiologies	Spontaneous survival rate
Hyperacute	1–7	Paracetamol (acetaminophen) toxicity ischaemia	36%
Acute	8–28	Viral	14%
Subacute	29 days to 12 weeks	Cryptogenic	7%

Although ALF is known to occur in patients without any pre-existing liver disease, most present as acute liver failure on underlying occult chronic liver disease. Acute decompensation in these patients may occur due to a precipitating event such as sepsis, upper GI bleeding or ischaemia, or with additional superimposed liver injury caused by alcohol, hepatotoxic drugs or hepatitis virus infection. Prognosis in this latter group is different from that of ALF (i.e. group with underlying occult chronic liver disease).

○ Differential diagnosis of acute liver failure

In developing countries, infections such as malaria, typhoid fever, leptospirosis and dengue fever can all present in complicated forms with febrile jaundice with encephalopathic features, and may mimic ALF. If these diseases are identified and treated early (Table 34.2) they have good prognosis, and must be kept in mind when evaluating a traveller to endemic countries; this is particularly true of *Plasmodium falciparum* malaria.

○ Causes of acute liver failure

Aetiologies of ALF vary from country to country, but serious drug-induced ALF predominates in most countries (see Table 34.2). Drugs are responsible for ALF in 19–75 per cent of all cases, hepatitis viruses in 4–36 per cent, and other aetiologies are found in 3–45 per cent of cases. Paracetamol (acetaminophen) is blamed in 60–75 per cent of drug-related cases in the UK, compared to 2–20 per cent in other countries, where 12–17 per cent of the drug-related cases of ALF are due to non-steroidal anti-inflammatory drugs (NSAIDs). Idiosyncratic drug reactions are responsible for 2–7 per cent of cases in the UK, and 12–17 per cent of cases elsewhere.

In Asian countries, 91–100 per cent of cases of ALF are caused by viruses; drugs are responsible for 0–7.4 per cent of cases, and other aetiologies are responsible for 0–1.5 per cent. Antituberculosis drugs are involved in most drug-related cases of ALF (1–7% of all cases); mushroom poisoning is responsible for 0.4 per cent. Paracetamol (acetaminophen) poisoning is rare in India.

In children, HAV is responsible for ALF in 10–71 per cent of cases, HEV in 2.7–25 per cent, HBV in 0–10.7 per cent, HCV in 0–2.5 per cent, HDV in 16.7 per cent, mixed infection in 10–22 per cent, non-A–E infections in 17.9 per cent, drugs in 5.5–7.5 per cent, and unknown aetiology in up to 22 per cent of cases.

In India, 25–32 per cent of fulminant hepatic failure (FHF) patients are pregnant, and more than 90 per cent of these cases are due to HEV.

Table 34.2 Aetiology survival rates and specific treatment for patients with ALF

Aetiology	Spontaneous survival rate	Specific treatment
Virus		
HBV/HDV	15–20%	Oral nucleosides
HEV	15–20%	Nil
HAV	50%	Nil
Rare virus		
HCV	Not known	Nil
CMV	Not known	Ganciclovir/valganciclovir
HSV	Not known	Acyclovir
EBV	Not known	Acyclovir
Metabolic		
Wilson's disease	5–10%	D-penicillamine plasmapheresis
Acute fatty liver of pregnancy	50%	Delivery of the baby
Autoimmune hepatitis	10%	Immunosuppressants/ steroids

continued

Table 34.2 *continued*

Aetiology	Spontaneous survival rate	Specific treatment
Ischaemic	30–50%	Resuscitations and volume replacement
Budd-Chiari syndrome	50–60%	Anticoagulation and TIPS
Malignant infiltration	0	Chemotherapy

HAV: hepatitis A virus; HBV: hepatitis B virus; HCV: hepatitis C virus; HDV: hepatitis D virus; HEV: hepatitis E virus; CMV: cytomegalovirus; HSV: herpes simplex virus; EBV: Epstein-Barr virus; INH: isonicotinylhydrazine, or isoniazid; PZA: pyrizinamide; TIPS: transjugular intrahepatic portosystemic shunt.

▷ Diagnosis

ALF is a complex syndrome which progresses rapidly. Time is the key issue in the management of patients. Any patient with severe acute hepatitis with prolonged prothrombin time by more than 4–6 seconds, or INR more than 1.5 and with altered sensorium, is immediately hospitalised with the diagnosis of ALF. Acute liver failure with coagulopathy (even without encephalopathy) should be hospitalised. In these patients with threatened ALF, avoidance of deleterious co-factors and early specific medical therapy is indicated. History-taking should be meticulous: see Table 34.3.

Table 34.3 Important points in history of patients with ALF

- History

  - Drug intake, including complementary and alternative medicines, quantity of drug consumed, associated alcohol consumption, immunosuppressed status or history of immunosuppressive medications
  - Recent travel to areas endemic for viral hepatitis
  - Intravenous drug abuse, sexual behaviour, tattooing and body piercing in the recent past.

- Symptoms

  - Anorexia, nausea, vomiting
  - General sense of not feeling well
  - Highly coloured urine and yellow sclera
  - Difficulty in concentrating, disturbed sleep rhythms, disorientation, confusion, tremor.

- Signs

    - Scleral icterus
    - Right upper quadrant tenderness
    - Flapping tremors
    - Ascites and/or oedema (in patients with Budd-Chiari syndrome).

Clinical examination

This should include (see Table 34.4):

1. assessment and documentation of mental status
2. stigmata of chronic liver disease
3. jaundice, right upper quadrant tenderness
4. measurement of liver volume.

Table 34.4 Stages of hepatic encephalopathy

Stage	Mental status	Physical signs
I	Conscious, orientated but with altered behaviours/speech/sleep	Flapping tremors, apraxia, incoordination
II	Increased drowsiness, confusion, inability to sustain concentration	Flapping tremors + brisk reflexes, dysarthria
III	Marked confusion, arousable but asleep	Extensor plantars, ataxia
IV	Coma, unable to test mental status	Decerebration

Initial laboratory evaluation

See Tables 34.5 and 34.6, and also include:

- blood group typing
- HIV status (implications for transplantation)
- amylase and lipase level
- pregnancy test if appropriate.

    Pulmonary artery catheterisation should be performed on all haemodynamically unstable patients.

Table 34.5 Initial work-up of patients with ALF

- CBC (complete blood count) including platelet count

- Serum bilirubin, SGOT, SGPT, alkaline phosphates, serum albumin, serum globulin, prothrombin time

continued

Table 34.5 *continued*

- Serum creatinine, electrolytes, magnesium, phosphates
- Arterial ammonia, arterial lactate
- Viral markers—HBsAg IgM, anti-HBc, IgM, anti-HAV IgM, anti-HEV
- Serology for hepatitis C, herpes simplex virus, cytomegalovirus and Epstein-Barr virus whenever clinically suspected
- Serum ceruloplasmin, serum copper, 24 hrs urinary copper and copper content of dry weight liver when Wilson's disease suspected
- ANA, ASMA. LKM1, M1 antibodies and liver biopsy when autoimmune hepatitis suspected
- Serum acetaminophen, drugs screening, blood alcohol and urine pregnancy test where appropriate
- Blood culture and urine culture
- Sonography of the abdomen, chest X-ray, ECG and CT brain scan.

Table 34.6 Parameters to be assessed several times a day

- Neurological assessment including eye signs
- Liver size
- Blood sugar
- Serum electrolytes
- For cerebral oedema:
  1. eye signs, rigidity
  2. blood pressure
  3. respiration
  4. external pressure monitoring.

Aetiology

To define aetiology, the following tests should be performed:

- liver biopsy via transjugular route is indicated in suspected autoimmune hepatitis (AIH)
- metastatic/malignant infiltration
- lymphoma or herpes simplex hepatitis.

The aim is to define treatable causes of acute liver failure (see Table 34.7, and Table 34.8 on page 378).

1. Serial measurements of mental status and clinical examination for liver span, ascites and worsening liver function; input-output charting,

cardiac monitoring, pulse oxymetry and central venous pressure (CVP) measurements should be carried out.

2. Coagulation parameters.

3. CBC including haemoglobin, platelet counts, haematocrit and WBC counts.

4. Metabolic panels including glucose, sodium, phosphate, potassium and magnesium.

5. Arterial blood gas analysis.

6. Daily bilirubin and aminotransferase levels.

7. Careful surveillance for infection by monitoring intracranial pressure (ICP):

   a) Clinical signs of elevated ICP such as hyper-reflexia, hypertonia, hypertension, bradycardia and irregular respirations are not present uniformly. Pupillary dilatation or signs of decerebration are late.

   b) ICP monitoring is used for the earliest detection of cerebral oedema; however, since it is an invasive procedure, it carries a risk of infection and bleeding, and the advantages of using ICP monitoring devices in determining outcome of ALF is not clear. It should be considered for patients being listed for transplantation. Patients requiring ICP monitoring can be selected by reverse jugular oxygen saturation (<55% or >80%). Continuous EEG monitoring and microdialysis techniques are emerging.

○ General management

There is no role for corticosteroids in the management of ALF.

Table 34.7 Management of acute liver failure

Grade 1–2 encephalopathy
• Admit patient in ICU, frequent monitoring of neurological status
• Quiet environment with minimal stimuli, avoid sedatives and hypnotics
• Continuous glucose infusion with regular blood glucose monitoring
• Keep strict watch on urine output, blood pressure and fever.

Grade 3–4 encephalopathy
• Elevate head end of the bed by 30 degrees
• Elective intubation if hypoxia, respiratory failure or protection of airways is necessary
• Can use propofol or midazolam for sedation
• Mannitol 0.4 g/kg body weight IV bolus 8-hourly for treatment of cerebral oedema if there are signs of persistent raised intracranial pressure
• Pentobarbital infusion 100 to 150 g bolus over 15 minutes followed by continuous infusion at the rate of 1 to 3 mg/kg
• If hypotension systolic BP <100 mm Hg, use dopamine or noradrenaline; vasopressin should be avoided
• If signs of ICP persist, adjusting blankets to keep the temperature less than 37°C.

continued

Table 34.7 *continued*

Management of renal failure
• Replace fluid if hypovolaemic, aggressive treatment of infection, vasopressor support and if required continuous venovenous haemofiltration
• Treatment of infections: if high index of suspension, start with broad spectrum antibiotics (third-generation cephalosporin or quinolone and vancomycin; avoid amino glycosides; if possible culture-guided selection of antibiotics)
• As well as antibiotic treatment continue to add empirical antifungals.

Management of coagulopathy
• Prophylactic use of fresh frozen plasma is unnecessary; FFP, platelet and cryoprecipitate should be reserved for actively bleeding patient or prior to planned invasive procedures. Recombinant factor VII is superior to FFP in clinically significant bleeding.

Cerebral oedema/intracranial hypertension

Cerebral oedema is the most commonly identifiable cause of death in fulminant hepatic failure (FHF), occurring in >75 per cent of FHF patients with grade 4 encephalopathy.

It is seen most commonly in patients with rapid onset of liver failure, and is unusual (<10%) in patients with late onset or sub-fulminant hepatic failure or coagulopathy, when invasive procedures are being undertaken or when volume overload is a concern.

Metabolic problems and nutrition

1. Frequent monitoring and expeditious correction of acid–base imbalance, hyperlactataemia, hyperthermia, hypercapnia, hypoglycaemia and electrolyte disturbances are recommended for all patients.
2. Enteral feeding should be started as soon as possible.
3. Parenteral feeding is an option when enteral feeding is contraindicated.
4. Protein restriction up to 60 g/day is reasonable.
5. Branched chain amino acid supplements have no proven benefit.

Haemodynamics and renal dysfunction

1. Maintenance of adequate intravascular volume and mean arterial pressure (MAP) of 50–60 mm Hg is recommended. Serial measurements of mean arterial pressure, filling status, cardiac output and state of oxygenation should be obtained. The pathophysiological basis of circulatory dysfunction is vasodilatation and increased cardiac output, leading to low mean arterial pressure.
2. Fluid resuscitation should preferably be done with a mixture of crystalloids and colloids similar to albumin. If using crystalloids, those containing dextrose should be chosen to help maintain euglycaemia. For patients who do not respond to fluid resuscitation, vasopressor support with

dopamine or noradrenaline should be used. Vasopressin or terlipressin should be avoided, as they may be harmful, and can increase intracranial pressure (ICP). The role of steroids for severe episodes of hypotension to improve adrenocortical insufficiency requires further large randomised trials.

3. To prevent renal failure, or in the presence of acute renal failure (ARF), nephrotoxic drugs including aminoglycosides and NSAIDs must be avoided, infection should be treated and nephrotoxic contrast agents whenever possible should be avoided (if used, *N*-acetyl-*L*-cysteine (NAC) may be helpful). Patients requiring dialysis for ARF should undergo continuous rather than intermittent renal replacement therapy, preferably continuous venovenous haemodialysis for better cardiovascular stability and neurological tolerance. Prostaglandins or NAC are not recommended for renal failure.

Liver support systems

Urgent liver transplantation (orthotropic or living-related) is indicated (UNOS status 1) in ALF with poor prognosis, except in patients with ongoing sepsis, or brain-dead patients.

Management of specific aetiologies

Acetaminophen hepatotoxicity, drug-induced hepatotoxicity, viral hepatitis

Refer to *Chaper 35: Acute hepatitis*.

Mushroom poisoning

Diagnosis: History of recent mushroom (*Amanita phalloides*) poisoning. Treatment: If GI symptoms are present, gastric lavage and activated charcoal via nasogastric tube.

1. Penicillin G is given IV 300 000 to 1 000 000 units/kg/day in known or suspected mushroom poisoning.
2. Silymarin in doses of 30–40 mg/kg/day either orally or IV for 3–4 days.
3. All such patients should be listed for transplantation, as it is often the only life-saving option.

Copper sulphate poisoning

D-penicillamine at 25 mg/kg/day is given until recovery, in addition to other measures.

Wilson's disease, autoimmune hepatitis and pregnancy

These conditions may occasionally result in acute liver failure.

Ischaemic hepatitis

This is a rare cause of acute liver failure.

Budd-Chiari syndrome (acute hepatic vein thrombosis)

This syndrome is an indication of liver transplantation if malignancy-associated hypercoagulability is excluded. Contraindications to liver transplantation in the setting of FHF should be identified as quickly as possible. These are:

1. Severe irreversible brain damage, cerebral perfusion pressure <40 mm Hg for >2 h, sustained elevation of ICP to >50 mm Hg.
2. Inability to oxygenate during anaesthesia due to ARDS or severe cardiopulmonary disease.
3. Evidence of multi-organ failure syndrome.
4. Septic shock.
5. Widespread mesenteric vein thrombosis.
6. Active alcohol or drug abuse.
7. Any other major complicating or lethal disorder (e.g. acquired immunodeficiency syndrome, severe depression).
8. Improving liver function; full recovery is expected if the patient survives the acute hepatic insult.

Table 34.8 Complications of acute liver failure

Complications	Incidence
Encephalopathy	100%
Cerebral oedema	50–80%
Coagulopathy (GI bleeding)	50%
Hypotension	50%
Respiratory failure	30–60%
Hypoglycaemia	40%
Electrolytes and acid base distribution	8–100%
Infection and sepsis	25–50%
Renal dysfunction	30–70%
Pancreatitis	10%
Portal hypertension	
Aplastic anaemia	

Summary

Acute liver failure is characterised by rapid deterioration of liver function resulting in coagulopathy and hepatic encephalopathy in patients without pre-existing liver disease. Drug reactions are the predominant cause in Western countries, and viral hepatitis infections in Asia. It is important that a multidisciplinary team manage patients in ALF.

Information for patients

Why does acute liver failure occur?

Acute liver failure (ALF) occurs when the liver loses it ability to function within a period of just a few days.

Are there any complications for someone with ALF?

ALF can cause many complications—increase in pressure in the brain leading to abnormal behaviour, coma and even death. ALF can also cause excessive bleeding, renal failure, respiratory failure and serious infections.

What causes it?

ALF can have many causes—viruses (hepatitis A, E and B), or overdose of drugs such as paracetamol (acetaminophen), or idiosyncratic reactions to anti-TB drugs, antibiotics or painkillers. Also herbal supplements, mushroom poisoning, autoimmune hepatitis, blockage of liver veins, metabolic diseases like Wilson's disease, or acute fatty liver of pregnancy. Rarely, cancer can cause it—and sometimes no apparent cause can be found.

What treatment would someone with ALF receive?

ALF is a medical emergency, and needs immediate hospitalisation in an intensive care unit. In most instances the patient would need a liver transplant.

Can ALF be prevented? How?

Yes. You can prevent acute liver failure by following these guidelines:

1. Be vaccinated against hepatitis.
2. Follow the instructions on the package insert of any medication you take, and don't exceed the recommended dose.
3. Avoid alcohol abuse, and whenever you go to your doctor inform them about all the medications you take, including herbal medicines and food supplements.
4. Avoid using illicit intravenous drugs.

Table 35.1 Causes of acute hepatitis

- Acute viral hepatitis
- Exacerbation of chronic viral hepatitis
- Non-viral liver disease

idiosyncratic drug reactions have emerged as the most frequent causes in recent studies (see Tables 35.1–35.3).

◇ Aetiology

Table 35.2 Causes of viral hepatitis

Hepatitis A, B, C, D or E viruses

Other viral causes:
  Herpes simplex
  Cytomegalovirus
  Epstein-Barr virus
  Yellow fever virus
  Adenoviruses
  Measles virus
  Varicella zoster
  Coxsackievirus
  Human immunodeficiency virus
  Non A to E viruses

Table 35.3 Common causes of non-viral hepatitis

Alcohol overuse

Non A to E hepatitis—putative, but uncharacterised viruses

Drug-induced liver injury

Direct hepatotoxicity:
  Hepatocellular damage and necrosis, usually caused by drugs or toxins
  Dose-dependent (e.g. paracetamol)

Idiosyncratic hepatotoxicity:
  Typically follows a sensitisation period of several weeks, or is due to a genetic predisposition; caused by, for example, isoniazid, methyldopa, mercaptopurine, lovastatin, pravastatin, dipyridamole, halothane

Cholestatic reactions and direct hepatotoxicity:
  May result from oral contraceptives or anabolic steroids; hypersensitivity to phenothiazine derivatives such as chlorpromazine, antibiotics, thyroid medications, antidiabetic drugs and cytotoxic drugs

Infectious agents:
  Spirochaetes (syphilis and leptospirosis), toxoplasma, Q fever, Rocky Mountain spotted fever

Metabolic and autoimmune disorders:
  Acute presentation of subclinical liver disease, such as autoimmune hepatitis and Wilson's disease

Ischaemic hepatitis:
  Due to poor cardiac output, hypotension and circulatory insufficiency

Non-alcoholic steatohepatitis:
  May present with raised serum aminotransferases

Pregnancy:
  Obstructive lesions such as gallstones may present as an acute hepatitis

◗ Clinical features

Acute viral hepatitis

The initial features of acute viral hepatitis are non-specific flu-like symptoms. Physical findings are usually minimal, apart from jaundice in one-third of cases, and tender hepatomegaly. The disease is more likely to be asymptomatic and anicteric in younger people.

   A small proportion of people with acute hepatitis progress to FHF, characterised by hepatic encephalopathy, oedema and bleeding. Acute liver failure is life-threatening and may require OLT.

Acute non-viral hepatitis

The clinical features of toxic and drug-induced hepatitis vary with the severity of liver damage and the causative agent. Specific toxins may induce specific symptoms. In FHF, the picture is similar for all causes, reflecting the hepatic injury and resulting organ failure. Even with optimal early management, however, many patients with acute liver failure (ALF) develop a cascade of complications that is often presaged by the systemic inflammatory response syndrome, which involves failure of nearly every organ system.

◗ Diagnosis of acute hepatitis

Diagnostic findings include elevations in liver enzymes, elevated white blood cell count (WBC) and, in some cases of drug-induced hepatitis, elevated eosinophil. A liver biopsy may help identify the underlying pathology, especially infiltration with WBCs and eosinophils.

○ Acute hepatitis A

Type A hepatitis is caused by the hepatitis A virus (HAV). Hepatitis A is endemic in all parts of the world. A high proportion of asymptomatic and anicteric infections occur; 80 to 90 per cent of children in developing countries have serological markers of past infection by the age of five years.

The incubation period of hepatitis A is between three and five weeks. HAV is spread by the faecal–oral route, most commonly by person-to-person contact, and infection is particularly common in conditions of poor sanitation and overcrowding.

Although hepatitis A is common in developed countries, the infection mainly occurs in small clusters. In places such as southern Europe and China where socioeconomic conditions and sanitation have improved, there has been a parallel increase in the mean age of hepatitis A infection.

Clinical features

Subclinical and anicteric infections are common, particularly in young children. Infection in adulthood results in acute icteric hepatitis in more than 70 per cent of cases. The risk of serious complication increases significantly with age.

Diagnosis

Hepatitis A antibody (anti-HAV) is always demonstrable early in the course of the infection. Serological diagnosis of recent infection can be established by demonstration of IgM antibody to hepatitis A.

Prevention and control

The spread of hepatitis A is reduced by taking simple hygienic measures. Human immunoglobulin will prevent or attenuate a clinical illness if given intramuscularly before exposure to the virus or early in the incubation period.

Highly immunogenic vaccines have become available. A single dose of vaccine may be offered to travellers, with the option of a booster dose six to 12 months later.

○ Acute hepatitis B

Refer to *Chapter 36: Hepatitis B infection*.

○ Acute hepatitis C

Refer to *Chapter 37: Hepatitis C infection*.

▷ Acute hepatitis D

Hepatitis delta virus (HDV) is now known to be a defective virusoid that requires a helper function from HBV for its propagation and transmission. HDV is coated with the surface antigen HBsAg of the hepatitis B virus, which is needed for release from and entry into the host hepatocyte.

The mode of transmission of hepatitis D is similar to parenteral spread of hepatitis B. The infection is important epidemiologically in southern Europe, the Middle East (particularly the Gulf States and Saudi Arabia), Japan and Taiwan, and in parts of Africa and South America; however, there is evidence that the prevalence of delta infection is declining in southern Europe. It has been estimated that 5 per cent of HBsAg carriers worldwide—approximately 15 million people—are infected with HDV.

Clinical course

Two major modes of delta hepatitis infection are known. In the first mode, a susceptible individual is co-infected with HBV and HDV, often leading to a more severe form of acute hepatitis caused by HBV. Epidemics with high mortality have been described in South America in association with severe hepatitis B. In the second mode of infection, an individual infected chronically with HBV becomes superinfected with HDV. This may accelerate the course of the chronic liver disease and cause overt disease in asymptomatic HBsAg carriers.

Diagnosis

Zuckerman et al. (2009) describe the laboratory diagnosis of HDV infection as follows:

> Specific serological tests are available to detecting antibodies to HDV—anti-HD IgM and anti-HD IgG—and for HDV RNA. HDgAg can be detected by immunohistochemical staining in the liver. Co-infection and superinfection can be distinguished by correlation of the results of these tests with those for markers of HBV infection.... Coexistence of anti-HBc in IgM with markers of HDV infection is a reliable indication of co-infection; anti-HD IgM becomes detectable, followed by anti-HD IgG. Markers of virus replication usually become undetectable during convalescence.
>
> Superinfection of HBV carriers with HDV frequently results in persistent HDV infection. HD viraemia is followed by an anti-HD IgM, and then IgG, response. Markers of HBV replication may be suppressed during acute HDV infection. Anti-HD IgM persists with HDAg and HDV RNA in serum in chronic delta hepatitis.[1]

QUICK FLICK 35

Management of HDV co-infection

The mainstay of treatment remains long-term interferon or PEG-interferon. Some patients become HDV RNA negative, or even HBsAg negative, and their histology improves. Patients with decompensated liver disease should be considered for transplantation, with prophylaxis against reinfection with HBV.

Prevention of HDV

Prevention and control measures of HDV are similar to those for HBV. Immunisation with hepatitis B vaccine protects against HDV.

◌ Acute hepatitis E

Acute hepatitis E is caused by the hepatitis E virus (HEV), a positive-sense single-stranded RNA virus with a 7.5 kilobase genome. HEV has a faecal-oral transmission route. Epidemic hepatitis, resembling hepatitis A but serologically distinct, was first reported on the Indian subcontinent and later in Central and South-East Asia, the Middle East, North Africa and Central America. Sporadic cases have been observed in developed countries among migrant labourers and travellers returning from these areas.

The average incubation period of six weeks is slightly longer than for hepatitis A. The infection is acute and self-limiting. Clinical disease mainly occurs in young adults, and high mortality rates (up to 20%) have been reported in the third trimester of pregnancy. The infection is spread by the ingestion of contaminated water and probably by food, but secondary clinical cases seem to be uncommon.

Clinical course

In general, the disease is self-limited. Cholestatic features are common, and may be prolonged. Liver biopsies obtained during the acute illness show portal inflammation and cytoplasmic cholestasis. An early observation was the high mortality (10–20%) in pregnant women due to fulminant hepatitis. Stool specimens may reveal 27–32 nm virus-like particles when tested by immune electron microscopy (IEM), but reverse transcriptase (RT)-PCR assay for HEV RNA is a more reliable method. Babies born to women with acute disease are at risk of vertical transmission and may also be at risk of perinatal morbidity: infant mortality of up to 30 per cent has been observed.

There are reports of reactivation of HEV in immunosuppressed patients with prolonged viraemia and liver injury.

Diagnosis

With the availability of recombinant antigens and synthetic peptides, serological assays have been developed to test for antibodies to hepatitis E virus (anti-HEV). IgM HEV is detected only infrequently at initial presentation, and disappears by three months after jaundice. IgG titres initially can be quite high, but tend to decrease over time. The diagnosis can be confirmed by RT-PCR on faecal material from acutely infected patients, and the serum also may be positive with a transient viraemia. Evidence of secondary intrafamilial spread is uncommon.

Management

Liver transplantation is indicated for fulminant hepatitis E if survival otherwise seems unlikely.

Prevention

Adult populations in endemic areas are susceptible to hepatitis E, with high attack rates in epidemics. A baculovirus-expressed HEV vaccine (spanning aa 112–607 of the ORF 2 protein of the Pakistan strain) has been tested in clinical trials and the initial data shows that the immune response protects against infection.

▷ Acute alcoholic hepatitis

Pure alcohol at the rate of 30 grams per day is regarded as 'safe'. Usually alcoholic hepatitis comes after a period of increased alcohol consumption. Alcoholic hepatitis can occur in patients with chronic alcoholic liver disease and alcoholic cirrhosis. Manifestations of liver damage range from fatty liver to end-stage cirrhosis, but the increasing number of cases presenting with an acute alcoholic hepatitis (AAH) is a cause for the greatest concern.

Alcoholic hepatitis is characterised by a variable constellation of symptoms: see Table 35.4.

Table 35.4 Symptoms of alcoholic hepatitis

- Feeling unwell

- Hepatomegly

- Ascites

- Modest elevation of liver blood tests

- Varies from mild liver inflammation to development of jaundice, prolonged prothrombin time, and liver failure

- Severe cases are characterised by either encephalopathy or elevated bilirubin and prothrombin time

- Significant mortaliy: 50% within 30 days of onset

Alcoholic hepatitis is evident pathologically by fatty change, cell necrosis and Mallory bodies. The role of endotoxins, tumour necrosis factor alpha, fibroblasts, and the immune response to altered hepatocyte proteins is being studied.

Treatment

The development of well-validated prognostic scoring systems (modified Maddrey's discriminant function, or the Glasgow alcoholic hepatitis score) makes it possible to select those patients with AAH who are most likely to respond to corticosteroids, but glucocorticoids and anti-tumour necrosis factor alpha (infliximab) are recommended only in severe AAH cases. The results of early pilot studies of a number of anti-TNF agents are encouraging.

There is ongoing debate regarding the utility and application of liver transplantation in severe AAH, and the need for a prior six-month period of alcohol abstinence.

Drug-induced hepatitis

Using a prospective, population-based French study with an annual estimated incidence of 13.9 cases of drug-induced liver injury (DILI) per 100 000 inhabitants, it has been extrapolated that nearly 44 000 individuals in the United States will suffer from DILI each year.[2]

Most adverse liver reactions are idiosyncratic, occurring in most instances anywhere from five to 90 days after the causative medication was last taken. The diagnosis of DILI is clinical, based on the patient's history, the probability of the suspect medication as a cause of liver injury, and exclusion of other hepatic disease. DILI can be hepatocellular (marked by a predominant rise in alanine transaminase), cholestatic (a predominant rise in alkaline phosphatase) or mixed liver injury. DILI has an incidence rate of 0.7–1.3 per 100 000. Acute liver failure is rare, but 13–17 per cent of all acute liver failure cases are attributed to idiosyncratic drug reactions. Response to drug withdrawal may be delayed up to a year in cholestatic liver injury, with occasional subsequent progressive cholestasis known as the vanishing bile duct syndrome. Overall, chronic disease may occur in up to 6 per cent of patients, even if the offending drug is withdrawn.

Antibiotics and NSAIDs are the most common cause of DILI. Statins rarely cause significant liver injury, whereas antiretroviral therapy is associated with hepatotoxicity in 10 per cent of treated patients. Multiple mechanisms of DILI have been implicated, including TNF-alpha-activated apoptosis, inhibition of mitochondrial function and neoantigen formation. Risk factors for DILI include age, sex and genetic polymorphisms of drug-metabolising enzymes such as cytochrome P450 (CYP). In patients with HIV the presence of chronic viral hepatitis increases the risk of antiretroviral therapy hepatotoxicity. It is hoped that the application of pharmacogenetics and proteomics will lead to accurate prediction of the risk of DILI (see Table 35.5).

Table 35.5 Drug-induced hepatitis

- Drugs can mimic all the patterns found in primary liver disease

- Acute hepatitis, with or without cholestasis, is the most common histological pattern (acetaminophen)

- Prolonged cholestasis and ductopaenia resembling primary chronic biliary disease can occur

- Most cases of DILI resolve on discontinuation of drug

- Recovery can take months

- Disease can progress despite drug withdrawal

- Drugs such as methotrexate can lead to chronic hepatitis and cirrhosis

- Minocycline, nitrofurantoin and methyldopa are implicated in autoimmune hepatitis

- Drug-induced steatohepatitis is well described (amiodarone and irinotecan)

- Other patterns: granulomatous hepatitis, vascular injury (e.g. sinusoidal obstruction syndrome), Ito cell lipidosis and neoplasms (e.g. adenomas)

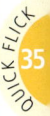

An elevated bilirubin level more than twice the upper limit of normal in patients with hepatocellular liver injury implies severe DILI.

DILI encompasses a spectrum of clinical disease ranging from mild biochemical abnormalities to acute liver failure (ALF). It accounts for approximately 20 per cent of acute liver failure in children and a higher percentage in adults. Although most patients experience milder drug hepatotoxic reactions such as hepatitis, cholestasis or asymptomatic enzyme elevation, it is important to recognise the potential for progression to ALF.

The most common cause of drug-induced ALF in children is acetaminophen (15% of all ALF in children in the UK and US), whereas other drugs such as antituberculosis and anticonvulsant therapy account for 5 per cent.

The pathogenesis of liver injury includes direct hepatotoxicity and idiosyncratic reactions for most drugs, although for others the mechanism of injury is assumed on the basis of clinical presentation and hepatic histological findings.

Although the frequency of drug-induced liver injury remains low, new data from the US Centers for Disease Control and Prevention confirms that acetaminophen hepatotoxicity accounts for 41 per cent of the approximately 1600 new acute liver failure cases annually. Among children with acute liver failure, acetaminophen was the second most common cause. Antimicrobials lead the list of non-acetaminophen causes of drug-induced liver injury. In Asia, herbal compounds are the most common causes of the condition (Table 35.6).

Table 35.6 Some commonly used drugs causing hepatitis

- Agomelatine (antidepressant)
- Allopurinol (hyperuricaemia)
- Amitriptyline (antidepressant)
- Amiodarone (antiarrhythmic)
- Azathioprine (immunosuppressant)
- Halothane (anaesthetic)
- Hormonal contraceptives
- Ibuprofen and indomethacin (NSAIDs)
- Isoniazid (INH), rifampicin (tuberculosis-specific antibiotics)
- Ketoconazole (antifungal)
- Loratadine (antihistamine)
- Methotrexate (immunosuppressant)
- Methyldopa (antihypertensive)
- Minocycline (tetracycline antibiotic)
- Nifedipine (antihypertensive)
- Nitrofurantoin (antibiotic)
- Paracetamol (analgesic)
- Phenytoin and valproic acid (antiepileptics)
- Troglitazone
- Antiretrovirals
- Some herbs and nutritional supplements

Clinical course

The clinical course is quite variable, depending on the drug and the patient's tendency to react to the drug. Hormonal contraception can cause structural changes in the liver. Amiodarone-induced hepatitis can be untreatable since the long half-life of the drug (up to 60 days) means that there is no effective way to stop exposure to the drug.

Statins can cause elevations of liver function blood tests, usually without indicating underlying hepatitis.

Lastly, human variability is such that any drug can be a cause of hepatitis.

Diagnosis

Drug-induced liver injury (DILI) from statins typically presents with an acute hepatocellular liver injury pattern, although mixed or cholestatic injury patterns have also been reported. Non-specific autoantibodies as well as clinical, laboratory and histological features of an autoimmune-like hepatitis may be present in some patients with statin hepatotoxicity.

Liver toxicity is one of the most relevant adverse effects of antiretroviral therapy. Efavirenz is considered a safer drug for the liver than nevirapine.

Pathology

Drugs can mimic all the patterns found in primary liver disease. Acute hepatitis, with or without cholestasis, is the most common histological pattern of DILI, and drugs such as acetaminophen are the leading causes of acute liver failure. Most cases of DILI resolve upon discontinuation of the drug, but recovery can take months. In some rare cases, the disease can progress despite drug withdrawal.

Drugs such as methotrexate can lead to chronic hepatitis and cirrhosis, while others such as minocycline, nitrofurantoin and methyldopa are implicated in autoimmune hepatitis. Prolonged cholestasis and ductopaenia resembling primary chronic biliary disease can occur. Drug-induced steatohepatitis is also an uncommon pattern, but is well described with drugs such as amiodarone and irinotecan.

In the presence of risk factors such as obesity and diabetes, some drugs—tamoxifen, oestrogens and nifedipine, for example—can precipitate or exacerbate steatohepatitis. Other observed patterns include granulomatous hepatitis, vascular injury (including sinusoidal obstruction syndrome), Ito cell lipidosis and neoplasms (adenomas, for instance).

○ Toxin-induced hepatitis

Mushrooms containing amatoxin cause hepatitis, including the Death Cap Mushroom (*Amanita phalloides*), the Destroying Angel (*Amanita ocreata*), and some species of *Galerina*. A portion of a single mushroom can be enough to be lethal (10 mg or less of α-amanitin).

Carbon tetrachloride (CCl_4) ('tetra', a dry cleaning agent), chloroform, trichloroethylene and all chlorinated hydrocarbons, cause steatohepatitis.

◗ Hepatitis caused by metabolic disorders

Some inherited metabolic disorders cause acute forms of hepatitis. Haemochromatosis and Wilson's disease can cause liver inflammation and necrosis and may present as acute hepatitis or FHF.

'Obstructive jaundice' is the term describing jaundice due to obstruction of the bile duct by gallstones or by external obstruction by cancer.

◗ Hepatitis caused by pregnancy

Pregnancy may result in acute hepatitis.

◗ Hepatitis caused by malignancy

Malignancy is an uncommon cause of acute liver failure.

◗ Ischaemic hepatitis

This is a rare cause of abnormal liver function.

◗ Hepatitis assocated with liver failure

Refer to *Chapter 34: Acute liver failure*.

◗ Prevention

Prevention of non-viral hepatitis

Patients should be educated about the risk of potentially hepatic drugs. Regular monitoring of liver function test and adherence to guidelines is especially important in patients with risk factors for antiretroviral-induced liver disease.

Genetic polymorphisms among enzymes involved in drug metabolism and types of human leukocyte antigens (HLA) may account for some of the differences in individual susceptibilities to drugs.

Prevention of hepatitis viral infection

Patients with chronic hepatitis B and C should be vaccinated, as appropriate, against hepatitis A and B. However, hepatitis A and B vaccinations are less effective in patients with advanced liver disease, or following liver transplantation. Several randomised, placebo-controlled trials have shown that reactivation of hepatitis B can be prevented by antiviral prophylaxis.

Summary

Acute hepatitis implies inflammation of the liver characterised by inflammatory cells in the tissue of the liver itself. It may be self-limiting, or it may progress to become fulminant hepatitis with liver failure, progressive fibrosis or cirrhosis. The causes are acute viral hepatitis, or exacerbation of chronic viral hepatitis, or non-viral liver disease.

The aetiologies vary from country to country: for example, paracetamol (acetaminophen) overdose and idiosyncratic drug reactions are major causes in Europe and the USA; in Asia and Africa, viral diseases are the predominant cause.

Alcohol is a major contributor to liver disease in many Western countries and is becoming more prevalent in Asia and India.

Other causes of acute hepatitis include pregnancy, autoimmune hepatitis, ischaemic hepatitis and metabolic disorders. Management is directed to the specific cause.

References

1. Zuckerman AJ, Banatvala JE, Griffiths P, Schoub B, Mortimer P, editors. Principles and practice of clinical virology. 6th ed. West Sussex: Wiley-Blackwell; 2009; pp. 308–9.

2. Bell LN, Chalasani N. Epidemiology of idiosyncratic drug-induced liver injury. *Semin Liver Dis*. 2009 Nov; 29(4):337–47.

QUICK FLICK 35

Recommended reading

Keeffe EB. Acute liver failure. In: McQuaid KR, Frieman SL, Grendell JH, editors. Current diagnosis and treatment in gastroenterology. 2nd ed. New York: Lange Medical Books/McGraw-Hill; 2003; p536–45.

Makin AJ, Wendon J, Williams RA. Seven year experience of severe acetaminophen-induced hepatotoxicity (1987–1993). *Gastroenterology*. 1995; 109:1907–16.

O'Grady JG, Schalm SW, Williams R. Acute liver failure: redefining the syndromes. *Lancet*. 1993 Jul 31; 342(8866):273–5.

Watanabe S, Arima K, Nishioka M, Yoshino S, Hasui H, Fujikawa M. Comparison between sporadic cytomegalovirus hepatitis and Epstein-Barr virus hepatitis in previously healthy adults. *Liver*. 1997 Apr; 17(2):63–9.

Chapter 36: Hepatitis B infection

A.A. Rani, M. Abdullah (Indonesia)

Key points

▶ Hepatitis B virus (HBV) infection is a global public health problem.
▶ Vaccination has resulted in a significant decrease in the incidence of acute hepatitis B.
▶ Hepatitis B remains an important cause of morbidity and mortality.
▶ Acute phase ranges from subclinical hepatitis to fulminant hepatitis.
▶ Chronic phase can be found as asymptomatic carrier state, chronic hepatitis, cirrhosis and hepatocellular carcinoma.
▶ Extrahepatic manifestations can occur in both acute and chronic HBV infection.
▶ The diagnosis of HBV infection is based on:
  – history and physical examination
  – laboratory findings: complete blood count, liver function tests, HBsAg, HBeAg, HBV DNA, anti-HBs antibody, anti-HBe antibody, anti-HBc antibody
  – abdominal ultrasound
  – liver biopsy (if needed).
▶ Therapy is indicated in patients with:
  – acute liver failure
  – cirrhosis with clinical complications
  – cirrhosis or advanced fibrosis with HBV DNA in serum
  – reactivation of chronic HBV after chemotherapy or immune suppression
  – infants born to women who are HBsAg-positive (immunoglobulin and vaccination).
▶ Therapy may be indicated in patients with immune-active phase but who do not have advanced fibrosis or cirrhosis (HBeAg-positive or HBeAg-negative chronic hepatitis)
▶ Therapy is not routinely indicated in patients with:
  – chronic HBV in the immune-tolerant phase (high levels of serum HBV DNA but normal serum ALT levels or little activity on liver biopsy)
  – inactive-carrier or low-replicative phase (low levels of or no detectable HBV DNA in serum and normal serum ALT levels)
  – latent HBV infection (HBV DNA without HBsAg).

▶ Recommended antiviral used in HBV infection:
  – interferon (interferon α-2b and peginterferon α-2a)
  – nukleosida or analogue nukleosida (lamivudine, adefovir, entecavir, tenofovir, telbivudine, clevudine).
▶ Goals of treatment for chronic HBV infection:
  – permanent suppression of HBV replication
  – HBeAg seroconversion and/or HBV-DNA suppression
  – ALT normalisation
  – prevention of hepatic decompensation
  – reduction or prevention of progression to cirrhosis and/or HCC
  – prolonging survival.

◐ Introduction

HBV infection is a global public health problem as it becomes the 10th leading cause of death worldwide. It is estimated that over two billion people have been infected with HBV resulting in 300 to 400 million carriers, 75 per cent of whom live in Asia or the Western Pacific. During their lifetime, 25 per cent of those individuals have a long-term risk of developing chronic active hepatitis, liver cirrhosis and primary hepatocellular carcinoma (HCC). Approximately 1.2 million people die annually because of HBV infection that results in complications caused by the interactions between the virus and the host immune response.

The implementation of effective vaccination programs in many countries has significantly decreased the incidence of acute hepatitis B. Despite the availability of HBV vaccines, the rate of HBV-related hospitalisations, cancers and deaths in the United States more than doubled in the first decade of the twenty-first century. As a result, hepatitis B remains an important cause of morbidity and mortality.

◐ Pathogenesis

HBV is transmitted by perinatal, percutaneous and sexual exposure, as well as by close person-to-person contact, presumably by open cuts and sores, especially among children in hyperendemic areas. The risk of developing chronic HBV infection after acute exposure ranges from 90 per cent in newborns of HBeAg-positive mothers to 25–30 per cent in infants and children aged under five years, and to less than 5 per cent in adults. Immunosuppressed persons are more likely to develop chronic HBV infection after acute infection.

The pathogenesis of hepatitis B is due to the interaction of the virus and the host immune system. The host immune responses of T cells and B cells to HBV peptide antigens (Ag) result in hepatic injury. Those responses include production of cytopathic and non-cytopathic cytokines along with activation and recruitment of non-HBV-specific innate immune effector leukocytes into the infected liver.

Four different stages have been identified in the viral life cycle of hepatitis B—these are immune tolerance, immune clearance, immune control and immune escape (Figure 36.1). The first stage is immune tolerance. The duration of this stage for healthy adults is approximately two to four weeks and represents the incubation period. For newborns, the duration of this period is often decades. Active viral replication is known to continue despite little or no elevation in aminotransferase levels and no symptoms of illness.

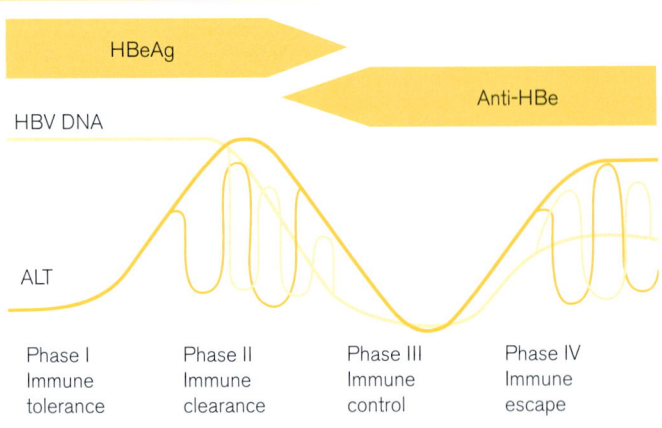

Figure 36.1 Natural history and phases of CHB

Source: Reproduced with the permission of the Gastroenterological Society of Australia (GESA).

In the second stage, known as immune clearance, an inflammatory reaction with a cytopathic effect occurs. HBeAg can be identified in the sera and a decline in the levels of HBV DNA is seen. The duration of this stage for patients with acute infection is approximately three to four weeks (symptomatic period). For patients with chronic infection, 10 years or more may elapse before cirrhosis develops.

In the third stage, the host can target the infected hepatocytes and the HBV. Viral replication no longer occurs and anti-HBe can be detected. The HBV DNA levels are lower or undetectable and aminotransferase levels are within the reference range. In this stage, an integration of the viral genome into the host's hepatocyte genome takes place. HBsAg can still be detected.

In the fourth stage, the virus cannot be detected and antibodies to various viral antigens have been produced. Different factors have been postulated to influence the evolution of these stages, including age, sex, immune status and co-infection with other viruses.

◗ Diagnosis

The diagnosis of hepatitis B infection is based on thorough clinical history, physical manifestations and laboratory findings.

History and physical manifestations

The spectrum of clinical manifestations of HBV infection varies in both acute and chronic disease. During the acute phase, manifestations range from subclinical or anicteric hepatitis to icteric hepatitis and, in some cases, fulminant hepatitis. Patients can present with anorexia, nausea, vomiting, low-grade fever, myalgia, fatigability, right upper quadrant and epigastric pain. In severe cases, hepatic encephalopathy, somnolence, disturbances in sleep pattern, mental confusion or coma can develop. During the chronic phase, manifestations range from an asymptomatic carrier state to chronic hepatitis, cirrhosis and hepatocellular carcinoma. Extrahepatic manifestations such as peripheral oedema, gynaecomastia, testicular atrophy and abdominal collateral veins (caput medusae) can occur in both acute and chronic phase.

Laboratory findings

During the acute phase of HBV infection, high levels of alanine aminotransferase (ALT) and aspartate aminotransferase (AST), in the range of 1000–2000 IU/mL, can be detected. Higher values are found in patients with icteric hepatitis. ALT levels are usually higher than AST levels. Alkaline phosphatase (ALP) levels may be elevated, but they are usually not more than three times the upper limit of normal (ULN). Albumin levels can be slightly low, and serum iron levels may be elevated. Several viral markers can be identified in the serum and the liver. HBsAg and HBeAg are the first markers that can be identified in the serum (see Table 36.1 overleaf). For patients who recover, seroconversion to anti-HBs and anti-HBe is observed. Patients with persistent HBsAg for longer than six months develop chronic hepatitis.

The chronic phase of HBV infection can be divided into chronic inactive and chronic active. Patients in the chronic inactive phase—known as healthy carriers—have normal AST and ALT levels. The markers of infectivity (HBeAg, HBV DNA) may be negative but HBsAg and anti-HBe can still be present in the serum. Patients in the chronic active phase have mild to moderate elevation of the aminotransferases (less than or equal to five times the ULN).

QUICK FLICK 36

Table 36.1 Serologic markers of HBV infection

HBsAg	> 6 months	> 6 months	> 6 months	> 6 months
HBeAg	+	+	–	–
Anti-HBe	–	Spontaneous seroconversion to anti-HBe may occur	+	+
ALT	Persistently normal	Persistently or intermittently elevated	Persistently normal	Persistently or intermittently elevated
HBV DNA	≥ 20 000 IU/mL	Persistently or intermittently ≥ 20 000 IU/mL	< 2000 IU/mL	Persistently or intermittently ≥ 20 000 IU/mL
Liver histology	Normal or mild hepatitis	Moderate–severe hepatitis ↓ Cirrhosis→	Normal or mild hepatitis Inactive cirrhosis	Moderate–severe hepatitis ↓ ←Cirrhosis

Source: Reproduced with the permission of the Gastroenterological Society of Australia (GESA).

The ALT levels are usually higher than the AST levels. HBV DNA levels are high during this phase.

Management

The detection of HBeAg and serum HBV DNA should be performed to determine if the patient should be considered for antiviral therapy (see Figure 36.2 on pages 400–3). Therapy is indicated in patients with acute liver failure, cirrhosis and clinical complications, cirrhosis or advanced fibrosis with HBV DNA in serum, reactivation of chronic HBV after chemotherapy or immunosuppression, and in infants born to women who are HBsAg-positive (immunoglobulin and vaccination). Therapy may be indicated in patients with immune-active phase who do not have advanced fibrosis or cirrhosis (HBeAg-positive or HBeAg-negative chronic hepatitis). Therapy is not routinely indicated in patients with chronic HBV in the immune-tolerant phase (high levels of serum HBV DNA but normal serum ALT levels or little activity on liver biopsy), inactive carrier or low-replicative phase (low levels of, or no detectable HBV DNA in serum and normal serum ALT levels), and latent HBV infection (HBV DNA without HBsAg).

The aims of treatment of chronic hepatitis B are to achieve sustained suppression of HBV replication and remission of liver disease. Clinically, the short-term goal of treatment is to achieve 'initial response' in terms of HBeAg seroconversion and/or HBV-DNA suppression, ALT normalisation, and prevention of hepatic decompensation; to ensure 'maintained/sustained response' to reduce hepatic necroinflammation and fibrosis during/after therapy. The ultimate long-term goal of therapy is to achieve 'durable response' to prevent hepatic decompensation, reduce or prevent progression to cirrhosis and/or HCC, and prolong survival. At the 2000 and 2006 NIH conferences on 'Management of Hepatitis B' it was proposed that responses to antiviral therapy of chronic hepatitis B be categorised as biochemical (BR), virologic (VR) or histologic (HR), and as on-therapy or sustained off-therapy.

Another important perspective on HBV treatment is the question of whether HBV infection is ever 'cured'. Chronic HBV exists in a very stable form in the hepatocyte known as covalently closed circular DNA (cccDNA) that has a very long intracellular half-life. There have been recent reports of antiviral effects (reduced cellular levels) by nucleoside or nucleotide analogues on cccDNA, including adefovir and entecavir. Clearance of this stable intracellular form of the HBV genome has not been shown conclusively with any antiviral agent and probably explains why HBV cannot be cured.

Interferon

Interferon is an appropriate treatment for people with chronic hepatitis B infection who have detectable virus activity, ongoing liver inflammation and no cirrhosis. Interferon is given for a finite duration (4–12 months).

Lamivudine

Lamivudine is effective for HBV infection in the dosage of 100 mg/day. The major problem with lamivudine is that a resistant form of hepatitis B virus frequently develops.

Adefovir

Resistance to adefovir is less likely to develop. Adefovir can suppress lamivudine-resistant HBV. Adefovir has been associated with kidney problems. The dosage used in HBV therapy is 10 mg/day, for at least one year.

Entecavir

Entecavir is more potent than lamivudine and adefovir. A dosage of 0.5 mg daily for patients who have no prior treatment and 1.0 mg daily for patients who have resistance to lamivudine, for at least one year, is required to achieve optimal result.

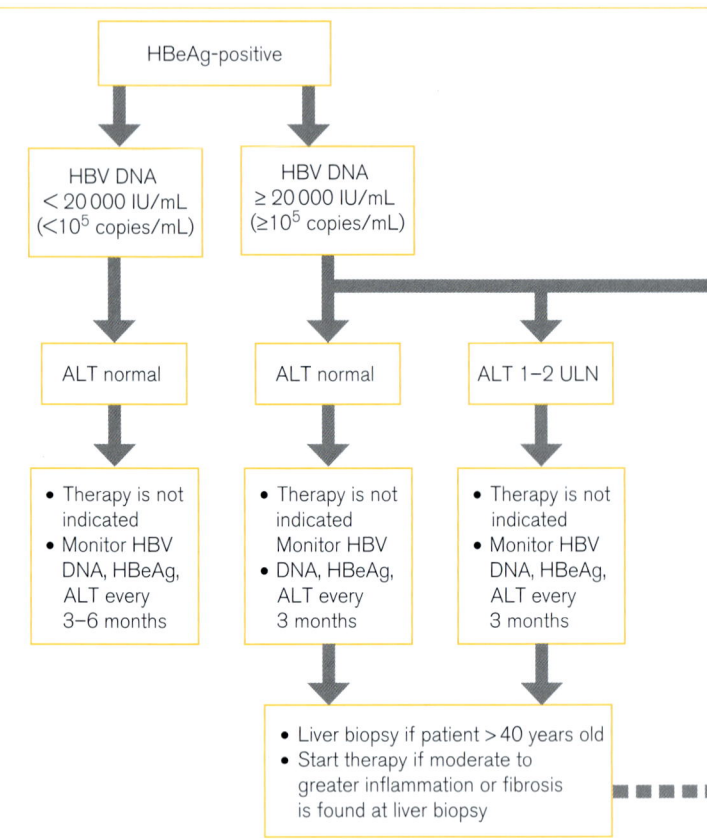

Figure 36.2 Algorithm of management of chronic hepatitis B

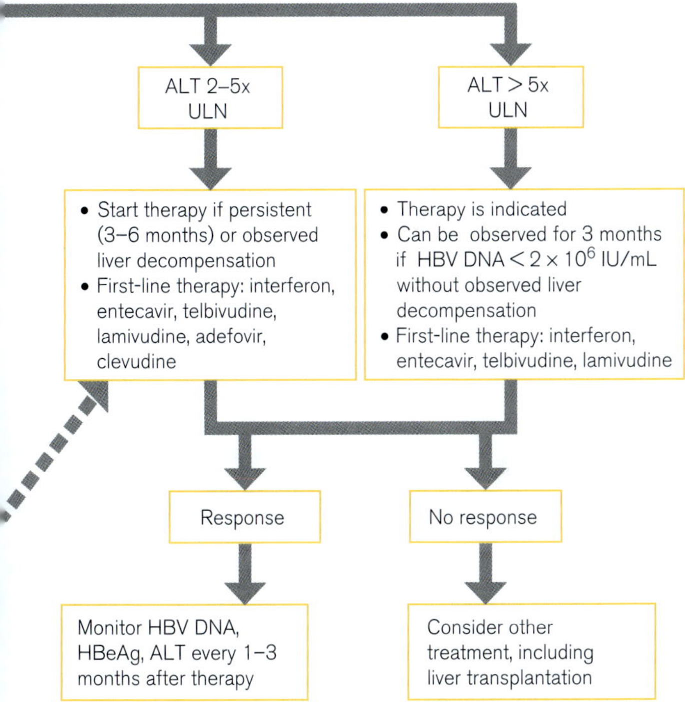

```
        ┌─────────────────┐         ┌─────────────────┐
        │   ALT 2–5x      │         │   ALT > 5x      │
        │     ULN         │         │     ULN         │
        └─────────────────┘         └─────────────────┘
```

- Start therapy if persistent (3–6 months) or observed liver decompensation
- First-line therapy: interferon, entecavir, telbivudine, lamivudine, adefovir, clevudine

- Therapy is indicated
- Can be observed for 3 months if HBV DNA $< 2 \times 10^6$ IU/mL without observed liver decompensation
- First-line therapy: interferon, entecavir, telbivudine, lamivudine

```
        ┌─────────────┐             ┌─────────────┐
        │  Response   │             │ No response │
        └─────────────┘             └─────────────┘
```

Monitor HBV DNA, HBeAg, ALT every 1–3 months after therapy

Consider other treatment, including liver transplantation

continued

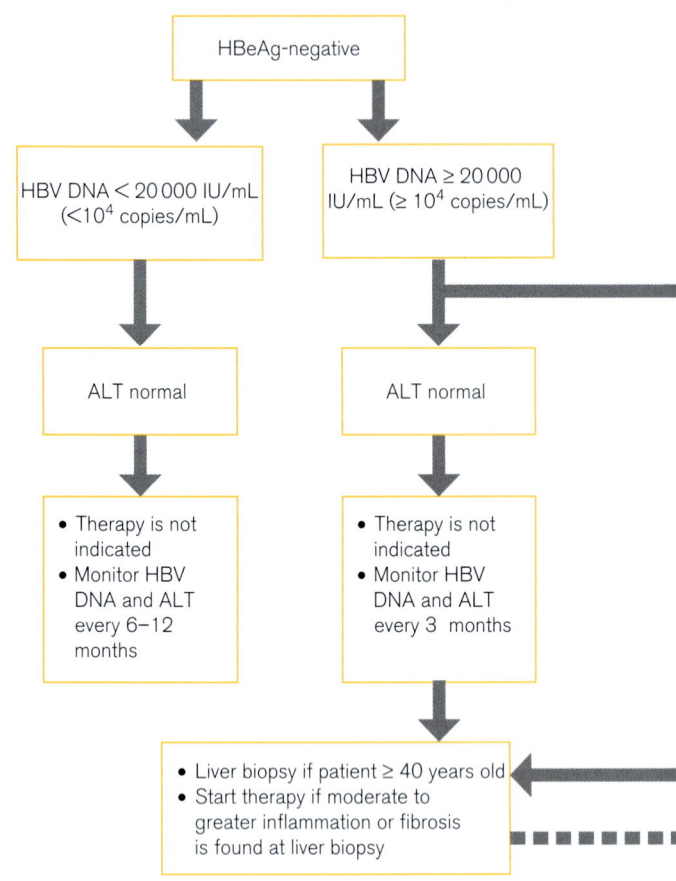

Figure 36.2 *continued*

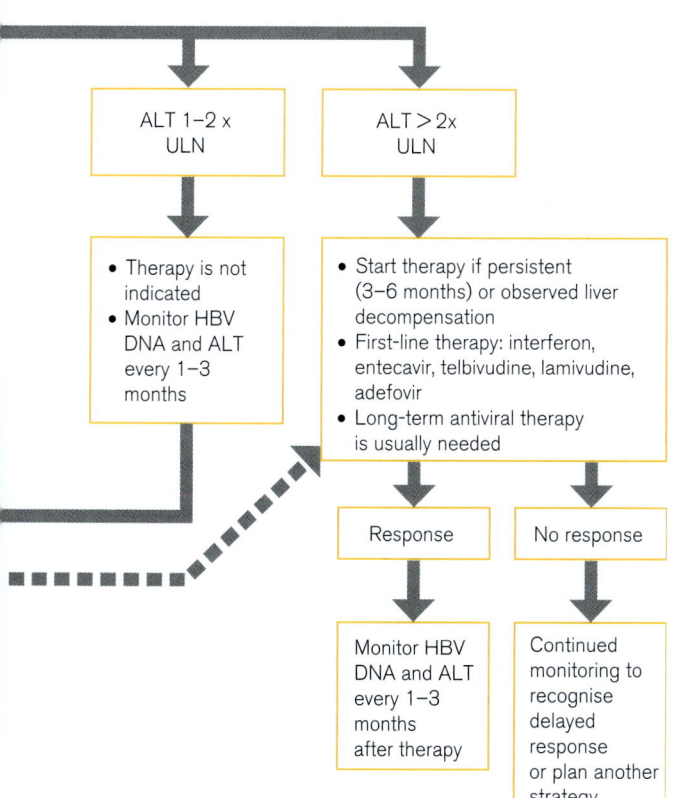

ALT 1–2 x ULN

ALT > 2x ULN

- Therapy is not indicated
- Monitor HBV DNA and ALT every 1–3 months

- Start therapy if persistent (3–6 months) or observed liver decompensation
- First-line therapy: interferon, entecavir, telbivudine, lamivudine, adefovir
- Long-term antiviral therapy is usually needed

Response

No response

Monitor HBV DNA and ALT every 1–3 months after therapy

Continued monitoring to recognise delayed response or plan another strategy

QUICK FLICK 36

Tenofovir

Tenofovir is more potent than adefovir and is effective as a first-line treatment in people who have not been treated with any antiviral drug and in patients who have hepatitis B virus that is resistant to lamivudine, telbivudine or entecavir.

Telbivudine

Telbivudine is slightly more potent than lamivudine. Unfortunately, it is associated with a high rate of resistance, similar to lamivudine.

Clevudine

Some Asian studies have shown that clevudine is well tolerated and has a potent and sustained antiviral effect without evidence of viral resistance during the treatment period in HBeAg-positive chronic hepatitis B.

Liver transplantation

Liver transplantation may be the only option for those who have developed advanced cirrhosis. Not all patients with cirrhosis are eligible. Only those with the most advanced cirrhosis and otherwise good medical and social conditions will be put on the transplant waiting list.

Summary

HBV infection is a global public health problem. It is estimated that over two billion people have been infected with HBV resulting in 300 to 400 million carriers, 75 per cent of whom live in Asia and or the Western Pacific. The spectrum of clinical manifestations of hepatitis B virus (HBV) infection varies in both acute and chronic disease. Diagnosis of HBV infection is based on clinical manifestations and laboratory findings. The HBV management, whether it is antiviral or transplantation, depends on the patient's condition.

Information for patients

How did I become infected?

The hepatitis B virus can be spread in from one person to another in several ways:

- contaminated needles
- sexual intercourse
- mother to infant
- close contact
- blood transfusion
- organ transplantation.

What are the symptoms?

The symptoms of hepatitis B differ during acute hepatitis and chronic hepatitis. Most infected people, even those with progressive disease, have no specific symptoms for many years. However, the absence of symptoms does not necessarily mean that the infection is under control. All persons who have chronic infection with hepatitis B are at increased risk of developing complications.

What are the symptoms of acute hepatitis B?

Symptoms of acute hepatitis B usually appear between one and four months after the person becomes infected. The first symptoms may be non-specific, and can include fever, skin rash, joint pain and inflammation, fatigue, loss of appetite, nausea, jaundice, or pain in the upper right abdomen. Some people have no symptoms at all. Acute hepatitis can be severe, with symptoms lasting for many weeks or months. Most people with acute hepatitis B spontaneously clear the infection.

Less commonly, acute hepatitis is life-threatening or fulminant. The only treatment for fulminant hepatitis is liver transplantation.

People who continue to harbour the virus are referred to as carriers. Liver damage associated with longstanding infection is referred to as chronic hepatitis.

What are the symptoms of chronic hepatitis B?

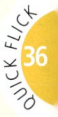

Chronic hepatitis B develops more commonly in people who are infected with the virus at an early age, such as at birth. The symptoms of chronic hepatitis B can vary widely and can last for many years. Many people who carry the virus have no symptoms at all; other people have symptoms of ongoing liver inflammation, such as fatigue and loss of appetite. Some people with chronic hepatitis B experience sudden, temporary worsening of symptoms.

Will I develop chronic hepatitis B?

The likelihood of acute hepatitis progressing to chronic hepatitis largely depends on a person's age at the time of infection. Chronic infection develops in about 90 per cent of children who are infected at birth, in 20 to 50 per cent of children who are infected between the ages of 1 and 5 years, and in fewer than 5 per cent of people infected during adulthood. If you develop chronic infection you should be evaluated by a physician who can discuss treatment options.

How can I maintain a healthy liver?

Here are some tips for maintaining liver health.

- Vaccinations
  1. Everyone with chronic hepatitis B should be vaccinated against hepatitis A unless they are known to be immune.
  2. Pneumococcal vaccine is recommended when HBV is diagnosed, and again at age 65.
  3. Influenza vaccination is recommended once per year, usually in autumn. Patients with liver disease should also receive standard immunisations.
- Liver cancer screening
  Regular screening for liver cancer is also recommended, particularly for older people, or those with cirrhosis, or if you have with a family history of liver cancer. In general, this includes a yearly or 2-yearly ultrasound examination of the liver, and a blood test for the alpha-fetoprotein (AFP) level.
- Diet
  No specific diet has been shown to improve the outcome in patients with hepatitis B. The best advice is to eat a normal healthy and balanced diet.
- Alcohol
  Alcohol should be avoided since it can worsen liver damage. All types of alcoholic beverages can be harmful to the liver. Patients with liver disease may develop complications even with small amounts of alcohol.
- Exercise
  Exercise is good for overall health and is encouraged, but it has no effect on the virus.
- Prescription and non-prescription drugs
  Many medications are broken down by the liver. Thus, it is always best to check with a healthcare provider or pharmacist before starting a new medication.

How can I prevent my family becoming infected?

Acute and chronic hepatitis B are contagious. Thus, people with hepatitis B should discuss measures to reduce the risk of infecting close contacts.

Recommended reading

Andreani T, Serfaty L, Mohand D, Dernaika S, Wendum D, Chazouillères O, Poupon R. Chronic hepatitis B virus carriers in the immunotolerant phase of infection: histologic findings and outcome. *Clin Gastroenterol Hepatol.* 2007 May; 5(5):636–41. Epub 2007 April 11.

Andy S, Ramsey C, Emmet B. Hepatitis B vaccines. *Infect Dis Clin N Am.* 2006; 20:27–45.

Anna S, Brian J. Chronic hepatitis B: updated 2009. AASLD practice guidelines. *Hepatology*. 2009; 50(3).

Asselah T, Lada O, Moucari R, Martinot M, Boyer N, Marcellin P. Interferon therapy for chronic hepatitis B. *Clin Liver Dis*. 2007; 11:839–49.

Belongia EA, Costa J, Gareen IF, Grem JL, Inadomi JM, Kern ER, McHugh JA, Petersen GM, Rein MF, Strader DB, Trotter HT. National Institutes of Health Consensus Development Conference Statement: Management of Hepatitis B. *Hepatology*. 2009 May; 49(5 Suppl):S4–S12.

Block TM, Guo H, Guo J-T. Molecular virology of hepatitis B virus for clinicians. *Clin Liver Dis*. 2007; 11(4):685–706.

Dienstag JL, Schiff ER, Wright TL, Perrillo RP, Hann HW, Goodman Z, Crowther L, Condreay LD, Woessner M, Rubin M, Brown NA. Lamivudine as initial treatment for chronic hepatitis B in the United States. *N Engl J Med*. 1999 Oct 21; 341(17):1256–63.

Digestive Health Foundation. Australian and New Zealand chronic hepatitis B (CHB) recommendations. Sydney: Gastroenterological Society of Australia; 2008 Oct.

Fung SK, Fontana RJ. Management of drug-resistant chronic hepatitis B. *Clin Liver Dis*. 2006 May; 10(2):275–302, viii.

Gish RG. Current treatment and future directions in the management of chronic hepatitis B viral infection. *Clin Liver Dis*. 2005; 9(4):541–65.

Hui CK, Leung N, Yuen ST, Zhang HY, Leung KW, Lu L, Cheung SK, Wong WM, Lau GK, Hong Kong Liver Fibrosis Study Group. Natural history and disease progression in Chinese chronic hepatitis B patients in immune-tolerant phase. *Hepatology*. 2007 Aug; 46(2):395–401.

Liaw YF, Leung N, Kao JH, Piratvisuth T, Gane E, Han KH, Guan R, Lau GK, Locarnini S, for the Chronic Hepatitis B Guideline Working Party of the Asian-Pacific Association for the Study of the Liver. Asian-Pacific consensus statement on the management of chronic hepatitis B: a 2008 update. *Hepatol Int*. 2008; 2(3):263–83.

Lok AS-F, McMahon BJ. Chronic hepatitis B: update 2009. *Hepatology*. 2009; 50(3):661–2.

National Institute of Health. Consensus Development Conference Statement, Management of Hepatitis B. Bethesda, Maryland USA; October 20–22, 2008.

QUICK FLICK 36

Yim HJ, Lok AS-F. Natural history of chronic hepatitis B virus infection: what we knew in 1981 and what we know in 2005. *Hepatology*. 2006 Feb; 43(S1):S173–81.

Yoo BC, Kim JH, Chung YH, et al. Twenty-four-week clevudine therapy showed potent and sustained antiviral activity in HBeAg-positive chronic hepatitis B. *Hepatology*. 2007 May; 45(5):1172–8.

Chapter 37: Hepatitis C infection

S. Nair, M. Bilal (USA)

Key points

▶ Hepatitis C is a worldwide health problem with life-threatening complications affecting about 200 million people.

▶ Hepatitis C virus (HCV) is an RNA virus of the Flaviviridae family. The replication process is error-prone resulting in heterogeneous viral genomes. The virus has six major genotypes. Genotypes 2 and 3 respond best to treatment.

▶ The primary source of infection is HCV-infected blood. Most common modes of transmission are blood or blood product transfusions and intravenous drug abuse.

▶ Acute infection with HCV is usually clinically silent. Chronic HCV infection is most commonly diagnosed in the setting of abnormal liver enzymes. Patients can have non-specific complaints like fatigue, arthralgias, myalgias or pruritis.

▶ Advanced disease can present with complications of portal hypertension, such as ascites, encephalopathy, gastrointestinal bleeding and even hepatocellular cancer.

▶ Eighty per cent of patients progress to chronic liver disease and related complications.

▶ Extrahepatic manifestations commonly include mixed cryoglobulinaemia, diabetes mellitus, membranoproliferative glomerulonephritis and porphyria cutanea tarda.

▶ The screening for hepatitis C is largely based on the detection of anti-HCV antibodies by serological assays.

▶ Detection of HCV RNA by polymerase chain reaction (PCR) technique confirms presence of active infection.

▶ Genotype testing should be done in all patients in whom treatment is a consideration.

▶ Liver biopsy can be helpful in appropriate patients.

▶ Patients should be carefully selected for HCV treatment.

▶ Standard treatment includes a combination of pegylated interferon and ribavirin. The duration of therapy is based on viral genotype and initial response.

▶ Patients should be regularly monitored during the treatment for side effects of therapy.

▶ Sustained viral response rates reach 80 per cent for genotypes 2 and 3 but only 50 per cent for genotype 1.

▶ Chronic hepatitis C and resultant end-stage liver disease are the most common indications for liver transplantation.

▶ Promising new therapies including protease inhibitors are on the horizon and soon will be available in the market.

⏾ Intoduction

Hepatitis C virus (HCV), first discovered in 1989, is an RNA virus of remarkable genetic variability and six major genotypes. Chronic infection with HCV can result in cirrhosis, portal hypertension and hepatocellular cancer (HCC). The high global burden of hepatitis C and related life-threatening complications call for a better understanding of the risk factors, preventative measures and management principles.

⏾ Epidemiology

An estimated 200 million (3.3%) people are infected with HCV worldwide. In the United States alone, about 4.1 million (1.6%) people are infected, accounting for 10 000 deaths and 2000 liver transplantations annually. There is a variance in the global prevalence of HCV, the highest prevalence being in South-East Asia and Africa, reaching an estimated 30–40 million.

⏾ Virology/pathology

HCV is a single-stranded, enveloped RNA virus of the Flaviviridae family. Viral replication occurs primarily in hepatocytes. HCV virus is classified into 6 major genotypes and, within these types, 40 different subtypes. In the United States, infections with genotype 1 are the most common (70%), followed by genotypes 2 and 3. Genotype 4 is more common in the Middle East and Egypt, genotype 5 in South Africa and genotype 6 in South-East Asia. Genotypes 1 and 4 have been associated with lower response rates to interferon compared to genotypes 2 or 3. The term 'quasispecies' refers to closely related yet heterogeneous isolates of the virus within an infected individual resulting from mutations during viral replication.

HCV virus itself is not cytopathic; the host's immune response plays a central role in the pathogenesis of hepatitis C. Severity of liver disease in HCV in terms of prognosis is usually determined by the amount of fibrosis seen in the liver biopsy. Fibrosis is typically referred to as stages I to IV inclusive. Stage IV is cirrhosis and any degree of fibrosis beyond stage II is considered to be advanced fibrosis.

◗ Modes of transmission

An HCV risk factor can be identified in about 90 per cent of patients upon careful questioning, leaving only about 10 per cent of sporadic cases. The primary source of transmission is infected blood or blood products. Intravenous drug abuse is now the chief mode of transmission in the United States. Monogamous sexual relationships carry a very low risk of HCV transmission; however partners should be tested for reassurance. Table 37.1 outlines the group of patients who should be screened for HCV.

Table 37.1 Persons for whom HCV testing is recommended

Current or past IV drug abuser
Persons who received blood products or organ transplants before 1992
Persons with conditions associated with high risk of HCV, e.g.: – HIV – haemodialysis – haemophiliacs receiving clotting factor concentrates before 1987 – unexplained abnormal aminotransferase
Children born to HCV-infected mothers
Healthcare workers after needle-stick injury or mucosal exposure to HCV-positive blood
Current sexual partners of HCV-infected persons

Source: Adapted from Centers For Disease Control and Prevention (CDC) and American Association for the Study of Liver Disease (AASLD) recommendations.

◗ Clinical features

HCV can cause both acute and chronic hepatitis. Acute infection is usually clinically silent and is seldom seen in clinical practice unless the patient is screened as a part of post-exposure follow-up. Acute liver failure secondary to an acute HCV infection is extremely rare. Chronic hepatitis is often found incidentally during evaluation of elevated transaminases. Most patients are asymptomatic; others have non-specific symptoms such as fatigue, arthralgias, paraesthesias, myalgias or pruritis. Symptom severity does not reliably relate to disease severity. Once liver disease progresses to cirrhosis, patients can present with complications of portal hypertension (ascites, upper gastrointestinal bleeding, encephalopathy). Fluctuating elevations in aminotransferases is the hallmark of chronic HCV infection. Usually serum ALT is more than serum AST, but as disease progresses to cirrhosis, serum AST becomes more than serum ALT. In addition, low or low-normal platelets in chronic HCV infection almost always suggest cirrhosis. It is noteworthy that about one-third of patients with chronic hepatitis C have normal aminotransferases. Patients can also have advanced liver disease with normal liver function tests.

○ Natural history

After acute infection, HCV persists in 80 per cent of patients and evolves into chronic infection (Figure 37.1). Progression to cirrhosis takes several decades, with about one-third of patients developing cirrhosis in 15–20 years. Several viral and host factors can contribute to accelerated progression, including male gender, aged over 40, obesity, alcohol intake, viral co-infections and marijuana use. Survival is generally not affected until cirrhosis develops. Death is caused by hepatic decompensation or by HCC. The risk of HCC is about 1 to 4 per cent per year after the development of cirrhosis. Chronic HCV infection can be associated with extra-hepatic manifestations (Table 37.2). Immune complex deposition is considered to be the primary underlying factor.

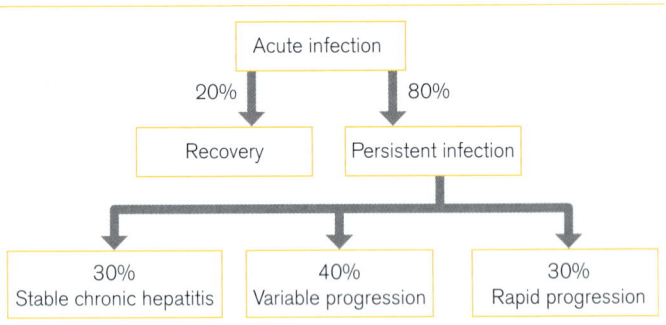

Figure 37.1 Natural history of HCV

Table 37.2 Extra-hepatic manifestations of HCV

Mixed cryoglobulinaemia
Diabetes mellitus
Membranoproliferative glomerulonephritis
Porphyria cutanea tarda

| Lichen planus |
| Autoimmune thyroid disease |
| Arthralgias |
| Non-Hodgkin's lymphoma |
| Leukocytoclastic vasculitis |

◊ Diagnosis

The screening of hepatitis C is largely based on the detection of anti-HCV antibodies by serological assays. Active infection is diagnosed by the presence of HCV RNA in the serum. Most patients with anti-HCV antibody have detectable RNA levels and hence active infection. HCV RNA can be detected by amplification techniques like polymerase chain reaction (PCR). PCR testing can be either qualitative or quantitative. Most clinicians prefer quantitative testing as it also helps in initiating and monitoring treatment. Qualitative testing, being more sensitive, is reserved for documentation of sustained viral response or to confirm diagnosis when a quantitative test is negative despite the presence of anti-HCV antibodies. Genotype testing should be done if treatment is a consideration. The issue of liver biopsy is controversial but it can help in assessing the degree of fibrosis and hence prognosis, which may impact on treatment decisions.

◊ Management (see Figure 37.2 overleaf)

Acute hepatitis C, if diagnosed in a timely manner, should be treated as there is a higher chance of response and eradication of the infection. Most patients in clinical practice, however, are chronically infected; the latter part of this chapter discusses treatment of chronic HCV infection.

Every patient with chronic hepatitis C should be evaluated for treatment. The main goal of treating HCV infection is to prevent the development of cirrhosis by sustained suppression of HCV. The treatment endpoint widely used in clinical practice is sustained virological response (SVR), defined as the absence of detectable viraemia 24 weeks after stopping treatment. Long-term follow-up data has shown that SVR is durable and that 99 per cent of patients remain undetectable for several years. Re-infection with HCV is possible in high-risk behaviour patients as there is no immunity. Patient who achieved SVR could also become reactivated if they receive immunosuppressive treatment such as liver transplantation.

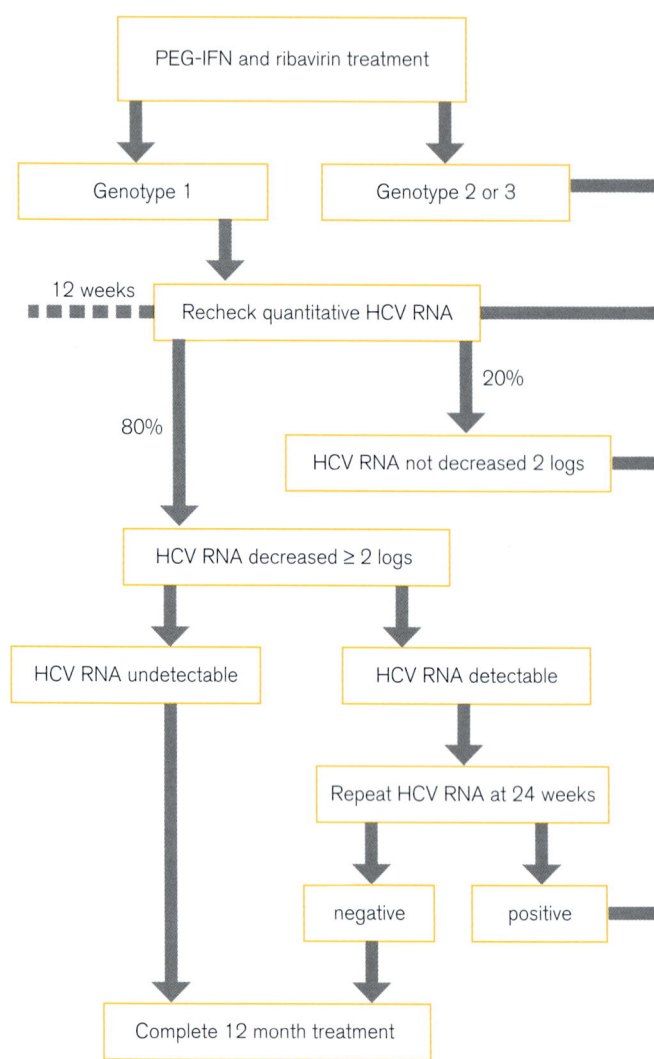

Figure 37.2 Algorithm for treatment of hepatitis C

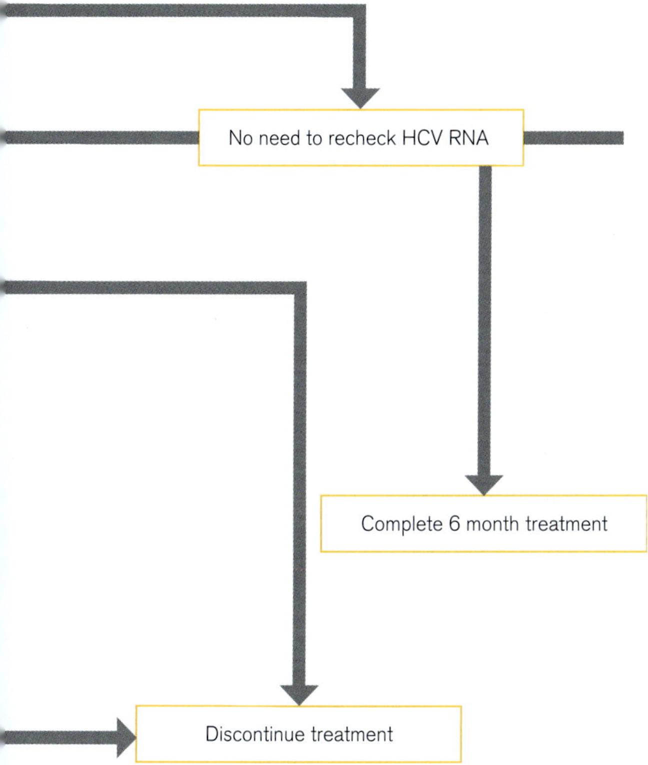

No need to recheck HCV RNA

Complete 6 month treatment

Discontinue treatment

QUICK FLICK
37

Standard treatment

The current standard treatment is a combination of pegylated interferon (PEG-IFN) once a week, and daily ribavirin. The dose of PEG-IFN α-2b (PEG Intron®, Schering Plough) is 1.5 µg/kg/week, and of PEG-IFN α-2a (PEGASYS®, Roche Pharmaceuticals), 180 µg/week subcutaneously. Ribavirin dosage is usually based on the patient's weight; higher doses have been shown to improve SVR. Ribavarin dosages in genotypes 1 and 4 are weight based, with 1000 mg/day for patients under 75 kg and 1200 mg/day for patients over 75 kg. In genotypes 2 and 3 a fixed dosage of 800 mg is administered.

Duration

In genotypes 2 and 3, the duration of treatment is 24 weeks. Genotype 1 treatment is guided by virological response during treatment as assessed by HCV RNA levels. The usual duration of treatment is 48 weeks.

Efficacy

The SVR rate with current treatment is 80–90 per cent for genotype 2 and 50 per cent for genotype 1 infection, and around 70–80 per cent for genotype 3 infection. Several factors have been found to decrease the response rate in genotype 1 infection. These include high viral load (defined as > 400 000 IU/mL), African American race, obesity (and high insulin resistance), fatty liver, presence of cirrhosis, older age, male gender, HIV infection and end-stage renal disease.

Side effects

Both PEG-IFN and ribavirin are associated with significant side effects (Table 37.3). Patients should be followed monthly for the first 3 months, then every 2–3 months until the end of treatment. Thyroid function should also be assessed every 12 weeks while on treatment.

Table 37.3 Treatment side effects

Side effect	Comments
1. Haematological	
• Anaemia	33% patients, mgmt: dose reduction (1st line), erythropoietin
• Neutropaenia	20% patients, mgmt: dose reduction (1st line), filgastrim (limit to ANC < 0.5×10^9/L, cirrhosis, immunosuppressed patient, HIV)
• Thrombocytopaenia	Mgmt: Dose reduction(1st line), eltrombopag
2. Flu-like symptoms	> 50% patients
3. Neuropsychiatric	2–31% patients

Side effect	Comments
4. Others	
• Respiratory	Dyspnoea, dry cough, interstitial pneumonia, BOOP
• Ophthalmologic	Cotton wool spots/haemorrhages, rarely CRAO, CRVO
• Glucose metabolism dysregulation	
• Dermatologic	Rash, hair loss
• Thyroid dysfunction	
• Autoimmune disease exacerbation, e.g. sarcoidosis	

Notes: ANC = absolute neutrophil count; BOOP = bronchiolitis obliterans organising pneumonia; CRAO = central retinal artery occlusion; CRVO = central retinal vein occlusion.

Selection of patients for treatment

Since the treatment regimen carries a potential risk of several complications, all patients should be meticulously assessed for treatment (see Tables 37.4 and 37.5, overleaf). The decision to treat a patient should be based on the risk of progression of untreated HCV, efficacy of treatment and potential toxicity from the treatment. The assessment of patients should be clinical, laboratory and/or histological. The clinical and laboratory assessment with the special relevance to HCV treatment are elaborated in Tables 37.4 and 37.5. In addition, all patients should be carefully screened for treatment contraindications (Table 37.6 overleaf).

Table 37.4 Clinical assessment

Clinical assessment	Comments
1. Co-morbid conditions	
a. Coronary artery disease, congestive heart failure	Ribavirin-associated anaemia can aggravate
	May be the life-limiting disease
b. Chronic obstructive pulmonary disease, uncontrolled HTN/DM	May be the life-limiting disease
c. Non-skin cancers	Potential contraindication
d. Psychiatric disorders (especially depression/suicide risk)	
e. Substance abuse (alcohol, drugs)	Establish abstinence prior to treatment
f. Autoimmune disorders (thyroid, DM, psoriasis, rheumatoid arthritis, Crohn's disease, etc.)	May exacerbate, should be well controlled, involve a specialist
2. Assess patient adherence (willingness)	Look for history of non-adherence
3. Ophthalmologic exam	Baseline in patient with risk factors, e.g. HTN, DM

Table 37.5 Laboratory tests

Test	Comments
HCV quantitative PCR	Low viral load, higher chance of response
Genotype	Predicts response likelihood (genotype 2 <3<4<1)
Complete blood count (CBC)	Interferon can cause cytopaenias and CBC should be closely followed
Renal function	Dose adjustment is needed for renal insufficiency. The response rate is low in patients with severe renal failure. *Ribavirin-induced haemolysis can be severe. Haemolysis can occur even in mild renal insufficiency.*
Hepatic synthetic function (albumin, bilirubin, INR)	Risk of decompensation of liver disease with treatment in patients with cirrhosis. Treatment is contraindicated in liver failure (Model for End Stage Liver Disease > 18). Not unreasonable to refer to a transplant centre.
Pregnancy test	All childbearing-age women should be tested (ribavirin is teratogenic). The use of two methods of contraception is recommended while taking ribavirin, and up to 6 months after stopping ribavirin.
Human immune deficiency virus (HIV)	Lower response rate, disease progression is higher.
Hepatitis B virus (HBV)	Co-infection is possible so all HCV patients should be screened and vaccinated if not immune.

Table 37.6 Contraindications for interferon treatment

Major uncontrolled depression

Solid organ transplant

Autoimmune disorders (can be exacerbated by interferon treatment)

Uncontrolled thyroid disease

Pregnancy or unwillingness to comply with contraception
Severe medical condition like uncontrolled HTN, DM, COPD, CAD, HF

Notes: HTN = hypertension; DM = diabetes mellitus, COPD = chronic obstructive pulmonary disease; CAD = coronary artery disease; HF = heart failure.

Source: Adapted from American Association for the Study of Liver Disease Recommendations, 2009.

Liver transplantation

Chronic HCV hepatitis is the most common indication for liver transplantation. Almost all patients develop recurrent disease after liver transplantation. Diagnosis should be based on HCV RNA testing as serological testing can be false negative given immunosuppression. Treatment is similar. Long-term survival is probably reduced as compared to patients undergoing liver transplantation for non-viral liver diseases.

Hepatocellualr carcinoma

Patients with HCV and cirrhosis are at a higher risk of developing HCC. Alfa fetoprotein may be normal in up to 40–50 per cent of HCC patients, thus ultrasound every 6–12 months should be used for screening. Screening is not routinely recommended for HCV patients in the absence of cirrhosis. HCC at earlier stages can be cured by liver transplantation.

Newer treatments

Several newer therapies are emerging targeting viral replication, viral entry and immune clearance. The most promising of these is a class of drugs called protease inhibitors, which target HCV serine proteases. Two drugs, telaprevir and boceprevir, are expected to be available by late 2011. Phase 3 clinical trials of these agents are completed and they are likely to increase the SVR rate by 20–30 per cent among genotype 1 patients. One of the biggest concerns about the new oral agents is the development of resistance. Eventually HCV could be treated with multiple potent oral agents alone, just like HAART regimen for HIV, but this ultimate goal is several years away.

QUICK FLICK

37

Summary

An estimated 200 million people are infected with HCV worldwide. HCV is an RNA virus of the Flaviviridae family and has six main genotypes. The primary source of chronic infection is HCV-infected blood. It is often found during evaluation of elevated transaminases. Advanced disease can present with the complications of portal hypertension. Eighty per cent of patients progress to chronic liver disease. Screening for HCV is usually by serology and is based on detection of anti-HCV antibodies, confirmed by PCR. Genotyping should be done, particularly if treatment is considered. Standard treatment includes a combination of pegylated interferon and ribavirin. Sustained viral response rates reach 80 per cent for genotypes 2 and 3, but only 50 per cent for genotype 1. Indication for liver transplant is usually end-stage liver disease.

Information for patients

What is hepatitis C?

Hepatitis C is a contagious infection of the liver caused by a virus. After acquisition some patients can clear the infection spontaneously but unfortunately most patients with hepatitis C eventually develop chronic liver disease which can be life-threatening.

How is hepatitis C acquired?

The main source of infection is the blood of an infected person. You can acquire hepatitis C if infected blood enters your blood. Before 1992, screening methods for detection of hepatitis C in blood were not available and hence blood transfusion was a major risk factor. Today, however, the biggest risk factor is sharing of needles for injecting intravenous drugs.

What can hepatitis C do to you?

Acute infection is usually clinically silent. About 10–15 per cent of patients can spontaneously clear the virus. Most patients will develop chronic disease. Chronic infection can cause non-specific complaints like fatigue, itching or muscle pains; however, most people are diagnosed incidentally during routine laboratory checks.

Is there a treatment?

Not all patients are treatment candidates. Eligible patients can be treated with weekly injections of pegylated interferon and daily ribavirin pills. The duration of therapy varies from 24–48 weeks. Treatment does not guarantee complete cure. There is no vaccine for prevention of hepatitis C yet.

What can patients do?

Patients with hepatitis C should follow up regularly with an experienced doctor. Alcohol should be avoided as it can cause additional liver damage. They should seek a doctor's opinion before taking any prescription pills, supplements or over-the-counter medications, as these can potentially harm the liver. They should check with their physician about getting vaccinated against hepatitis A and hepatitis B.

Recommended reading

Di Bisceglie AM, Shiffman ML, Everson GT, Lindsay KL, Everhart JE, Wright EC, Lee WM, Lok AS, Bonkovsky HL, Morgan TR, Ghany MG, Morishima C, Snow KK, Dienstag JL. Prolonged therapy of advanced chronic hepatitis C with low-dose peginterferon. *N Engl J Med*. 2008 Dec 4; 359:2429–41.

Feld JJ, Hoofnagle JH. Mechanism of action of interferon and ribavirin in treatment of hepatitis C. *Nature*. 2005 Aug 17; 436:967–72. doi:10.1038/nature04082 Insight.

Ghany MG, Strader DB, Thomas DL, Seeff LB, American Association for the Study of Liver Diseases. Diagnosis, management, and treatment of hepatitis C: an update. *Hepatology*. 2009 Apr; 49(4):1335–74.

Hezode C, Forestier N, Dusheiko G, Ferenci P, Pol S, Goeser T, Bronowicki JP, Bourlière M, Gharakhanian S, Bengtsson L, McNair L, George S, Kieffer T, Kwong A, Kauffman RS, Alam J, Pawlotsky JM, Zeuzem S. Telaprevir and peginterferon with or without ribavirin for chronic HCV infection. *N Engl J Med*. 2009 Apr 30; 360(18):1839–50.

McHutchison JG, Everson GT, Gordon SC, Jacobson IM, Sulkowski M, Kauffman R, McNair L, Alam J, Muir AJ. Telaprevir with peginterferon and ribavirin for chronic HCV genotype 1 infection. *N Engl J Med*. 2009 Apr 30; 360:1827–38.

QUICK FLICK 37

Chapter 38: Non-alcoholic fatty liver disease

E.V. Gomez, E.A. Soler, A.Y. Garcia (Cuba)

Key points

- ▶ NAFLD has a worldwide distribution. Its prevalence in non-Western countries is increasing. Prevalence of NAFLD in the general population is approximately 20 per cent.
- ▶ Obesity, type 2 diabetes, hyperdyslipidaemia and insulin resistance are frequently associated with NAFLD.
- ▶ It has become the most common form of chronic liver disease worldwide.
- ▶ The disease is increasingly diagnosed in children and adolescents.
- ▶ Non-alcoholic steatohepatitis (NASH) is considered to be the most severe form of NAFLD and may progress to cirrhosis, liver failure and hepatocellular carcinoma (HCC), leading to liver-related death.
- ▶ Most patients are asymptomatic at the time of diagnosis. Mildly to moderately elevated serum levels of aminotransferase are often the only finding.
- ▶ Ultrasonography shows a diffuse increase in liver echogenicity that reveals fatty infiltration.
- ▶ Liver biopsy with histological examination is the 'gold standard' for confirming and staging NAFLD.
- ▶ The goal of the management is to halt the progression of the disease and to correct underlying risk factors such as hypertension, diabetes, hyperdyslipidaemia and metabolic syndrome.
- ▶ Avoid or minimise alcohol consumption and drugs known to cause steatohepatitis.
- ▶ Improvement of insulin resistance with lifestyle intervention based on a hypocaloric diet and exercise is the mainstay for the prevention and treatment of NAFLD.
- ▶ Bariatric surgery is reserved for patients with associated obesity-related co-morbidities.
- ▶ Liver transplantation may be required for patients with decompensated cirrhosis or liver cancer.
- ▶ There is no universally accepted pharmacological treatment.
- ▶ Pharmacological treatment should be considered in patients at the highest risk of developing complications (NASH and metabolic syndrome).
- ▶ Thiazolidinediones may be the preferred option for patients with type 2 diabetes and NAFLD.

▶ The use of antioxidants may show particular promise in combination with lifestyle modification or thiazolidinediones.

◑ Introduction

Non-alcoholic fatty liver disease comprises a wide spectrum of pathological conditions ranging from simple hepatic steatosis to non-alcoholic steatohepatitis (NASH), which is characterised by the presence of concomitant necroinflammatory changes and/or fibrosis, and cirrhosis, in the absence of significant alcohol consumption defined as two standard drinks a day (140 g of ethanol/week) for men and one standard drink a day (70 g of ethanol/week) for women. Once cirrhosis is present, hepatocellular carcinoma (HCC) may also develop.

◑ Epidemiology: prevalence and worldwide impact

NAFLD has a worldwide distribution. Its prevalence in the general population is approximately 20 per cent; however, there are geographic regions with a very high prevalence, such as North and South America, much of the Asia–Pacific, the Middle East and Europe. The prevalence of NAFLD in non-Western countries is increasing, in part because of the globalisation of Western diet and altered socioeconomic circumstances. Population-based screening studies using serum liver tests or ultrasonography suggest an apparent prevalence of approximately 22 per cent, ranging from three to 33 per cent in the general population and up to 80 per cent in the morbidly obese. A recent study based on ultrasonography reported a prevalence of NAFLD of 29 per cent among healthy Japanese adults. The prevalence of NASH, the most serious form of NAFLD, has not been adequately elucidated as a liver biopsy is needed to confirm the diagnosis; however, recent studies have reported a prevalence of approximately 3 per cent in the general population and 30 per cent in obese individuals. There is an alarming increased prevalence of NAFLD in children and adolescents that appears to be associated with overweight and obesity. The overall prevalence of NAFLD in children is 2.6 per cent, but prevalence in obese children increases up to 53 per cent.

NAFLD has been shown to be independently associated with obesity, type 2 diabetes or glucose intolerance, hypertriglyceridaemia, low HDL cholesterol and insulin resistance, as well as globally associated with the presence of metabolic syndrome. The presence of NASH is strongly associated with central, but not overall, obesity.

Population-based studies suggest that NAFLD is probably more common in men, particularly men under the age of 50 years, and may be somewhat higher in Caucasian populations.

Also, NAFLD is one of the most common causes of elevated liver enzymes and chronic liver disease in Western and non-Western countries alike.

○ Natural history and clinical features

Although simple steatosis appears to be a less progressive stage of NAFLD, there is no conclusive scientific evidence to consider it as a benign form of NAFLD. On the other hand, NASH is considered to be the most aggressive form of NAFLD. It may progress to cirrhosis, liver failure and HCC, which lead to liver-related death. Subjects with NAFLD have a higher risk of all-cause mortality than the general population. This may be explained by an increased risk of death secondary to liver, cardiovascular and neurovascular disease as a result of the underlying metabolic syndrome. The mortality rate in patients with NAFLD is similar to or worse than that for cirrhosis associated with hepatitis B or C. More advanced stages of NAFLD appear to be associated with older age, type 2 diabetes or glucose intolerance, obesity, hypertension, insulin resistance and AST/ALT ratio above 1. The histological pattern of simple steatosis is indicative of the slow progression of the disease with a 4 per cent risk of developing cirrhosis over a median follow-up of approximately eight years, in contrast to 8 per cent of patients with NASH who may develop cirrhosis in approximately five years.

Most patients with NAFLD are asymptomatic; however, clinical symptoms and signs including fatigue, discomfort in the right upper quadrant and hepatomegaly are present at the time of diagnosis. In addition, patients frequently have clinically significant co-morbidities (Table 38.1) such as type 2 diabetes, obesity and hyperdyslipidaemia, well known to coexist with NAFLD. Clinical findings of portal hypertension, hyperbilirubinaemia, thrombocytopaenia and hypoalbuminaemia may suggest the presence of cirrhosis (Table 38.2).

Table 38.1 Co-morbidities associated with NAFLD

• Metabolic syndrome*	• Gout
• Dyslipidaemia	• Hypothyroidism
• Obesity	• Hypopituitarism
• Type 2 diabetes mellitus	• Obstructive sleep apnoea
• Polycystic ovary syndrome	

* Based on adult treatment panel III (abdominal obesity, BP $\geq$ 130/85, triglycerides
   > 250 mg/dL, HDL < 40 mg/dL for men and < 50 mg/dL for women, and fasting blood
   glucose $\geq$ 110 mg/dL).

Table 38.2 Clinical features and laboratory abnormalities at the time of diagnosis

Symptom or sign	Frequency (%)
Asymptomatic	60
Fatigue or malaise	35
Discomfort in the right upper quadrant	35
Hepatomegaly	20
Splenomegaly not related to portal hypertension	4
Pruritus	4
Laboratory abnormalities	
ALT > 30 IU/L	60
AST > 30 IU/L	50
AST/ALT ratio < 1*	80
Alkaline phosphatase > 200 IU/L	50
γ-glutamyltransferase > 30 IU/L	50

*   AST/ALT ratio increases with advanced fibrosis and/or alcohol consumption.

○ Diagnosis

The presence of NAFLD is frequently associated with a family or personal history of obesity, type 2 diabetes or glucose intolerance, hypertension, dyslipidaemia and metabolic syndrome.

Metabolic syndrome and insulin resistance are present in most patients with NAFLD; nevertheless, it is important to exclude secondary causes of hepatic steatosis that can be corrected by specific aetiologic treatment (Table 38.3).

Table 38.3 Causes of NAFLD

Primary	Metabolic syndrome is the most frequent cause of NAFLD
Secondary	
• Drugs	Corticosteroids, synthetic oestrogens, calcium channel blockers, protease inhibitors, tamoxifen, tetracycline, amiodarone, valproate, methotrexate, aspirin, cocaine

continued

Table 38.3 *continued*

• Nutritional	Total parenteral nutrition, protein-calorie malnutrition, rapid weight loss, bariatric surgery, starvation, short bowel syndrome
• Metabolic or genetic	Acute fatty liver of pregnancy, lipodystrophy, dysbetalipoproteinaemia, Weber-Christian syndrome, Wolman's disease
• Others	Small bowel bacterial overgrowth, HIV, chronic hepatitis C, chronic inflammatory disorders, toxins (*Amanita phalloides* mushroom, petrochemicals)

NAFLD is most often suspected in an asymptomatic subject who is found to have elevations in liver tests, such as alanine aminotransferase (ALT) or aspartate aminotransferase (AST), or an abnormal ultrasonographic finding suggestive of fatty liver. Otherwise, hepatomegaly might be the only sign detected during routine physical examination even with normal liver test results. Mildly or moderately elevated liver enzyme levels are often the only laboratory abnormality. Liver tests do not usually discriminate between simple steatosis and NASH. Ultrasonography shows a diffuse increase in the echogenicity of the liver when compared with the echogenicity of the kidney. Ultrasonography is an excellent and cheap method for detecting hepatic steatosis; however, it is less sensitive at detecting minimal steatosis (< 20%), or in the case of obese patients. Physical examination for patients with NAFLD should include anthropometric measurements (BMI, waist circumference and waist-to-hip ratio) to characterise the degree (mild, moderate or severe) and the nature (central or peripheral) of obesity. In patients without pre-existing type 2 diabetes, fasting blood glucose, insulin levels, haemoglobin A1c, and insulin resistance by calculating HOMA-IR or QUICKI should be evaluated. A HOMA-IR value greater than 3 is considered to be clinically significant. A fasting lipid profile should be obtained. Usually, hypertriglyceridaemia and low values of HDL cholesterol are recorded in patients with NAFLD.

All patients with NAFLD should be examined for the presence of co-morbidities such as hypothyroidism, hypopituitarism, obstructive sleep apnoea and polycystic ovary syndrome.

Liver biopsy is the 'gold standard' for the diagnosis, grading and staging of NAFLD (see Figure 38.1 on pages 428–9). It is the only way to distinguish between simple steatosis and NASH, or to stage the degree of fibrosis. It should be performed in patients at high risk of fibrosis progression, such as those with diabetes, obesity, age more than 45 years and AST/ALT ratio higher than 1.

NAFLD can be divided into two well-defined categories. Histological confirmation of simple steatosis requires a minimum of 5 per cent of steatosis. NASH may exhibit macro/microvesicular steatosis, lobular inflammation, cellular ballooning and zone 3 fibrosis that is predominantly pericellular and/or perisinusoidal. Recently, a NAFLD activity score (NAS), that evaluates only features of active injury, has been proposed to identify patients with a histological diagnosis of NASH (Table 38.4). Individuals whose NAS is above 5 are diagnosed as having NASH.

Table 38.4 Histological scoring system for grading and staging NAFLD

Histological finding	Score
Grading	
• Steatosis	0–3
• Lobular inflammation	0–3
• Hepatocellular ballooning	0–2
Staging	
• Fibrosis	0–4

Source: Adapted from Kleiner et al. (2005). The scoring system comprises four histological features that are evaluated semi-quantitatively.

Current non-invasive clinically available tests lack accuracy and reliability. Screening for varices and HCC should be performed in cirrhotic patients.

The NAFLD activity score (NAS) includes only features of active injury (steatosis, lobular inflammation and ballooning) that are potentially reversible in the short term.

Cases with a NAS in the range 0–4 are considered inconclusively diagnosed as NASH.

Cases with a NAS of 5 or more are diagnosed as NASH.

Fibrosis is evaluated independently of NAS.

◯ Management

The goal of management is to halt the progression of the disease and to improve co-morbidities. The correction of underlying risk factors such as hypertension, diabetes, hyperdyslipidaemia and metabolic syndrome may reverse or reduce neuro/cardiovascular risk as well as improve NAFLD. All patients with NAFLD should stop or minimise alcohol consumption and drugs known to cause steatohepatitis. Lifestyle modification based on a hypocaloric diet and exercise is the mainstay for inducing weight loss in overweight or

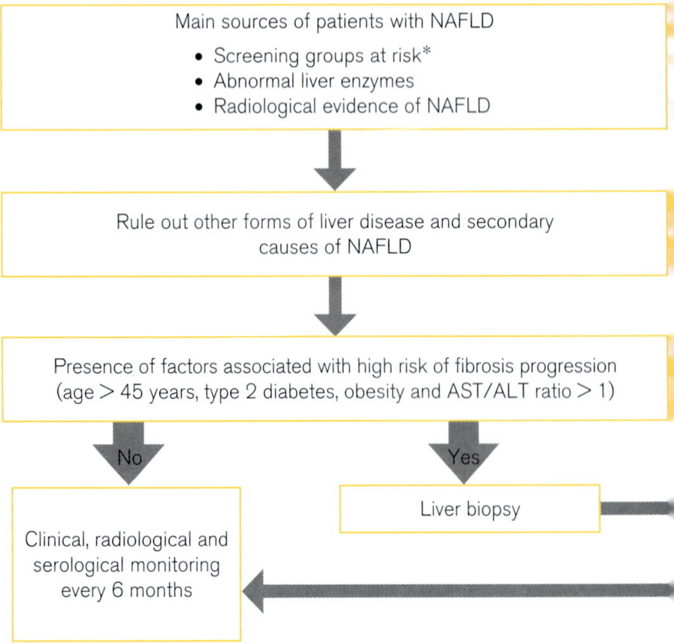

Main sources of patients with NAFLD

- Screening groups at risk*
- Abnormal liver enzymes
- Radiological evidence of NAFLD

Rule out other forms of liver disease and secondary causes of NAFLD

Presence of factors associated with high risk of fibrosis progression (age > 45 years, type 2 diabetes, obesity and AST/ALT ratio > 1)

No

Yes

Liver biopsy

Clinical, radiological and serological monitoring every 6 months

Figure 38.1 Algorithm for the diagnosis and management of NAFLD

*   Metabolic syndrome, obesity, type 2 diabetes or glucose intolerance, hypertension, gout and dyslipidema.

obese patients with NAFLD. Evidence shows that comprehensive lifestyle modification based on a hypocaloric diet alone or combined with exercise for 6 to 12 months not only induces sustained and moderate weight loss, but also improves aminotransferase levels and insulin sensitivity, reduces steatosis and inflammation, and reverses hepatic fibrosis. However, weight loss should be gradual because rapid weight reduction has been associated with the exacerbation of liver injury.

```
                    ┌──────────────────────┐   ┌──────────────────────┐
                    │   Simple steatosis   │   │        NASH          │
                    │         or           │   │         or           │
                    │      NAS ≤ 4         │   │      NAS ≥ 5         │
                    │  Potentially benign  │   │Potentially progressive│
                    └──────────────────────┘   └──────────────────────┘
                                                            │
                                                            ▼
                                               ┌──────────────────────┐
                                               │Consider specific treatment│
                                               └──────────────────────┘
```

QUICK FLICK 38

No clear recommendation on diet composition can be made; however, a hypocaloric and low-fat (<10% of saturated fat) diet, normal in carbohydrates (50–60%) and proteins (≈15%), tends to ameliorate features of metabolic syndrome and NAFLD. Physical exercise itself improves insulin resistance and may modify liver fat content. It is recommended to perform at least five sessions per week of moderate aerobic exercise (walking or jogging) for 30–45 minutes. Several expert panels have recommended that obese individuals attempt to lose 10 per cent of their initial weight because this is associated with the reduction of obesity-related health complications such as NAFLD.

Bariatric surgery is reserved for patients with associated obesity-related co-morbidities who failed to lose weight despite repeated nutritional counselling.

Liver transplantation may be required for patients with decompensated cirrhosis or liver cancer.

◗ Pharmacological treatment (see Table 38.5)

There is no universally accepted pharmacological treatment due in part to the lack of adequately powered randomised trials with sufficient duration and adequate endpoints. Pharmacological treatment should be considered in patients at the highest risk of developing complications (NASH and metabolic syndrome) (see Figure 38.2). The significant association of NASH with insulin resistance and metabolic syndrome is the rational basis for treatment with weight-reducing programs and/or insulin-sensitising agents. However, insulin sensitisers such as thiazolidinediones (TZDs) and biguanides (metformin) are not yet ready for routine treatment of NAFLD. A recent meta-analysis reported that administration of metformin in non-diabetic patients leads to the normalisation of serum aminotransferase as compared with dietary modification; however, its favourable effect on hepatic histology may not be robust. On the other hand, TZDs improve hepatic histology in patients with NASH, in particular steatosis. Their favourable effect on liver histology and liver biochemistries disappears on their discontinuance, suggesting that long-term

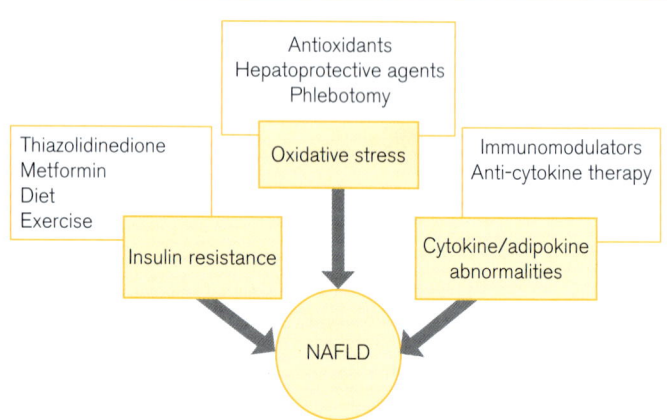

Figure 38.2 Pathophysiologically targeted treatment of NAFLD

treatment is needed to maintain their therapeutic benefits. Moreover, a recent study raised the possibility that TZDs alone without lifestyle intervention may not be so effective (Figure 38.3).

TZDs may be the preferred option for patients with type 2 diabetes and NAFLD. Long-term use with pioglitazone is preferred because it may have a more favourable cardiovascular risk profile than rosiglitazone.

Lipid-lowering agents have not clearly shown a beneficial effect.

Hepatoprotective or antioxidant agents provide limited evidence of effectiveness.

Particular promise may exist in the use of antioxidants in combination with lifestyle modification or TZDs. A recent study has reported that the combination of Viusid (an antioxidant 'cocktail') with hypocaloric diet and exercise for six months has a beneficial effect on hepatic histology, particularly steatosis and inflammation.

Table 38.5 Therapeutic modalities for NAFLD and associated co-morbidities

Type 2 diabetes or glucose intolerance	
• Metformin	All patients
• Pioglitazone	Antioxidants or hepatoprotective agents
• Rosiglitazone	Vitamins C and E
Obesity (BMI < 35 kg/m^2)	Viusid
• Weight loss (low-carbohydrate vs low-fat diet)	Sylimarin
	Omega-3 fatty acids
• Orlistat	Ursodeoxycholic acid
• Sibutramine	Betaine
• Rimonabant	Tocopherol
Obesity (BMI > 35 kg/m^2)	Iron depletion
• Bariatric surgery	N-acetylcysteine
Dyslipidaemia	Silybin
• Gemfibrozil	SAMe
• Clofibrate	• Anti-TNF regimens
• Atorvastatin	• Pentoxifylline
Hypertension	Probiotics
• Losartan	

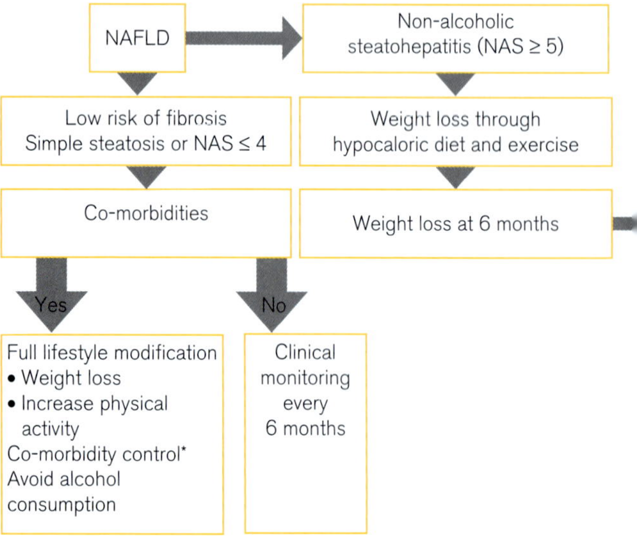

Figure 38.3 Algorithm for the individualised and optimised treatment of NAFLD

*   Consider long-term treatment with pioglitazone or metformin if presence of metabolic syndrome or type 2 diabetes; antihyperlipidaemic agents if evidence of hyperlipidaemia; and angiotensin-converting enzyme (ACE) inhibitors if existence of hypertension.

†   Consider long-term treatment with pioglitazone if high risk of cardiovascular events.

Summary

Non-alcoholic fatty liver disease (NAFLD) is one of the most common causes of chronic liver disease with a worldwide distribution. NAFLD comprises a wide spectrum of pathological conditions ranging from simple hepatic steatosis to steatohepatitis in the absence of significant alcohol consumption. It is usually associated with insulin resistance and features of metabolic syndrome. Prevalence in non-Western countries is increasing, in part because

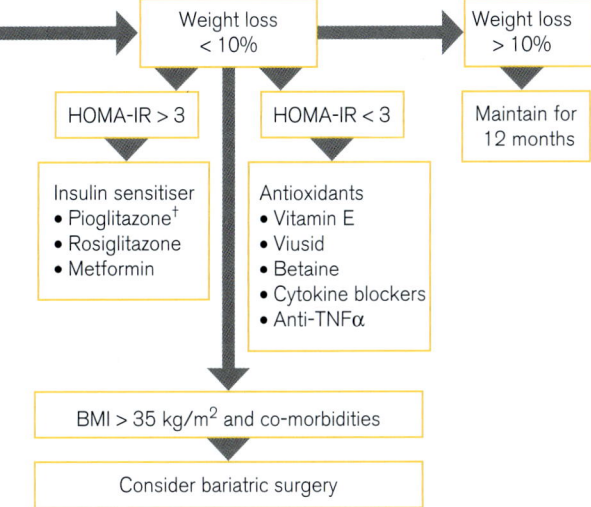

of the globalisation of the Western diet. Steatosis alone appears to be a less progressive form of NAFLD; however, NASH may progress to cirrhosis, liver failure and HCC, which lead to liver-related death.

Most patients are asymptomatic at the time of diagnosis. Liver biopsy with histological examination is the 'gold standard' for confirming and staging NAFLD. It should be performed in patients at high risk of advanced fibrosis. Improvement of insulin resistance with lifestyle intervention based on a hypocaloric diet and exercise is the mainstay for the prevention and treatment of NAFLD. Pharmacological treatment should be considered in patients at the highest risk of developing complications (NASH and metabolic syndrome). Insulin sensitisers such as thiazolidinediones and biguanides are not yet available for routine treatment of NAFLD. Particular promise may exist in the use of antioxidants in combination with lifestyle modification or thiazolidinediones. Liver transplantation may be required for patients with decompensated cirrhosis or liver cancer.

Information for patients

What is non-alcoholic fatty liver disease?

Non-alcoholic fatty liver disease, or NAFLD, is a common, often 'silent', and progressive liver disease. It resembles alcoholic liver disease, but occurs in people who drink little or no alcohol. The major feature of NAFLD is fat in the liver; however, it may be associated with inflammation and fibrosis, and then it is called NASH (non-alcoholic steatohepatitis). Most people with NAFLD have no symptoms and are unaware that they have a liver problem. Nevertheless NASH, a progressive form of NAFLD, may cause severe liver damage that leads to more advanced stages of the disease, including cirrhosis, where the liver is seriously damaged, ending in failure to perform its vital functions and incapable of working properly.

NAFLD is directly associated with a clinical condition called metabolic syndrome, which is characterised by the presence of obesity, hypertension, type 2 diabetes or glucose intolerance, hypertrygliceridaemia and low values of high-density lipoprotein. We must not forget that NAFLD appears to be the clinicopathological complication of an obesity-related inappropriate lifestyle.

NASH is usually an asymptomatic and 'silent' disease; however, symptoms or signs such as fatigue, discomfort in the right upper quadrant and hepatomegaly may be present at the early stages of the disease.
The progression of NAFLD can take years, even decades, and leads to the end-stage of liver disease: liver cirrhosis. At the end-stage of liver cirrhosis, fluid retention, muscle wasting, cramps, bleeding from the intestines and liver failure may be present. Liver transplantation is the only treatment for advanced cirrhosis with liver failure.

How is diagnosis performed?

NAFLD is most often suspected in asymptomatic subjects who are found to have elevations of liver test results, such as alanine aminotransferase (ALT) or aspartate aminotransferase (AST), or an abnormal ultrasonographic finding suggestive of fatty liver. Secondary causes of liver disease, such as alcohol abuse, viral hepatitis or medication, should be excluded. The only means of proving a diagnosis of NASH and separating it from simple fatty liver is liver biopsy. NASH is present when the histological examination shows fat along with inflammation and/or fibrosis.

What is the recommended treatment?

The goal of the treatment is to halt the progression of the disease and improve co-morbidities. The correction of underlying risk factors such as hypertension, diabetes or glucose intolerance, hyperdyslipidaemia and metabolic syndrome may reverse or reduce neuro/cardiovascular risk as well as improve NAFLD.

There is no universally accepted specific treatment for NAFLD; however, there are important recommendations that should be followed by people with NAFLD:

- Stop or minimise alcohol consumption.
- Avoid unnecessary medication, particularly drugs known to cause steatohepatitis.
- If overweight or obese, reduce weight through a healthy balanced diet and increased physical activity.

These standard recommendations are also helpful for other conditions such as cardiovascular disease, diabetes and metabolic syndrome.

Sustained and moderate weight loss for six months can improve liver test results in patients with NASH and may reverse histological features of NAFLD, including fibrosis.

Experimental studies are evaluating antioxidants such as vitamins C and E, betaine and Viusid for NAFLD; however, whether these substances help treat the disease has not been completely elucidated yet. Another experimental approach to treating NASH is the use of insulin sensitiser drugs—even in people without diabetes. The objective of this medication is to make the body more sensitive to insulin and thus reduce liver injury in patients with NASH. Methodologically well-designed studies of this medication, including metformin and rosiglitazone, have been carried out.

QUICK FLICK
38

Reference

Kleiner DE, Brunt EM, Van Natta M, Behling C, Contos MJ, Cummings OW, Ferrell LD, Liu YC, Torbenson MS, Unalp-Arida A, Yeh M, McCullough AJ, Sanyal AJ. Nonalcoholic steatohepatitis clinical research network. Design and validation of a histological scoring system for nonalcoholic fatty liver disease. *Hepatology*. 2005; 41:1313–21.

Recommended reading

Aithal GP, Thomas JA, Kaye PV, Lawson A, Ryder SD, Spendlove I, Austin AS, Freeman JG, Morgan L, Webber J. Randomized, placebo-controlled trial of pioglitazone in nondiabetic subjects with nonalcoholic steatohepatitis. *Gastroenterology*. 2008; 135:1176–84.

Farrell GC, Larter CZ. Nonalcoholic fatty liver disease: from steatosis to cirrhosis. *Hepatology*. 2006; 43(2 Suppl 1):S99–S112.

Loomba R, Sirlin CB, Schwimmer JB, Lavine JE. Advances in pediatric nonalcoholic fatty liver disease. *Hepatology*. 2009; 50:1282–93.

Vilar Gomez E, Rodriguez De Miranda A, Gra Oramas B, Arus Soler E, Llanio Navarro R, Calzadilla Bertot L, Yasells Garcia A, Del Rosario Abreu Vazquez M. Clinical trial: a nutritional supplement Viusid, in combination with diet and exercise, in patients with nonalcoholic fatty liver disease. *Aliment Pharmacol Ther*. 2009 Nov 15; 30:999–1009.

Vuppalanchi R, Chalasani N. Nonalcoholic fatty liver disease and nonalcoholic steatohepatitis: selected practical issues in their evaluation and management. *Hepatology*. 2009; 49:306–17.

Zivkovic AM, German JB, Sanyal AJ. Comparative review of diets for the metabolic syndrome: implications for nonalcoholic fatty liver disease. *Am J Clin Nutr*. 2007; 86:285–300.

Chapter 39: Alcoholic liver disease

S.M. Riordan, P. Chang (Australia)

Key points

- Alcohol is the most frequently used hepatotoxin worldwide.
- The prevalence of alcoholic liver disease varies in different countries.
- The term 'alcoholic liver disease' refers to pathology for which other possible causes have been excluded.
- Fatty liver develops in at least 90 per cent of heavy alcohol drinkers. Only 10–35 per cent develop alcoholic hepatitis, and 5–15 per cent develop cirrhosis.
- Gender, genetics and nutritional status probably influence the risk of the more severe forms of alcohol-related liver disease.
- An important co-factor in progressive liver injury is hepatitis C viral infection.
- Continued abstinence from alcohol and correction of any nutritional deficiencies are important management strategies.
- Alcoholic liver disease is the second most common indication for liver transplantation in the Western world.

◗ Introduction

Alcohol is the most frequently used hepatotoxin worldwide. The prevalence of alcoholic liver disease varies from country to country according to geographic patterns of alcohol intake. A substantial increase in per capita alcohol ingestion in some Asian countries has been demonstrated in recent years, in comparison to stable levels of intake in many Western countries. Excessive alcohol consumption is defined by an intake in excess of 28 units per week in men and 21 units per week in women, where one unit of alcohol is approximately 10 grams, equivalent to a glass of wine, a single measure of spirits or half a pint of beer. These limits take the liver as the organ at risk, as opposed to other organs such as the brain and heart, which may have lower safety limits. Nonetheless, the daily intake of alcohol resulting in liver damage in individual subjects is highly variable.

The term 'alcoholic liver disease' should be reserved for pathology for which other possible causes have been excluded, in the setting of excessive alcohol use and, preferably, in association with confirmatory changes on liver biopsy. Liver pathology related to alcohol is generally considered in three forms: fatty liver, alcoholic hepatitis and cirrhosis. These entities are not mutually exclusive and do not represent discrete stages of alcoholic liver disease. Although fatty liver will develop in at least 90 per cent of heavy alcohol drinkers, it is notable that only 10 to 35 per cent will develop alcoholic hepatitis and 5 to 15 per cent will develop cirrhosis. A range of co-factors including gender, genetics and nutritional status probably influence the risk of developing these more severe forms of alcohol-related liver disease: for example, alcoholic liver disease occurs at lower levels of exposure in women and individuals of Hispanic origin. Nonetheless, none of these currently identified co-factors, either singly or in combination, can completely explain why only a minority of individuals who ingest potentially toxic amounts of alcohol progress to more severe forms of alcohol-related injury. An important co-factor in progressive liver injury is concurrent hepatitis C viral infection.

�‣ Clinical features

Fatty liver related to alcohol is common but probably under-diagnosed, with the steatosis often being attributed to other causes such as obesity, hyperlipidaemia and diabetes mellitus. Alcoholic fatty liver is frequently asymptomatic. Soft, non-tender hepatomegaly is a common clinical finding. Peripheral stigmata of chronic liver disease are typically absent. Portal hypertension is an uncommon complication.

Patients with acute alcoholic hepatitis often complain of anorexia, nausea, vomiting, diarrhoea and general weakness. They are often malnourished and pyrexial. Jaundice is a frequent clinical finding. Spider naevi are also common. Tender hepatomegaly is evident in most patients. Hepatic bruits may be audible. Ascites and encephalopathy are also evident in a substantial proportion of cases. The latter must be distinguished from Wernicke's encephalopathy, hypoglycaemia and delirium tremens.

Alcoholic cirrhosis is often asymptomatic. Consequently, presentation is commonly with a complication, such as ascites or variceal bleeding related to portal hypertension, encephalopathy from liver failure or hepatocellular carcinoma. Alternatively, cirrhosis may be diagnosed following further investigation of abnormal liver function tests found during the course of investigation for other purposes. Although some peripheral stigmata of chronic liver disease, such as parotid enlargement and Dupuytren's contracture, are more commonly observed when alcohol is the causative factor, no single physical finding or combination of findings is specific for this aetiology.

◯ **Diagnosis**

Laboratory abnormalities

The serum aspartate aminotransferase (AST) level is typically raised only two to six times normal in patients with liver disease related to alcohol. Alanine aminotransferase (ALT) levels are often normal or only mildly elevated. Levels of AST in excess of 500 IU/L or levels of ALT more than 200 IU/L suggest an aetiology other than alcohol. An AST/ALT ratio greater than two is evident in around 70 per cent of patients, although this ratio is of greater discriminatory value in non-cirrhotic patients. A disproportionate increase in gamma glutamyl transferase (GGT) may be apparent. Macrocytosis may also be evident. A combination of a raised GGT in association with elevated mean corpuscular volume has sensitivity in the order of 40 per cent for an alcoholic aetiology. Serum carbohydrate-deficient transferrin levels are a more accurate marker, but not in widespread clinical use. A polyclonal hyperglobulinaemia with elevations in both immunoglobulin G and immunoglobulin A may be seen, but as with other laboratory tests, is not specific for an alcoholic cause of liver disease. Neutrophilia is common in patients with alcoholic hepatitis, in whom the possibility of coincident infection must be excluded.

Role of liver biopsy

Liver biopsy is particularly helpful in establishing the diagnosis of alcohol-related liver disease, since up to around 25 per cent of patients with alcohol abuse are found to have another, unrelated aetiology for their liver disease. Liver biopsy is also helpful in diagnosing cirrhosis in those patients without suggestive clinical, laboratory or imaging features. Histological assessment is particularly useful in those patients who continue to have abnormal liver function tests despite a period of abstinence from alcohol of at least three months. As the clinical diagnosis is not always accurate, consideration should also be given to liver biopsy in those patients with a presumptive diagnosis of alcoholic hepatitis in whom corticosteroid or anti-cytokine therapy, as discussed below, is being contemplated.

Imaging

Imaging studies, such as with ultrasound, computed tomography or magnetic resonance imaging, are important for suggesting fatty change, with moderate sensitivity and specificity. The liver may be enlarged in the case of fatty liver or alcoholic hepatitis. Established cirrhosis is marked by the findings of a reduced liver volume and an irregular liver outline. Enlargement of the caudate lobe is often evident. Evidence of a patent umbilical vein and intra-abdominal varices, along with splenomegaly and ascites, suggests

associated portal hypertension. Assessment for the possibility of a focal abnormality to suggest complicating hepatocellular carcinoma is also important.

Endoscopy

Upper gastrointestinal endoscopy is useful in patients with alcoholic hepatitis or cirrhosis to screen for the possibility of gastro-oesophageal varices or other portal hypertensive changes, with the aim of instituting primary prophylaxis against gastrointestinal bleeding. Endoscopy has both diagnostic and therapeutic value in an alcoholic patient with active upper gastrointestinal bleeding.

▷ Management

Continued abstinence from alcohol is generally all that is required in patients with alcohol-related fatty liver. At the other end of the severity spectrum, those with cirrhosis may additionally require treatment of complications, such as variceal bleeding, liver failure and hepatocellular carcinoma. Cirrhotic patients should be enrolled in surveillance programs to detect gastro-oesophageal varices and hepatocellular carcinoma at asymptomatic stages. Specific nutrient deficiencies and protein calorie malnutrition are common in patients with alcoholic liver disease; the latter is significantly associated with risk of complications, including infection, encephalopathy and ascites. It is clear that long-term aggressive nutritional support is necessary in this group. Nutritional assessment should be an ongoing process. In addition to correction of any specific nutrient deficiencies, dietary intakes in the order of 1.5 g/kg for protein and 40 kcal/kg for energy are indicated. Further increases in dietary protein and energy intakes during intermittent acute illnesses are required to reverse protein calorie malnutrition in this group.

The approach to management of acute alcoholic hepatitis is influenced by factors that predict mortality. Relevant scoring systems include the Maddrey discriminant function, the model for end-stage liver disease (MELD) score and the Glasgow alcoholic hepatitis score. The first of these is the most widely used index: discriminant function = 4.6 (prothrombin time – control time) + (serum bilirubin in µmol/L ÷ 17.1). Values of 32 and above are associated with an in-hospital mortality rate of around 40 per cent, compared to around 10 per cent in those with a discriminant function of less than 32 and, as discussed below, have been used to select patients for further therapeutic intervention. A MELD score of 21 or more (based on parameters including the serum bilirubin and creatinine values and international normalised ratio) is also taken as a marker of poor prognosis. Along with nutritional support, interest has centred upon the possible benefit of anti-inflammatory or anti-cytokine therapy, using corticosteroids or pentoxifylline, respectively. These treatments have been shown to be effective in improving short-term survival in those patients with severe alcoholic hepatitis (Figure 39.1).

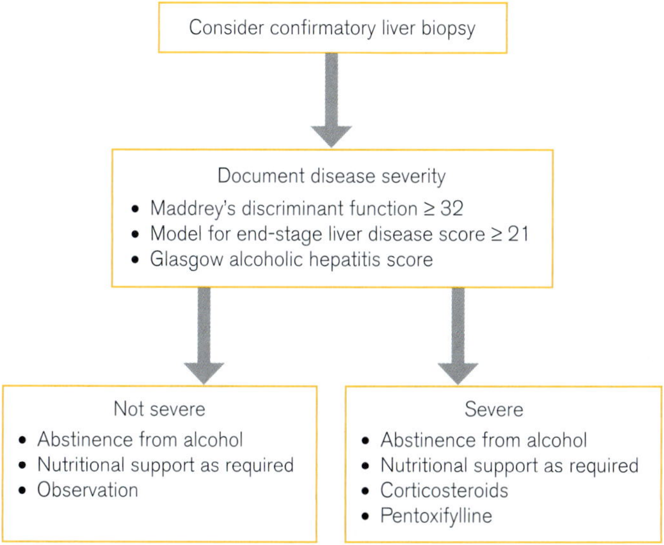

```
┌─────────────────────────────────────┐
│  Consider confirmatory liver biopsy  │
└─────────────────────────────────────┘
                   │
                   ▼
┌─────────────────────────────────────┐
│       Document disease severity      │
│  • Maddrey's discriminant function ≥ 32
│  • Model for end-stage liver disease score ≥ 21
│  • Glasgow alcoholic hepatitis score │
└─────────────────────────────────────┘
          │                   │
          ▼                   ▼
┌──────────────────┐  ┌──────────────────┐
│    Not severe    │  │      Severe      │
│ • Abstinence from alcohol │ • Abstinence from alcohol
│ • Nutritional support as required │ • Nutritional support as required
│ • Observation    │  │ • Corticosteroids │
│                  │  │ • Pentoxifylline  │
└──────────────────┘  └──────────────────┘
```

Figure 39.1 Management of alcoholic hepatitis

Corticosteroids

Corticosteroid therapy is the most studied of these treatment modalities for alcoholic hepatitis. An analysis of recent placebo-controlled randomised trials, restricted to patients with a Maddrey discriminant function of at least 32, demonstrated a significantly higher survival rate at 28 days in corticosteroid-treated patients compared to those receiving placebo (85% vs 65%; P = 0.001). Based on this data, about five patients would need corticosteroid treatment to prevent one death. Corticosteroid therapy is contraindicated in patients with active infection.

Anti-cytokine therapy

Treatment with pentoxifylline, which reduces synthesis of the pro-inflammatory cytokine, tumour necrosis factor-alpha (TNF-α), has been shown in a double-blind, prospective, randomised trial in patients with

QUICK FLICK 39

severe alcoholic hepatitis, as suggested by a Maddrey discriminant function of at least 32, to be associated with a significantly reduced in-hospital mortality compared to placebo (46% vs 24%), predominantly as a consequence of a reduced incidence of complicating hepatorenal syndrome. The difference in mortality between the two groups suggests that 4.7 patients would need to be treated to prevent one death, which is comparable to the situation with corticosteroid therapy described above.

Two small uncontrolled pilot studies have suggested the possible benefit of infliximab, a monoclonal antibody against TNF-α, in patients with alcoholic hepatitis. Nonetheless, a randomised controlled trial in which infliximab was used in combination with prednisolone compared to prednisolone alone was terminated prematurely because of a significantly higher mortality rate, related to infection, in the infliximab-treated group.

Liver transplantation

Alcoholic liver disease is currently the second most common indication for liver transplantation for cirrhosis in the Western world. In selected patients with end-stage cirrhosis, transplantation may be highly effective, with post-transplant outcomes similar to those in patients transplanted for non-alcoholic causes of cirrhosis. Most units insist that the patient should have been abstinent from alcohol for at least six months, allowing time for both dependency issues to be addressed and any recovery in liver function, such that transplantation may no longer ultimately be required, to begin to occur. Rates of recidivism at three to five years after transplantation ranging from around 10 to 50 per cent have been documented. The role of liver transplantation in acute alcoholic hepatitis is currently unresolved.

Summary

Alcohol is the most frequently used hepatotoxin worldwide. The term 'alcoholic liver disease' should be reserved for pathology for which other possible causes have been excluded, in the setting of excessive alcohol use and, preferably, in association with confirmatory changes on liver biopsy. An important co-factor in progressive liver injury is concurrent hepatitis C viral infection. Anti-inflammatory or anti-cytokine therapy, using corticosteroids or pentoxifylline, respectively, have been shown to be effective in improving short-term survival in those patients with severe alcoholic hepatitis. In selected patients with end-stage cirrhosis, transplantation may be highly effective, with post-transplant outcomes similar to those in patients transplanted for non-alcoholic causes of cirrhosis.

Recommended reading

Lucey MR. Management of alcoholic liver disease. *Clin Liver Dis*. 2009; 13:267–75.

O'Shea RS, Dasarathy S, McCullough AJ. Alcoholic liver disease. *Am J Gastroenterol*. 2010; 105:14–32.

O'Shea RS, Dasarathy S, McCullough AJ, Practice Guideline Committee of the American Association for the Study of Liver Diseases, Practice Parameters Committee of the American College of Gastroenterology. Alcoholic liver disease. *Hepatology*. 2010; 51:307–28.

QUICK FLICK 39

The possible value of other serum markers, such as des-γ carboxyprothrombin and fucosylated AFP, is currently unresolved.

The sensitivity of ultrasound for small HCCs is comparable to that of other non-invasive modalities such as dynamic computed tomography (CT) and magnetic resonance imaging (MRI). Sensitivity of ultrasound for nodular HCCs 1.1 to 3.0 cm in diameter is 95 per cent, although the detection rate by each of these techniques is substantially reduced when the tumour diameter is less than 1 cm. Over 90 per cent of solid lesions detected by ultrasound in cirrhotic patients enrolled in screening/surveillance programs are subsequently confirmed to be HCCs, the differential diagnosis including haemangiomas, regenerative nodules, focal fatty change and metastases. There are no firm guidelines established concerning the optimum surveillance interval. Nonetheless, surveillance every six months is a rational approach, based on data from China in which the median doubling time of HCCs was found to be almost four months and the time taken for tumour diameter to increase from 1 cm to 3 cm was not less than five months. A recent multicentre study performed in France found that increasing the frequency of surveillance ultrasonography to every three months did not improve performance.

HCC arising in an otherwise normal liver tends to occur in younger patients. Fibrolamellar HCC is one such variant and tends to carry a better prognosis than other varieties of HCC. Liver function tests are less often abnormal in this group and serum AFP levels are not usually elevated, even in the presence of large tumours. Furthermore, the lack of association with underlying chronic liver disease or chronic HBV carriage mitigates against an effective screening program for this tumour.

Further investigation

Further imaging is necessary in patients with elevated serum AFP levels but negative hepatic ultrasonography. Although the sensitivity of ultrasound for small HCCs is, in general, comparable to that of other non-invasive imaging modalities, areas immediately below the diaphragm can be relative blind spots. Furthermore, diffuse HCCs, isoechoic with the non-tumorous hepatic parenchyma, may be difficult to detect. The next imaging investigation of choice is contrast-enhanced CT or MRI. Relative advantages of the latter modality are that it does not involve the use of ionising radiation or iodinated contrast. Hepatic arteriography is required if no lesion is evident on non-invasive imaging. Sensitivity of hepatic arteriography for small HCCs is improved by modifications such as CT scanning seven to ten days after the intra-hepatic arterial injection of lipiodol, an iodised oil retained in HCC rather than normal hepatocytes (lipiodol-CT), or, especially, microbubble-enhanced sonographic angiography (MESA). CT during arterial portography

(CTAP) may be necessary to detect the relatively small proportion of HCCs which are hypovascular. Patients in whom no lesion is definable by any of these imaging modalities should be followed by hepatic ultrasonography with or without MRI at three-monthly intervals. The possibility of an unrelated germ-cell tumour must be excluded.

Establishing the diagnosis of HCC and tumour staging

The presence of a solid mass on ultrasound or other imaging in association with a serum AFP level above 1000 ng/mL in a patient with histologically proven cirrhosis provides strong presumptive evidence of HCC. Confirmation of the diagnosis and staging, including determination of the size and number of tumour foci and the possibility of vascular invasion, can usually be obtained by contrast-enhanced dynamic CT or MRI, based on the demonstration of typical arterial neovascularity. Hepatic arteriography may occasionally be required but it is uncommon. The arteriographic diagnosis of HCC is based on the presence of typical arterial neovascularity with irregular vascular dilatation, vessel proliferation, tumour stain, venous threads and streaks, pooling of contrast medium and arteriovenous shunting. High velocity Doppler signals reflecting arteriovenous shunting are evident in over 80 per cent of patients with large HCCs, 4 cm in diameter, and are specific for this disorder. In the case of small tumours not detectable on routine hepatic arteriography, characteristic abnormalities on MESA and lipiodol-CT have positive predictive values for HCC of 100 per cent and over 90 per cent, respectively.

The role of percutaneous biopsy for early tissue confirmation of HCC is controversial, as this procedure carries a small but definite risk of tumour dissemination along the needle tract, thereby precluding potentially effective local treatment. Many centres adopt the policy that percutaneous biopsy should be performed only if angiography is non-diagnostic or the patient is known to have extrahepatic disease. In this latter setting, it is appropriate to proceed directly to histological diagnosis.

Extrahepatic spread, most commonly to local lymph nodes, the thorax and bone, tends to occur relatively late in the course of the disease but must be excluded in any patient in whom potentially curative local therapy is contemplated. Abdominal and thoracic CT or MRI and radionuclide bone scanning play important roles in this aspect of the staging process.

Assessment of hepatic functional reserve

Determination of whether or not underlying cirrhosis is present is of paramount importance in assessing hepatic functional reserve and, therefore, in evaluating the risk of hepatic decompensation following

treatments such as partial hepatic resection, as discussed below. Consideration of a number of additional parameters has been proposed for further risk evaluation in patients shown to be cirrhotic, including the residual hepatic volume after planned resection as measured by CT scanning, the indocyanine green and bromosulphthalein retention rates and the hepatic venous pressure gradient. A raised pre-operative serum bilirubin level and the pre-operative presence of significant portal hypertension—defined by a hepatic venous pressure gradient in excess of 10 mm Hg—are important predictors of post-operative hepatic decompensation. Consideration of Child's class alone is inadequate for selecting patients for hepatic resection, as unresolved deterioration in hepatic function subsequently occurs in more than 50 per cent of otherwise unselected Child's A patients.

○ Management

Possible treatment options for HCC may be categorised as local (for disease confined to the liver) or systemic (for disease with extrahepatic spread) (see Figure 40.1). The further indications, contraindications and efficacies of these treatments are discussed below. It must be emphasised that, with the exception of OLT, anti-HCC treatment may not modify the overall prognosis of patients with decompensated hepatic function, in whom survival is often determined by the underlying advanced cirrhosis rather than progression of the complicating tumour.

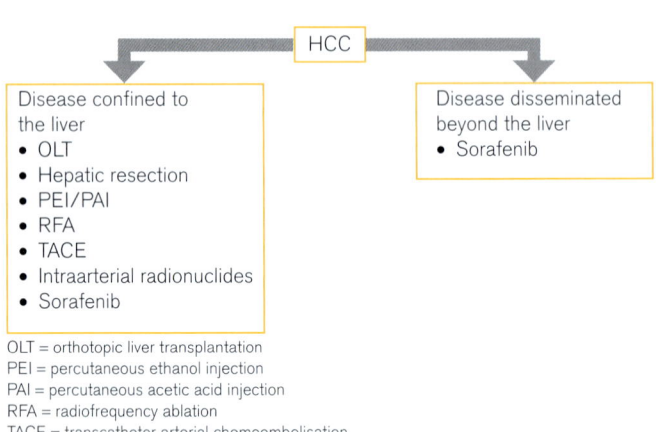

HCC

Disease confined to the liver
- OLT
- Hepatic resection
- PEI/PAI
- RFA
- TACE
- Intraarterial radionuclides
- Sorafenib

Disease disseminated beyond the liver
- Sorafenib

OLT = orthotopic liver transplantation
PEI = percutaneous ethanol injection
PAI = percutaneous acetic acid injection
RFA = radiofrequency ablation
TACE = transcatheter arterial chemoembolisation

Figure 40.1 Possible management options for hepatocellular carcinoma (HCC)

Therapeutic options for HCC confined to the liver

Orthotopic liver transplantation (OLT)

In patients with HCC complicating cirrhosis, OLT is the only treatment which can possibly both cure the tumour and remove the pre-malignant potential of the cirrhotic liver, and it may be the only feasible option that favourably influences overall survival in patients with advanced degrees of underlying liver dysfunction. Excellent results may be obtained when OLT is restricted to patients with a single HCC at least 5 cm in diameter, or with three or fewer tumour nodules at least 3 cm in diameter, in the absence of vascular invasion or extrahepatic spread. Low rates of tumour recurrence and survival comparable to that of patients transplanted without HCC have been recorded in these settings. Modalities such as PEI, TACE and RFA, as discussed below, can be effective at limiting tumour growth that might otherwise render the patient untransplantable during time spent on a waiting list for OLT.

Over 50 per cent five-year tumour-free survival has been reported in patients transplanted for the fibrolamellar variant of HCC, even those with large and/or multifocal tumours not amenable to resection. OLT is the treatment of choice in this group.

Partial hepatic resection

Partial hepatic resection is feasible in cirrhotic patients who have a solitary HCC less than 5 cm in diameter in an anatomically suitable (not central) location, provided hepatic functional reserve is adequate and disease is confined to the liver with no macroscopic evidence of vascular invasion.

Overall, only about 20 per cent of patients in Asian countries and fewer than 10 per cent in the West are finally deemed to be suitable candidates for hepatic resection after careful pre-operative assessment. When only patients with HCCs detected in screening/surveillance programs are considered, 43 to 81 per cent in Asian countries and 7 to 50 per cent in the West are ultimately operable. Prior embolisation of the portal vein branch supplying the segment to be resected with a mixture of fibrin, thrombin and lipiodol can be used to increase pre-operative hepatic functional reserve and, hence, the number of patients in whom hepatic resection may be appropriate.

Five-year survival following hepatic resection for HCC is in the order of 45 per cent in non-cirrhotic patients and 30 to 60 per cent in patients with underlying cirrhosis. In well-compensated patients, survival is predominantly limited by the high rate of tumour recurrence (33% by one year, 50% by two years and over 60% by three years). In both Asia and the West, most (68–96%) recurrences are found in the remnant liver rather than in extrahepatic sites. These are predominantly new HCCs, rather than previously unrecognised satellite lesions. Multivariate analysis has demonstrated that disease-free survival following resection for HCC is inversely related to the degree of necroinflammatory activity in the remnant

liver. In patients with chronic hepatitis C virus-related cirrhosis, risk of HCC is substantially reduced among those who achieve a sustained virological response to interferon therapy compared with non-responders (relative risk of HCC development of 0.35), especially when combination treatment with ribavirin is used (relative risk of HCC development of 0.25). Maintenance therapy with interferon does not reduce HCC risk among cirrhotic patients who do not respond to anti-viral treatment.

Percutaneous ethanol injection (PEI) and acetic acid injection (PAI)

PEI is appropriate for patients with a single HCC less than 5 cm in diameter or up to three tumour nodules each 3 cm or less in size, especially if superficially located. Contraindications to PEI include ascites, uncorrectable coagulopathy and extrahepatic dissemination. PEI is not useful in patients with larger tumours, as the diffusion of ethanol is limited by not only the texture of the tumour parenchyma but also the presence of septa, which isolate portions of the tumour and prevent the homogeneous distribution of ethanol within it.

Up to 79 per cent of three-year survival rates have been reported with PEI, depending on the size and number of HCC foci treated and underlying Child's classification. A cohort study comparing PEI with hepatic resection in patients with HCCs 4 cm or less in diameter found similar overall four-year survival, despite less rigorous patient selection in those treated with PEI. Consequently, PEI is becoming increasingly used both in Asia and the West as an alternative to hepatic resection in patients with small, resectable HCCs for whom OLT is not available or otherwise contraindicated, especially in view of its lower associated morbidity and cost. Acute procedure-related pulmonary hypertension, due to disturbances in nitric oxide synthesis and endothelial dysfunction, may occur. Available data suggest that PAI is of comparable efficacy to PEI. Similar rates of tumour recurrence to those occurring after hepatic resection have been reported. As with percutaneous biopsy, needle tract seeding is a possible but uncommon complication of PEI, a finding with important implications if this technique is used with curative intent or as a bridging procedure while awaiting OLT.

Radiofrequency ablation (RFA)

RFA is widely applied for the local ablation of liver malignancies up to 3 cm in diameter. Recent advances have focused on an improved design of devices, with the aim of increasing the ablation zone. A meta-analysis of randomised controlled trials suggests that RFA is superior to PEI with regard to three-year overall survival and cancer-free survival rates, and tumour response, in cirrhotic patients with small HCCs. A significantly reduced risk of local HCC recurrence was also apparent in the RFA-treated group. A comparable survival rate to that following resection has been reported in potentially operable cirrhotic patients with a single tumour focus up to 2 cm in diameter.

Intrahepatic arterial-based therapies

These include TACE and the injection of radionuclides (^{131}I-labelled lipiodol, ^{188}Re-labelled lipiodol or ^{90}Y-labelled microspheres). TACE, which combines targeted chemotherapy and temporary hepatic arterial embolisation with particulate matter such as gelfoam, is an option for patients with HCCs confined to the liver, including large or centrally located tumours not amenable to other local treatments. Emulsifying the chemotherapeutic agent(s) with lipiodol prolongs the contact time between anti-cancer drugs and tumour cells and is associated with improved efficacy of TACE. Use of drug-eluting beads is an emerging alternative strategy. Main portal vein occlusion is a contraindication to TACE. Many centres also exclude patients with Child's C cirrhosis on the premise that prognosis would remain poor even if the HCC was successfully ablated, and since the procedure carries a risk of further hepatic decompensation consequent to transient ischaemia of the non-tumorous liver. Most patients experience transient fever and right upper quadrant pain following TACE. Other uncommon side effects include liver abscess, renal failure and neutropaenic sepsis.

Tumour ablation rates following repeated sessions of TACE are substantially higher for HCCs smaller than 4 cm in diameter than for larger tumours. Multivariate analysis has identified tumour size, along with underlying liver function, as important factors influencing survival following this form of treatment. A survival advantage has been documented compared to patients receiving no anti-HCC therapies. Limited published experience suggests that pre-operative TACE to reduce tumour bulk may improve the post-operative outcome in patients with HCCs considered borderline for resection.

The intra-arterial injection of radionuclides is a potentially attractive alternative hepatic arterially-delivered therapy to TACE, especially in patients with portal vein thrombosis, in whom the latter is contraindicated. Reports of efficacy are currently limited, although several recent studies performed in small cohorts of patients with unresectable, non-metastatic HCC suggest comparable efficacy and toxicity to those following TACE.

Therapeutic options for HCC disseminated beyond the liver

Sorafenib, an oral multikinase inhibitor that targets Raf kinase and tyrosine kinases, leading to both anti-proliferative and anti-angiogenesis effects, has recently emerged as a promising treatment for patients with inoperable HCC, including those with tumour spread beyond the liver. A meta-analysis of randomised controlled trials suggests a 37 per cent improvement in overall survival rate and a 79 per cent prolongation in time to tumour progression. Although these findings translate to only a modestly prolonged survival time, in the order of a few months, the prospect of this and other

molecular-targeted therapies currently undergoing preliminary assessment, either alone or in combination, has brought new hope to the management of this otherwise untreatable group.

Systemic chemotherapy with a variety of agents, including doxorubicin, epirubicin, mitoxantrone, cisplatin and etoposide, either alone or in combination, has historically been used in patients with HCC disseminated beyond the liver. However, the response rate is in the order of only 15 per cent or less and the value of systemic chemotherapy has never been confirmed in controlled trials. Consequently, this form of treatment has no accepted role in the management of HCC.

Summary

HCC is among the most common cancers worldwide. There is a high prevalence in Asia and sub-Saharan Africa; however, detection rates are increasing in Western countries. The range of potentially effective treatments available includes OLT, hepatic resection, percutaneous ethanol injection, percutaneous acetic acid injection, radiofrequency ablation and the hepatic arterial injection of radionuclides.

It is essential that a reliable screening and surveillance program is instituted aimed at detecting small tumours at an asymptomatic stage in groups at an increased risk of HCC development. Sorafenib, an oral multi-kinase inhibitor that targets Raf kinase and tyrosine kinases, has recently emerged as a drug that is associated with improved modest survival in patients with advanced HCC.

Recommended reading

Cabrera R, Nelson DR. Review article: the management of hepatocellular carcinoma. *Aliment Pharmacol Ther*. 2010; 31:461–76.

Colombo M. Screening and diagnosis of hepatocellular carcinoma. *Liver Int*. 2009; 29:143–7.

Forner A, Reig ME, de Lope CR, Bruix J. Current strategy for staging and treatment: the BCLC update and future prospects. *Semin Liver Dis*. 2010; 30:61–74.

Gusani NJ, Jiang Y, Kimchi ET, Staveley-O'Carroll KF, Cheng H, Ajani JA. New pharmacological developments in the treatment of hepatocellular cancer. *Drugs*. 2009; 69:2533–40.

Shih ST, Crowley S, Sheu JC. Cost-effectiveness analysis of a two-stage screening intervention for hepatocellular carcinoma in Taiwan. *J Formos Med Assoc*. 2010; 109:39–55.

Chapter 41: Hepatic imaging

J. Chaganti (Australia)

Key points

▶ Hepatic steatosis can be diffuse or focal, and varying radiology of steatosis can resemble focal liver lesions.

▶ Chronic parenchymal damage leads to cirrhosis and one of the sequelae is regenerating nodules. Dysplastic nodules are regenerative, with atypical features.

▶ Transformation into HCC is associated with neoangiogenesis. Imaging correlate of neoangiogenesis is enhancement with contrast during the arterial phase.

▶ The nodule within nodule sign is highly suggestive of malignant transformation in regenerative nodules.

▶ Tailored imaging protocols are necessary to characterise benign focal liver lesions.

▶ Transient hepatic attenuation differences (THAD): unique dual blood supply to the liver can lead to differential perfusion in different diseases during the arterial phase of the scan and can mimic tumour morphology.

○ Introduction

Imaging of the liver has progressed rapidly as with other areas of imaging in the past decade. Simultaneous advancement in the imaging technologies has heralded better anatomical delineation of the lesion as well as characterisation. Each of these modalities has become complementary to the others, facilitating more effective characterisation of the lesion. The introduction of contrast in the imaging paradigm has further enhanced the ability to identify and characterise the lesions. Technological improvement and usage of the work station environment has undoubtedly produced the additional benefit of interrogating the disease in many phases and in different orthogonal planes.

This chapter discusses the role of individual imaging modalities in determining the specificity and sensitivity of:

- hepatic steatosis imaging and quantification, and fatty sparing
- cirrhosis and lesion characterisation
- benign focal hypervascular lesions

- hepatic vascular and perfusion disorders
- diffusion-weighted imaging of the liver.

◯ Hepatic steatosis

Fatty liver is the most common cause of chronic liver disease worldwide. The key histological feature of fatty liver disease is hepatic steatosis. The current diagnostic standard of reference for assessing the steatosis is liver biopsy which has the disadvantages that (a) it is invasive, (b) sampling errors occur and (c) it is not appropriate for screening or evaluating treatment response. Diagnosing steatosis is a challenge in living liver donors and not being able to do so has an adverse prognostic implication.

The accumulation of triglyceride in the hepatocyte appears to occur in the centre of the lobule (around the central vein) rather than at the periphery. Consequently steatosis tends to be more pronounced around the portal triads in the initial stages. In some cases, the steatosis tends to progress to steatohepatitis (inflammation, cell injury and fibrosis) and then cirrhosis, although this latter step is uncommon.

Imaging

Ultrasound (US)

The echogenicity of normal liver equals or minimally exceeds that of renal cortex or spleen. The intrahepatic vessels are sharply demarcated and diaphragms are well delineated. Fatty liver may be diagnosed if the echogenicity of liver exceeds the renal cortex or spleen or if there is loss of definition of intrahepatic vasculature and diaphragms. In milder forms of steatosis there is mild diffuse increase in echogenicity. In moderate steatosis there is obscuration of portal vessels; in severe steatosis there is posterior attenuation of the sound and visualisation of diaphragms is precluded. It has been shown that this posterior attenuation of the sound beam roughly corresponds to 30 per cent or more of steatosis. Evaluation of steatosis in patients with hepatitis can be difficult due to accompanying inflammation and fibrosis. Recent innovations in the United States using artificial neural networks and computerised analysis of liver texture by indices of ultrasonic backscatter appear to be sensitive in assessment of diagnosis of early steatosis. Hepatic steatosis can induce changes in the Doppler wave forms in both hepatic arterial and venous systems. Hepatic arterial resistance appears to show a significant drop with increasing levels of hepatic steatosis.

Computed tomography (CT)

Steatosis results in reduced attenuation of the liver and can be measured by CT units. Enhanced CT has a limited role in the diagnosis of steatosis.

Comparing the CT units of the skeletal muscle with the liver appears to be more sensitive than comparing with the spleen. In the qualitative evaluation of steatosis, the splenic liver attenuation ratio or difference can be taken to grade the steatosis. In healthy people, the attenuation difference of the spleen is 8–10 units less than for the liver. It has been reported that a liver:spleen attenuation difference greater than −10 HU was highly predictive of hepatic steatosis.

Dual peak kilovoltage (kVp) CT and dual-source CT, which was introduced subsequently, appear to be more sensitive for diagnosing steatosis.

Magnetic resonance imaging (MRI)

MRI appears to be more sensitive in the diagnosis and quantification of steatosis. Breath-hold gradient echo (GRE) with both in-phase and out-of-phase is the sequence of choice to assess the steatosis. This sequence was further optimised to quantitative measurement of fat fraction in the liver by applying dual flip angle to resolve the ambiguity of the dominant constituent.

Patterns of steatosis

Diffuse

Major causes of diffuse hepatic steatosis are alcoholic liver disease and non-alcoholic steatohepatitis (NASH). The latter cause has emerged as a distinct entity, and diagnosis is currently based on liver biopsy. In the evaluation of potential liver donors, MR is used as a one-stop shop to assess the hepatic fat content, vascular variations and volume of right and left lobes, as well as looking for any incidental parenchymal pathologies. It is generally accepted that mild-degree steatosis (<30%) is acceptable for living-related liver transplantation.

Focal steatosis

Both focal fat sparing and focal steatosis present with atypical image morphology and may resemble tumours. In most cases, however, they have characteristic locations such as gall bladder fossa, medial segment near falciform ligament, subcapsular regions and porta hepatis. These focal areas of fatty infiltration and fatty sparing are attributed to anomalous small veins entering into the liver and communicating with the pancreatico-duodenal, cholecystic and gastric venous systems as well as other small venous systems around the liver. These areas appear as wedge-shaped or geographic in configuration, with lack of mass effect, normal vascular structures coursing through the area, enhancement similar to or less than the normal liver parenchyma and stability over time.

Multifocal steatosis

In some cases there are confluent areas of fatty infiltration that may resemble a mass. The exact aetiology is unknown.

The imaging features of such mass-like morphology still carry the same radiology of focal fatty lesions, and out-of-phase MR clinches the diagnosis.

Perivascular steatosis

This is a recently described entity which is mostly seen in alcoholic patients. Periportal and perivenular fatty infiltration can be observed independently or in combination. MR shows a signal drop and CT shows areas of hypodensity following the course of hepatic vasculature.

Perilesional and subcapsular steatosis

Perilesional steatosis has been shown to occur around insulinoma metastasis. It is thought to represent the local effect of insulin in the liver parenchyma. Like steatosis elsewhere it appears as a hypodense area on CT, a hypointense area on out-of-phase T-1 and echogenic on US.

Patients who are diabetic and receiving insulin through peritoneal dialysis have also shown characteristic steatosis along the subcapsular surface, which could be due to the local action of insulin.

Intratumoral steatosis

Fat deposition within the lesion can be intracellular (microscopic) or macroscopic. The intracellular lipid areas are seen as steatosis and appear dark on out-of-phase T-1 imaging on MRI. This finding is not uncommon in HCC, hepatic adenomas and regenerating nodules, but rarely in FNH.

Fat sparing

Focal fat sparing is also attributed to haemodynamic disturbances, similar to focal fat deposition. Contrary to focal fat deposition, these areas appear as hyperdense relative to the surrounding fatty liver on CT, and echogenic on US. MR, however, can characterise these lesions, showing a signal similar to that from normal parenchyma. When focal fat sparing occurs around a tumour it can mask liver lesions on CT. Peritumoral and perilesional fat sparing has been described around haemangiomas, metastasis and HCC. One recent study reported that perilesional fat sparing was observed most frequently around metastasis. The aetiology for this is postulated as due to decreased portal flow.

Conclusion

Presentation of multifaceted steatosis can be a diagnostic challenge and can mimic focal liver lesions. Diffuse steatosis can lead to steatohepatitis

and cirrhosis. Although the current diagnostic standard of reference is liver biopsy, newer imaging methods are increasingly employed to obviate the need for this.

Cirrhosis

Cirrhosis is a consequence of chronic diffuse parenchymal injury of the liver parenchyma. The resulting healing process is by diffuse fibrosis and nodular regeneration. The imaging features of cirrhosis include irregular contours, atrophy of some segments (usually seg-4), peripheral atrophy and hypertrophy of the caudate lobe and left lobe. Presence of portal hypertension is a helpful associated finding.

Cirrhotic liver can develop regenerating nodules which over time may change into dysplastic nodules and finally transform into hepatocellular carcinoma. The regenerating nodules are proliferations of hepatocytes surrounded by fibrosis; depending upon their size they are classified as micronodular (< 3 mm) or macronodular (> 3 mm). Dysplastic nodules are regenerative nodules with atypical cellular features but without definite malignant change.

Blood supply of the cirrhotic liver is different from that of the normal liver. This is due to global reduction of portal venous supply, which is compensated by increased arterial flow. Most of the regenerative nodules receive blood supply from the portal vein initially but this slowly changes from the portal to the hepatic artery, as for the rest of the liver in cirrhosis. With progressive increase in dysplasia the regenerating nodules develop neoangiogenesis. The new arteries so developed are unpaired and do not have accompanying portal veins or biliary ducts. Consequently these nodules can be identified on the imaging as hypervascular lesions in the arterial phase.

Imaging

US, CT and MRI have all been shown to be valuable in the detection of cirrhosis. MRI has proven to be far superior to other modalities in the detection of parenchymal abnormalities and the associated complications.

Contrast agents in MRI

Gadolinium chelates produce T-1 shortening (bright signal) and has dynamic behaviour similar to iodinated contrast agents. These agents are routinely used in the evaluation of neoangiogenesis in a suspected dysplastic nodule/HCC. Superparamagnetic iron oxide (SPIO) is an agent used to assess the liver parenchyma, being selectively taken up by Kupffer cells to produce a significant signal drop on T-2 weighted imaging.

MRI features of cirrhosis

Normal liver parenchyma is intermediate-intense on T-1 and hypointense on T-2. The cirrhotic liver appears more heterogeneous on MRI. The heterogeneity is due to the loss of the normal cellular arrangement and deposition of fibrous tissue, glycogen, fat and other ions.

In the milder form, the cirrhotic liver presents with granular appearance due to small regenerative nodules mixed with fibrosis.

Large areas of fibrosis can appear as pseudomasses and may cause some alarm. This fibrous tissue is typically dark on T-1 but carries a high signal on T-2; differentiating this from HCC is important, as they both carry high signal on T-2. Confluent fibrosis has a predilection for seg-4, and associated capsular retraction is not generally seen with HCC. Fibrosis shows gradual accumulation of contrast over time and these features generally are helpful in differentiating HCC from fibrosis.

Nodules in cirrhosis

Regenerative nodules are typically small (< 1 cm); they are either isointense or hypointense on T-2 and generally do not enhance more than the surrounding liver parenchyma. In comparison, dysplastic nodules have varying morphology. They are typically hyperintense on T-1 and hypointense on T-2, although this is not always true: dysplastic nodules show signal intensities varying from hypointense on T-1 to hyperintense on T-2, or they can be hypointense on all sequences.

Haemosiderin is observed in both dysplastic and regenerative nodules, and is responsible for characteristic signal loss. Malignant transformation in the siderotic nodules causes a characteristic 'nodule within nodule' image signified by a high signal central focus on T-2 which is hypervascular and does not take up SPIO. These siderotic nodules are also seen in the spleen (Gamna-Gandy bodies) and generally measure 6–8 mm.

Hepatocellular carcinoma

Hepatocellular carcinoma nodules are typically hypointense on T-1 and high signal on T-2, but this can vary. While well-differentiated HCCs are circumscribed lesions similar to regenerative or dysplastic nodules, they become more complex and mosaic in appearance as they lose the differentiation. They may carry intracellular lipid and characteristically show loss of signal on out-of-phase T-1. A haemorrhage is yet another cause for mosaic appearance and not commonly observed in HCC, and practically never seen in regenerative or dysplastic nodules. Haemorrhages appear as a high signal on both in-phase and out-of-phase T-1 GRE sequences (cf intracellular fat). Calcification is rare in HCC but, when present, shows as a loss of signal on all sequences.

Vascular invasion is a consistent finding in advanced HCC and should be differentiated from bland thrombus, which is not an uncommon association with cirrhosis. Tumour thrombus generally shows enhancement characteristics similar to that of primary tumour—that is, enhancement in the arterial phase—while bland thrombus does not enhance. Expansion of the portal vein is another feature of tumour-related thrombus.

Most HCCs are hypervascular and best assessed in the late arterial phase. They may also contain a fibrous pseudocapsule which, like any other fibrous tissue, enhances over time.

In one analysis comparing various modalities in the diagnosis of HCC, MRI was found to have a sensitivity of 98 per cent when combined with SPIO and gadolinium contrast agents, 93 per cent with CT arterioportography (CTAP) and 87 per cent with gadolinium only.

Benign focal hepatic lesions

Benign hepatic lesions are often encountered during an unrelated imaging evaluation. These tumours have a specific imaging morphology, and prior knowledge of these features will help to avoid more invasive diagnostic methods. Benign tumours are classified according to cell of origin into hepatocellular, cholangiocellular or mesenchymal adenomas.

Hepatic adenoma

Hepatic adenomas are rare benign tumours of the liver. They are often solitary, and typically occur in females. Histologically they contain well-differentiated hepatocytes. They lack bile ducts and portal triads, which are important histological features differentiating them from FNH. Kupffer cells are rarely present. Rarely these tumours may degenerate into hepatocellular carcinomas.

Sonography is not characteristic. They may be hypoechoic or hyperechoic but typically they are heterogenous and show increased vascularity. On CT these lesions appear isodense to the liver and show moderate enhancement with contrast in the arterial phase, with wash-out similar to liver parenchyma. MRI shows similar findings, with intensity similar to liver parenchyma on both T-1 and T-2. Because of the dilated sinusoids with scanty connective tissue, they are prone to haemorrhaging, which appears as bright areas in both in-phase and opposed-phase imaging. Although these tumorous enhancements appear to be brisk, they are not as hypervascular as FNH. They may have a pseudocapsule which may or may not show delayed enhancement.

Adenoma cells may be filled with glycogen and fat. This intracellular lipid gives a characteristic low signal on opposed-phase imaging. The presence of intracellular lipid is seen in 35 to 77 per cent of hepatic adenomas.

Focal nodular hyperplasia

This common benign tumour of the liver is second only to haemangioma in frequency of occurrence. It appears predominantly in young asymptomatic women and is often discovered incidentally. FNH consists of aggregates of hepatocytes that are circumscribed by fibrous septa containing bile ducts and mononuclear inflammatory cells. These biliary structures are sequestrated from the main ductal system. Kupffer cells are present in greater abundance than in the surrounding liver tissue. FNH is thought to be due to a proliferative response to an underlying vascular malformation.

- On sonography, the image morphology is typically not classical, appearing as solid tumour with some central flow. The findings on sonography are often very subtle.
- CT demonstrates a mildly hyperdense lesion to the surrounding parenchyma, which shows brisk homogenous enhancement with visualisation of large feeding vessels and an early wash-out. Delayed images show enhancement of the central scar. The scar enhancement is typical with lack of early arterial enhancement and persistent delayed enhancement. This distinguishes FNH from other scar-containing lesions such as fibrolamellar HCCs and haemangiomas.
- On MRI, FNH is hypointense relative to the liver on T-1 and isointense to relatively hyperintense on T-2. A central scar is classically present and is hypointense on T-1 and hyperintense on T-2. The signal intensity of scar tissue is due to blood vessels, bile ducts and oedema with myxomatous tissue. The scar tissue shows delayed enhancement. Dynamic contrast demonstrates enhancement identical to CT, with lesions becoming hypointense in the portal phase. FNH can sometimes show a hyperintense signal in equilibrium-phase imaging. If a liver mass is indeterminate on routine gadolinium contrast studies, hepatocyte-specific contrast agents may help to confirm the hepatocellular origin of the tumour. Gadobenate dimeglumine (Gd-BOPTA) is one such hepatocyte-specific contrast: FNH appears isointense to hyperintense on 1–3 hour delayed studies. The enhancement characteristics can change occasionally and can be either patchy or ring-like.

Haemangioma

Cavernous haemangiomas are the most common benign tumour of the liver, occurring in up to 7 per cent of the general population. They arise from the endothelial cells that line the blood vessels and consist of multiple, large vascular channels lined by a single layer of endothelial cells. It seems that haemangiomas rarely occur in cirrhotic livers as the fibrotic process of cirrhosis inhibits their development. They are rarely large tumours, measuring less than 3 cm. When they become larger than 5 cm they are referred to as 'giant' haemangiomas. Haemangiomas are often solitary but multiple haemangiomas can occur in the same patient up to 50 per cent of the time. There appears to be an increased frequency in their occurrence with FNH.

Imaging of the haemangiomas can be diverse. Sonography is considered to be the most cost-effective imaging modality; however, CT and MRI are required to specify the diagnosis.

- On sonography the typical haemangioma appears as well-circumscribed, uniformly hyperechoic lesions. This increased echogenicity is considered to be due to multiple interfaces between the walls of cavernous spaces. Posterior acoustic enhancement, when present in haemangiomas, appears to be well correlated to hypervascularity on angiography. Atypical features of haemangioma include heterogeneity in echotexture, and a small percentage of haemangiomas are completely hypoechoic. Colour flow studies are generally regarded as insensitive. Sonographic contrast media have shown increased specificity in the diagnosis of haemangiomas.

- On CT, haemangiomas are typically less dense than surrounding liver parenchyma and show characteristic dynamic contrast enhancement. During the arterial-dominant phase they show puddles/nodular peripheral enhancement and show progressive centripetal fill that is considered pathognomonic for haemangiomas. Small haemangiomas may not follow this pattern of enhancement, more often showing dense homogenous enhancement in the arterial phase that may mimic HCC or FNH, but the delayed wash-out pattern of haemangiomas differentiates these conditions.

  Rarely, haemangioma may not show any enhancement and is attributed to hyalinisation. This form of haemangioma poses a diagnostic challenge. Giant haemangiomas may be associated with a central scar. This scar tissue, unlike that associated with FNH, is due to thrombosis and does not enhance with contrast.

- MRI is more specific and sensitive than other imaging modalities. Typical MRI features of haemangioma are hypointense septated lesion on T-1, and on T-2 show a very high signal which is identical to CSF/bile signal with increased echo time—referred to as the 'light bulb sign'. Enhancement characteristics are similar to CT, with peripheral puddling of contrast in the arterial phase and persistence of contrast in the late portal phase. This contrast enhancement typically lasts for about five minutes.

  Haemorrhage and myxomatous degeneration give a cystic appearance to haemangiomas. They may also demonstrate fluid levels. MRI is more sensitive than CT and has 100 per cent sensitivity, 92 per cent specificity and 97 per cent accuracy.

- Nuclear imaging: red blood cell-tagged technetium-99m (^{99m}Tc) scintigraphy with single photon emission computed tomography (SPECT) scanning allows specific diagnosis of haemangiomas.

Nodular regenerative hyperplasia (NRH)

NRH is an uncommon entity with diffuse nodularity of the liver associated with Budd-Chiari syndrome, myeloproliferative disorders, collagen vascular disorders and drugs. The pathogenesis of these nodules is not definitively known. At pathology, NRH lesions closely resemble FNH.

On MRI these lesions appear hypointense on T-1 and remain hypointense on T-2. Dynamic contrast-enhanced studies show the lesions as enhancing multiple, small, similar-sized nodules with rapid wash-out and becoming isointense to the liver in the late arterial phases. This is useful for differentiating from HCC, which become isointense to the liver only in the equilibrial or portal phase.

Hypervascular metastasis

Typical enhancement characteristics of metastasis are intense enhancement in the arterial phase and wash-out in the portal phase. These findings are identical to many other tumours in the liver. Without a prior history, the characterisation of a given hypervascular lesion can sometimes be difficult.

The common causes of hypervascular metastasis are carcinoid tumours, neuroendocrine tumours, renal cell carcinomas, melanomas and sarcomas.

One of the characteristic finding in metastasis from insulinomas is perilesional lipid which produces signal drop on out-of-phase imaging. On T-2 weighted imaging, most of the metastases are intensely bright, a feature that distinguishes them from hepatocellular carcinoma.

◑ Hepatic vascular and perfusion disorders

The unique dual blood supply to the liver makes it a challenging organ to assess, more so due to changing flow dynamics. Changes in arterial pressures can occur due to arterial abnormalities or portal abnormalities or a combination of these. They can be seen in various spectra of conditions that affect the liver. Such changes may result in selective diversion, resulting in some areas being over-perfused and other areas being less perfused. This leaves areas of the liver showing different contrast enhancement in the arterial phase. Knowledge of these haemodynamic changes is crucial not only in the identification of the cause of such differences but also in avoiding the pitfall of incorrectly concluding that an area is abnormal.

Broadly these disorders can classified as either those occurring due to diffuse increase in the arterial flow, or those occurring due to focal lesions. Discussion of these is beyond the scope of this chapter; the reader is referred to the recommended reading list for more information.

Peliosis hepatis

This is a rare benign disorder of the liver that causes sinusoidal dilatation and multiple blood-filled lacunae. Although the exact aetiology is not known, it is widely considered to be due to chronic wasting disorders and malignancies. Bacillary peliosis is reportedly caused by *Bartonella henselae* infection in patients with HIV.

CT typically shows the lesion as hypoattenuating on non-contrast studies and varying enhancement patterns with contrast. Enhancement of peliosis can be homogeneous or can be progressive filling. When opacification is progressive it can be either centrifugal or centripetal filling, which is seen during the portal phase. When thrombosis occurs in the cavernous spaces it can appear as non-enhancing nodules.

○ Diffusion-weighted imaging of the liver

The expanding role of MR for liver disorders has seen an exciting new development: the introduction of diffusion-weighted imaging (DWI). This technique has been the cornerstone of brain disorder diagnosis and is now becoming increasingly used for characterising liver lesions.

The principle of diffusion imaging is based on the random movement of protons in the water in the body. Any condition that arrests or reduces this multidirectional random motion enhances the signal on the diffusion-weighted image. This restriction can be quantified by measuring the apparent diffusion coefficient (ADC), the numbers so derived then being used to characterise a lesion, and also to assess its response to therapy.

Summary

MRI appears to be superior to CT, CTAP, US and PET in both sensitivity and specificity in the diagnosis of both diffuse and focal lesions of the liver. Proper protocols play a pivotal role when using MRI and thorough knowledge of the pulse sequences and proper application are crucial for optimum results.

Recommended reading

Anderson SW, Kruskal JB, Kane RA. Benign hepatic tumors and iatrogenic pseudotumors. *Radiographics*. 2009; 29:211–29.

Başaran C, Karcaaltincaba M, Akata D, Karabulut N, Akinci D, Ozmen M, Akhan O. Fat-containing lesions of the liver: cross-sectional imaging findings with emphasis on MRI. *Am J Roentgenol*. 2005; 184:1103–10.

Cassidy FH, Yokoo T, Aganovic L, Hanna RF, Bydder M, Middleton MS, Hamilton G, Chavez AD, Schwimmer JB, Sirlin CB. Fatty liver disease: MR imaging techniques for the detection and quantification of liver steatosis. *Radiographics*. 2009; 29:231–60.

Colgrande S, Centi N, La Villa G, Villari N. Transient hepatic attenuation differences. *Am J Roentgenol*. 2004; 183:459–64.

Guthrie JA. Cirrhosis and focal liver lesions: MRI findings. *Imaging*. 2004: 16:351–63.

Hamer OW, Aguirre DA, Casola G, Lavine JE, Woenckhaus M, Sirlin CB. Fatty liver: imaging patterns and pitfalls. *Radiographics*. 2006; 26:1637–53.

Hussain S, Reinhold C, Mitchell D. Cirrhosis and lesion characterisation at MR imaging. *Radiographics*. 2009; 29:1637–52.

Hussain SM, Semelka RC. Hepatic imaging: comparison of modalities. *Radiol Clin N Am*. 2005; 43:929–47.

Karcaaltincaba M, Akhan O. Imaging of hepatic steatosis and fatty sparing. *Eur J Radiol*. 2007; 61:33–43.

Prasad SR, Sahani D, Saini S. Cavernous hemangioma of the liver. *eMedicine*. 2009 1–19. Available from http://emedicine.medscape.com/gastroenterology.

Silva AC, Evans JM, McCullough AE, Jatoi MA, Vargas HE, Hara AK. MR imaging of hyper vascular liver masses: a review of current techniques. *Radiographics*. 2009; 29:385–402.

Taouli B, Koh DM. Diffusion weighted MR imaging of the liver. *Radiology*. 2010; 254:47–66.

Torabi M, Hosseinzadeh K, Federle MP. CT of nonneoplastic hepatic vascular and perfusion disorders. *Radiographics*. 2008; 28:1967–82.

Chapter 42: Gallstones and their sequelae

R. Tandon (India)

Key points

▶ Most acquired inflammatory diseases of the of the biliary tract in adults are the sequalae of gallstones.

▶ Incidence of gallstone disease shows considerable geographic and regional variation.

▶ The type of gallstones may also change with time: the predominant type of gallstones in Japan at present are rich in cholesterol whereas in the past they were pigment stones.

▶ Only 18 per cent of patients with gallstones develop symptoms.

▶ Dyspepsia is not a symptom of gallstones.

▶ Clinical syndromes include acute cholecystitis, choledocholithiasis, acute cholangitis, biliary pancreatitis, gallstone ileus and acute acalculous cholecystitis.

▶ Ultrasound examination of the abdomen is the preferred imaging modality. MRCP is an excellent method for demonstrating stones in the common bile duct.

▶ ERCP is used predominantly only when a therapeutic intervention is to be done.

▶ Asymptomatic gallstones are generally left alone.

▶ Laparoscopic cholecystectomy has almost completely replaced conventional cholecystectomy for surgical removal of the gall bladder.

Introduction

Gallstones form the hub of biliary tract diseases. Most acquired inflammatory diseases of the biliary tract in adults are sequelae or complications of gallstones.

Epidemiology

Gallstone disease is a major health problem worldwide, particularly in adult populations. The incidence of gallstone disease shows considerable geographical and regional variation. In the United States, approximately 10 to 15 per cent of adults have gallstones.[1] In Latin American countries, the prevalence of gallstones is even higher—up to 50 per cent in women. In India there is a large variation in gallstone prevalence in different communities: about 6 to 8 per cent in North Indian Punjabis and 1 or 2 per cent in South Indians.[2–4] Such marked ethnic variation raises the strong possibility that genetic factors play a role in the pathogenesis of gallstones.[5]

With increasing affluence and altered lifestyles, however, gallstone prevalence has been shown to increase in the same population. The type of gallstones may also change with time; thus the predominant type of gallstones in Japan at the present time is cholesterol-rich, whereas in the past pigment stones predominated.[1] Migration studies have shown that ethnic groups acquire the prevalence rates of gallstones of the community into which they move. All these observations point clearly to the aetiological role played by environmental factors, including dietary habits. Thus, both genetic predisposition and environmental factors act together to produce gallstones.

Gallstones are more common in women than men at all ages. The incidence of gallstones increases steadily and persistently with advancing age and with that the possibility of their becoming symptomatic also increases. Overall, however, only 20 per cent of patients with gallstones ever develop symptoms throughout their life. At the same time, the incidence of problems related to old age—diabetes, coronary artery disease, hypertension, cerebrovascular disease and chronic obstructive lung disease—also increase, adding to the morbidity and mortality associated with gallstones. Mortality associated with cholecystectomy is 1 in 50 (2%) in gallstone patients older than 50, compared to 1 in 5000 (0.02%) in younger patients.

Natural history of gallstones

Gracie and Ransohoff (1982) followed-up a cohort of asymptomatic gallstone patients for 20 years, and showed that only 18 per cent of them developed symptoms, the first of which were usually mild.[6]

The course of the disease is much more severe for gallstone patients who have had biliary colic even once, however. They may have a recurrence rate of symptoms as high as 38 to 50 per cent per year.[7]

○ Clinical presentation

Biliary colic is the most common and also the most characteristic symptom of gallstone disease. It is episodic, usually located in the right upper quadrant of the abdomen with radiation to the back or right shoulder, and lasts 15 minutes to two hours. If such a pain persists more than six hours, acute cholecystitis or pancreatitis should be suspected. It is important to appreciate that dyspepsia is not a symptom attributable to gallstones, as it occurs in patients with other diseases as often as in those with gallstones.

Occasionally, one or more gallstones may block the cystic duct and cause acute cholecystitis, or slip out of the cystic duct and block the common bile duct causing jaundice and/or cholangitis, or go further down and block the small intestine to produce gallstone ileus. These clinical syndromes are discussed below briefly.

Acute cholecystitis

This condition presents with biliary colic of more than six hours duration. It may be associated with signs of systemic illness such as fever, nausea and vomiting, and abdominal wall tenderness in the right upper quadrant. These patients may have an elevated white blood cell count and ultrasound findings of a thickened gall bladder wall or free intra-abdominal fluid surrounding the gall bladder. Most of them resolve within two days with intravenous fluids, antibiotics and analgesics and undergo an elective cholecystectomy after two to three months. Some may show signs of perforation, however, and may have to undergo surgery immediately. Laparoscopic cholecystectomy is the standard operation; 'conversion' to open surgery is more likely in the elderly than in young patients. Because elderly patients can have gangrene of the gall bladder without appearing seriously ill, early surgery should be considered in all elderly patients with cholecystitis. If the risk of surgery is felt to be prohibitive, an ultrasound-guided drainage tube can be placed under local anaesthetic to decompress the gall bladder (cholecystostomy) in patients who require urgent drainage of the gall bladder.

Choledocholithiasis

The risk of common bile duct stones increases substantially with age. When bile duct stones do not obstruct the bile duct, patients may have symptoms that are indistinguishable from biliary colic, or may be asymptomatic.

QUICK FLICK

42

Symptoms of choledocholithiasis caused by biliary obstruction include intermittent upper abdominal or back pain and jaundice. Patients may notice dark urine or pale stools, and may be icteric on physical examination. In the elderly, it is important to exclude malignant causes of obstructive jaundice, such as pancreatic or gall bladder cancer or other periampullary malignancies.

Ultrasound of the abdomen usually demonstrates dilated bile ducts, but may not detect the stone in the bile duct. Other diagnostic modalities include endoscopic retrograde cholangiopancreatography (ERCP), magnetic resonance cholangiopancreatography (MRCP) and endoscopic ultrasound (EUS).

In some patients choledocholithiasis is diagnosed intraoperatively when an intraoperative cholangiogram is done. Patients with obstructive jaundice or other evidence suggestive of choledocholithiasis should have an ERCP, with sphincterotomy and extraction of the bile duct stones. Following common bile duct clearance most patients should undergo cholecystectomy to avoid future problems with an intact gall bladder, except in the elderly where the remaining lifespan is limited.

Acute cholangitis

Choledocholithiasis predisposes patients to bacterial infection of the bile, or acute cholangitis. The cardinal manifestations are fever, jaundice and right upper quadrant abdominal pain (Charcot's triad). This can proceed rapidly to septic shock if not recognised and treated promptly. Laboratory investigations typically show leukocytosis, and elevated serum bilirubin and transaminases. Ultrasound of the abdomen may show bile duct dilatation and stones or 'sludge'. The initial management should include resuscitation with intravenous fluids and administration of antibiotics. That is followed by emergent decompression of the biliary tract by ERCP with sphincterotomy and stone extraction. In very sick patients with haemodynamic instability or altered coagulation parameters, placement of a nasobiliary tube through ERCP may suffice to tide over the critical period. Occasional patients may require percutaneous transhepatic cholangiography (PTC) to achieve biliary decompression and common bile clearance.

Biliary pancreatitis (*see* Chapter 29: Acute pancreatitis)

Gallstone ileus

Gallstone ileus is mechanical small bowel obstruction caused by one or more large gallstones that erode through the gall bladder wall into the duodenum or pass through the normal route of common bile duct. Although rare among the general population, it is not uncommon in elderly patients. Patients with gallstone ileus commonly present with signs and symptoms of intestinal obstruction (crampy abdominal pain, vomiting, abdominal distension). Plain abdominal radiographs show findings of a small bowel obstruction and gas in the biliary tree. Patients with gallstone ileus require an urgent laparotomy with removal of the gallstones impacted in the small intestine (enterolithotomy).

Pathogenesis

Gallstones are of two types:

- Cholesterol gallstones: those with more than 50 per cent of their dry weight as cholesterol. These are formed from bile that is supersaturated with cholesterol.
- Pigment gallstones: those that have less than 20 per cent of their dry weight as cholesterol. These are formed from bile that is supersaturated with unconjugated bilirubin.

There may be combinations of these. Depending on the predominance of the precipitated component, the stone may be treated as cholesterol or pigment gallstone.[1, 3]

Cholesterol gallstones are predominant in Northern India and in Western countries (80%), and pigment gallstones predominate in Southern India. The cause for this difference is not known but diet may be a factor.

Diagnosis

Since most gallstones (75%) are radiolucent, plain film X-ray of the abdomen is of little use. Ultrasound examination is the preferred imaging modality if gallstones are suspected, with greater than 95 per cent sensitivity and 99 per cent specificity.

Oral cholecystography had traditionally been the method of visualising radiolucent gallstones but now is mainly used to determine the patency of the cystic duct—an important prerequisite for treating gallstones with oral bile acids or lithotripsy (see below).

Computed tomography (CT) scanning helps in assessing the density of the stones but not in detecting any stones missed by other tests.

For demonstrating stones in the common bile duct, ERCP was the 'gold standard' but has been almost completely replaced by magnetic resonance cholangiopancreatography (MRCP), a good non-invasive imaging modality. ERCP is now mainly used for therapeutic intervention in the bile duct—for example, papillotomy or stone extraction.

Acute cholecystitis is best diagnosed by scintigraphy.

◯ **Management**

Since only 20 per cent of gallstones ever become symptomatic, asymptomatic gallstones are generally left alone and treated expectantly except in special circumstances—for example, a patient who is posted to a place where medical facilities are not readily available, or a patient who is carrying a gallstone larger than 3 cm, or who has multiple small stones; in both of these latter situations the complications are reportedly high. Symptomatic patients should, on the other hand, be treated as soon as it becomes clear that the symptoms are attributable to gallstones. The chances of recurrence of symptoms and/or complications are high in such patients; cholecystectomy appears to be the best treatment as it eliminates the chances of re-formation of gallstones and their sequelae. Cholecystectomy is a safe procedure with an overall mortality of 0.1 to 0.6 per cent and a morbidity of 10 to 30 per cent; however, both of these rates increase with age or concomitant disease, or when the procedure is accompanied by common bile duct exploration.

Selection of patients for surgery should be done carefully as cholecystectomy performed for an abdominal pain/discomfort arising from an organ other than the gall bladder may result in persistence of the pre-operative discomfort—a condition termed 'post-cholecystectomy syndrome'. It is best to wait for the appearance of a definite indication of gall bladder disease, such as acute cholecystitis or biliary colic, before surgery is undertaken.[9]

Laparoscopic cholecystectomy

Since its introduction in 1980s, laparoscopic cholecystectomy ('lap chole') has almost completely replaced conventional cholecystectomy because it is associated with less post-operative pain, faster recovery and shorter hospital stay. Indeed, it is done as a day care procedure at many centres, with the operation taking only 30 to 45 minutes.

The complications of lap chole are comparable with those in conventional cholecystectomy. In five or six per cent of patients, the procedure has to be converted into conventional open cholecystectomy.[10, 11]

Acute cholecystitis, difficulties with the anatomy in Calot's triangle and adhesions have been the main reasons for conversion besides difficulties in establishing pneumoperitoneum.[11]

Acute acalculous cholecystitis

Acute cholecystitis mainly occurs in association with gallstones, but may do so even in the absence of gallstones (acalculous cholecystitis), predominantly in elderly males; this is in contrast to calculous cholecystitis which occurs in all age groups. Common factors that predispose to acute acalculous cholecystitis are prolonged fasting, immobility and haemodynamic instability

or vascular insufficiency. In the setting of trauma, septic shock or vasculitis there is vascular insufficiency which in turn results in ischaemic and chemical injury to the gall bladder epithelium. These conditions tend to occur more often in the elderly, with attendant atherosclerotic changes in cystic artery and mesenteric circulation, and predispose them to acalculous cholecystitis. Infection of the gall bladder is a secondary phenomenon in this condition.

The typical symptoms of calculous cholecystitis, such as pain in the right upper quadrant, fever, tenderness and leukocytosis, may be absent in this condition. Unexplained fever may often be the only lead to the diagnosis. The course of this entity is fulminant; more than 50 per cent of these patients have suffered serious complications such as gangrene and perforation of the gall bladder by the time the diagnosis is made. Thus, in an elderly patient at risk, a high index of suspicion for biliary tract sepsis is essential. The mortality rates of acute acalculous cholecystitis range from 10 to 50 per cent, far in excess of that in patients with calculous cholecystitis (less than 1%).

Diagnosis is confirmed by abdominal ultrasonography, CT or hepatobiliary scintigraphy. The features suggesting acalculous cholecystitis at ultrasonography are thick gall bladder wall (> 4 mm), sonographic Murphy's sign and pericholecystic collection in the absence of gallstones. CT can also reveal intramural gas and sloughing of the mucosa.

Supportive medical care should include antibiotics and restoration of haemodynamic stability. The definitive therapy of acute acalculous cholecystitis is urgent laparotomy and cholecystectomy, but this is not possible, primarily because of haemodynamic instability and an underlying debilitating condition. Surgical or ultrasound-guided cholecystostomy are useful alternatives as life-saving procedures.

Emphysematous cholecystitis

This condition is mainly seen in the elderly and in diabetics. It is associated with the presence of gas in the wall or lumen of the gall bladder and the biliary tract. The clinical presentation is similar to acute cholecystitis and the diagnosis is made by demonstration of gas in the biliary system. An urgent cholecystectomy is required under cover of adequate antibiotics, preferably penicillin plus an aminoglycoside. The most common gas-forming bacteria in bile are *Clostridia* and *Escherichia coli*.

Xanthogranulomatous cholecystitis

This condition is characterised by an irregularly thickened gall bladder wall with poorly demarcated yellow nodules of varying size which on microscopy are seen to comprise foaming histiocytes and chronic inflammatory cells. The clinical features are those of chronic cholecystitis. Ultrasonography shows a thickened sonolucent gall bladder wall containing finely echogenic non-shadowing material. Fifty per cent of these patients have gallstones and about 15 per cent develop carcinoma.

Porcelain gall bladder

Porcelain gall bladder is a condition characterised by extensive calcification on the gall bladder mucosa, visible on X-rays, caused by calcium carbonate deposition. Carcinoma develops in almost all such gall bladders which should therefore be surgically removed.

Torsion of the gall bladder

This is a rare condition that mainly occurs in the elderly. The patient presents with acute abdominal pain, nausea and vomiting without any fever, jaundice, rigidity or mass in the right upper quadrant. Pre-operative diagnosis is difficult but a high index of suspicion in an aged patient should help. Gallstones may or may not be present. Management is by early cholecystectomy.

Biliary ascariasis

In the developing countries helminthiasis is common. In regions such as the Kashmir Valley, where infection of the gut with *Ascaris lumbricoides* is prevalent, adult worms may migrate to the biliary tract and cause biliary colic. Biliary stones may develop subsequently over the egg or cuticle of the worm, either in the intrahepatic biliary ducts or the gall bladder. Although any associated biliary stones should be treated just like stones in other situations, treatment of *Ascaris* infection can pose problems when present in the biliary tract.

An attempt is generally made to pull the worm out alive from the biliary tract using a Dormia basket passed through an endoscope, then treat the parasite in the gut with piperazine or pyrantel palmoate. If the parasite dies high up within the biliary tree, it may become somewhat difficult to extract, but if left inside it will become a source of repeated infection.

Other infections

Clonorchis sinensis, *Fasciola hepatica* and *Opisthorchis viverrini* are well known in East Asian countries to infect the biliary tract and to introduce ascending bacterial infection which may result in stone formation in the intrahepatic biliary ducts as well as the gall bladder. Intrahepatic ductal stones present with recurrent cholangitis—so-called 'oriental cholangitis'—pose a difficult therapeutic challenge. Management is initially by a combination of antibiotics and endoscopic removal of the biliary stones, often at repeated sessions, but ultimately by surgical resection of the part of the liver carrying a large number of intraductal stones.

Hyperplastic cholecystosis

This term includes a variety of degenerative and non-inflammatory hyperplastic conditions involving the gall bladder mucosa and muscle. The conditions are adenomyomatosis, cholesterolosis, neuromatosis, lipomatosis, fibromatosis and calcified gall bladder. It is doubtful if any of these produce symptoms.

Haemobilia

Haemobilia should be suspected whenever jaundice and/or upper gastrointestinal bleeding occurs in combination with pain in the right upper quadrant of the abdomen, particularly if the common causes of bleeding have not been found. Trauma, intrahepatic stones, hepatocellular carcinoma, erosion of the cystic artery by a gallstone, haemorrhagic cholecystitis, cancer of the gall bladder and post-operative conditions are among the common causes of haemobilia.

Perforation of the gall bladder

This is extremely rare, but may occur more commonly in the aged because of delayed surgical intervention.

Miscellaneous conditions

Acute cholecystitis due to Cytomegalovirus may occur in immunosuppressed states such as AIDS and in post-liver transplant patients, and in systemic diseases such as sarcoidosis, tuberculosis, systemic lupus erythematosus, polyarteritis nodosa and giant cell arteritis, and also following hepatic arterial infusion of floxuridine.

Summary

Gallstones are the cause of most of the acquired diseases of the biliary tract. The incidence of gallstone disease shows considerable geographical and regional variation. The incidence is greater in women than in men. The hallmark of clinical presentation is biliary colic. The various clinical syndromes are acute cholecystitis, choledocholithiasis, acute cholangitis, biliary pancreatitis, acute acalculous cholecystitis and gallstone ileus. Ultrasound examination is the preferred imaging modality. ERCP is used predominantly for therapeutic intervention. Laparoscopic intervention is the surgical therapy of choice.

References

1. Nakayma F. Cholelithiasis: causes and treatment. 1st ed. Tokyo: Igaku-Shoin Ltd; 1997.

2. Khuroo MS, Mahajan R, Zargar SA, Javid G, Sapru S. Prevalence of biliary tract disease in India: a sonographic study in adult population in Kashmir. *Gut*. 1989; 30:201–5.

3. Tandon RK. Studies on the pathogenesis of gallstones in India. *Ann Natl Acad Med Sci (India)*. 1989; 25:213–22.

4. Tandon RK, Thakur VS, Basak AK, Lal K, Jayanthi V, Nijhawan S. Pigment gall bladder stones predominate in South India. *Indian J Gastroenterol*. 1994; 13(Suppl 1):A18(A–E 6).

5. Lammert F, Wasmuth HE, Matern S. Molecular genetics of gallstone formation: human association studies and comparative genomics. In: Adler G, Fuchs M, Blum HE, Stange EF, editors. Gallstones: pathogenesis and treatment. Dordrecht, Boston, London: Kluwer Academic Publishers, 2004:28–39.

6. Gracie WA, Ransohoff DF. The natural history of silent gallstones: the innocent gallstone is not a myth. *N Engl J Med*. 1982; 307:798–800.

7. Friedman GD, Raviola CA, Fireman B. Prognosis of gallstones with mild or no symptoms: 25 years of follow-up in a health maintenance organisation. *J Clin Epidemiol*. 1989; 42:127–36.

8. Friedman LS, Roberts MS, Brett AS, Marton KI. Management of asymptomatic gallstones in the diabetic patient: a decision analysis. *Ann Intern Med*. 1988; 109:913–9.

9. Tandon RK. Management of gallstones: therapeutic options. In: Wahal PK, editor. Medicine update (APICON- 94). Bombay: Association of Physicians of India 1994; X17–X21.

10. Strasberg SM, Hertl M, Soper NJ. An analysis of the problem of biliary injury during laparoscopic cholecystectomy. *J Am Coll Surg*. 1995 Jan; 180(1):101–25.

11. Shamiyeh A, Wayand W. A 14-year analysis of laparoscopic cholecystectomy: conversion—when and why? *Surg Laparosc Endosc Percutan Tech*. 2007 Aug; 17(4):271–6.

Chapter 43: Neoplasms of the gall bladder and biliary tracts

R.K. Tandon, D. Singhal (India)

Key points

▶ Proximal biliary tract cancers demand a high degree of technical expertise for management.

▶ MRI with MRA with MRCP is the one-stop investigation modality of choice.

▶ Surgical resection with negative margins is the only treatment option consistent with long-term survival.

▶ The main symptoms needing palliative management include pruritus and cholangitis.

▶ Endoscopic stenting with SEMS is preferred for biliary drainage.

▶ Percutaneous biliary drainage with internal stenting reportedly outperforms EBD.

▶ Only 15–20 per cent of all periampullary carcinomas are resectable.

▶ Contrast-enhanced spiral CT scan of whole abdomen with (preferably) 3 mm sections is preferred for staging.

▶ Side-viewing endoscopy and lesion biopsy may be routinely performed.

▶ Pre-operative ERCP and biliary drainage is indicated only for definite indications.

▶ Diagnostic laparoscopy is replaced by high quality CT scan if available.

▶ Pancreatoduodenectomy (PD) is the only curative option for resectable lesions.

▶ The current mortality at specialised centres is 1–5 per cent and morbidity is 40–60 per cent.

▶ The most common complication following PD is delayed gastric emptying.

▶ The most dangerous complication following PD is leak from pancreato-enteric anastomosis.

▶ Endoscopic stenting (biliary/duodenal) or surgical double bypass are acceptable palliative procedures.

◗ Introduction

Benign neoplasms include gall bladder polyps and ampullary adenomas. Carcinomas may involve the entire biliary system and involve the distal or the proximal biliary system.

Any mucosal projection into the lumen of the gall bladder is referred to as a polyp. Adenomyomatosis of the gall bladder that is localised to the fundus may produce a hemispheric projection into the lumen resembling a polyp. Such a lesion is called an adenomyoma, although it is not neoplastic in origin.

Adenomas are not common; their incidence is only about 0.15 per cent of all resected gall bladder specimens. It is not known what percentage, if any, develops into cancer. Polyps larger than 1.2 cm may contain malignant cells and hence should be observed carefully. Current management policy is to follow-up all polyps ultrasonically and to recommend surgery only if they are seen to be increasing in size.

Benign tumours of the ampulla of Vater

These tumours are uncommon and are usually discovered during upper GI endoscopy; sometimes they may present with biliary obstruction or occult or overt GI bleed.

A simplified classification of these tumours based on their origin is as follows:

- Mucosa: Solitary polyps (commonest) or part of various polyposis syndromes such as familial adenomatous polyposis
- Submucosa: Neural tumours, lymphoma or lipoma
- Muscularis mucosa or propria: Gastrointestinal stromal tumours (GIST), leiomyoma.

For tumours arising from the deeper layers, at upper GI endoscopy the ampulla appears bulging with normal overlying mucosa. In such a situation, endoscopic ultrasound may establish the diagnosis by demonstrating the gut layer from which the lesion is arising and showing other sonologic characteristics.

The great majority of these lesions can be effectively managed by either endoscopic polypectomy or submucosal resection. The larger tumours not amenable to currently available endoscopic techniques may be managed with transduodenal local resection. The long-term prognosis of benign ampullary tumours is excellent.

Carcinomas of the distal bile duct and ampulla of Vater

Carcinomas arising within 2 cm of the ampulla of Vater (i.e. the head of the pancreas, ampulla, distal common bile duct and descending duodenum) are collectively referred to as 'periampullary carcinomas'. Most of these tumours (approximately 75%) are adenocarcinomas. In published Western reports, pancreatic carcinomas predominate (50–70%), with 15 to 20 per cent incidence of ampullary carcinoma and 10 per cent incidence both of carcinomas of the distal common bile duct and descending duodenum. By contrast, ampullary cancer appears to predominate in India. Although the presentation, investigation and surgical treatment of the periampullary carcinoma are similar, location of the primary tumour is one of the important prognostic factors for perioperative and long-term outcome (see below).

In the following sections the diagnostic work-up, treatment and outcome of these tumours are briefly discussed.

Clinical presentation

The common symptoms and signs of periampullary carcinoma are presented in Tables 43.1 and 43.2.

Table 43.1 Common symptoms of periampullary carcinoma

Symptom	Incidence (%)
Weight loss	90
Jaundice	82
Pain	72
Anorexia	60
Dark urine	60
Pale stools	60
Pruritis	24

Table 43.2 Common signs of periampullary carcinoma

Signs	Incidence (%)
Jaundice	85
Palpable liver	80
Palpable gall bladder*	25
Ascites	14
Mass	13

* Courvoisier's sign is positive in only a quarter of the patients.

The differentiating features of the various periampullary carcinomas are presented in Table 43.3.

Table 43.3 Differential diagnosis of periampullary carcinoma

Carcinoma of the head of the pancreas
  Age: usually 6th–7th decade
  Pain epigastrium ++
  Loss of weight, anorexia, jaundice common

Ampullary carcinoma
  Age: 5th decade
  No pain
  Intermittent jaundice (due to periodic sloughing of the tumour)
  Intermittent fever with chills (bactibilia due to periodic sloughing of the tumour)

Carcinoma of the duodenum
  Age: 4th–5th decade
  Gastric outlet obstruction common
  Melaena common
  Jaundice late event

Carcinoma of the distal common bile duct
  Age: usually 6th–7th decade
  Painless, progressive jaundice

The initial clinical examination should always include assessment of factors that would preclude resection:

- left supraclavicular lymph node enlargement
- presence of ascites
- poor performance status
- severely compromised cardiopulmonary function.

Objective and initial assessment

Periampullary carcinomas are aggressive tumours that are usually in an advanced stage at the time of presentation in most patients (precluding curative resection). Moreover these tumours occur predominantly in the elderly population who often have significant co-morbidities. Consequently only 15 to 20 per cent of all patients are fit for pancreatoduodenectomy; others are suitable only for palliative therapy.

Thus, the objectives of managing a patient with suspected periampullary carcinoma are:

- Establish the diagnosis.
- Assess fitness for major surgery.
- Meticulous preoperative staging so that only the patients with a curative intent should undergo exploration.
- Appropriate palliation for the remaining patients. Whether the strategy adopted is of endoscopic or surgical palliation would depend predominantly on the available local expertise.

Diagnosis

For a patient suspected to have a periampullary carcinoma on the basis of clinical history and examination, abdominal ultrasonography (USG) should be the initial investigative procedure. This test confirms mechanical obstruction as the cause of jaundice, provides information about the level of obstruction (supracystic or infracystic) and initial assessment of the stage of the disease (ascites and liver metastasis). A complete visualisation at USG is possible in up to 90 per cent patients and is defined as visualisation of head, neck, body and tail of pancreas and that of superior mesenteric vein (SMV), portal vein (PV) and SMPV confluence. A normal pancreatic anatomy is described as uniform texture, echogenicity equal to that of liver, and pancreatic duct (PD) size of 3 mm in the head and 2 mm in the body of pancreas.

When there are no contraindications for resection on USG of the abdomen, a triple-phase contrast-enhanced (oral and intravenous) CT scan of the whole abdomen with 3 mm sections is done as the next investigation for pre-operative staging at most centres. The pancreatic head lesion is typically seen as a hypodense mass with distortion of the normal contour. The obstruction of PD and common bile duct gives rise to the 'double duct sign' (see Figure 43.1 overleaf). The CT criteria for resectable tumour are absence of extrapancreatic disease (liver or peritoneal metastasis, gross lymphadenopathy), patent SMPV confluence and no direct extension to superior mesenteric artery or coeliac axis.

Recently MR with MRCP has been proposed as the investigation of choice for staging. The advantages of this modality are detection/exclusion of carcinoma in focal enlargement of the head of the pancreas and avoiding understaging (better characterisation of liver and peritoneal lesions).

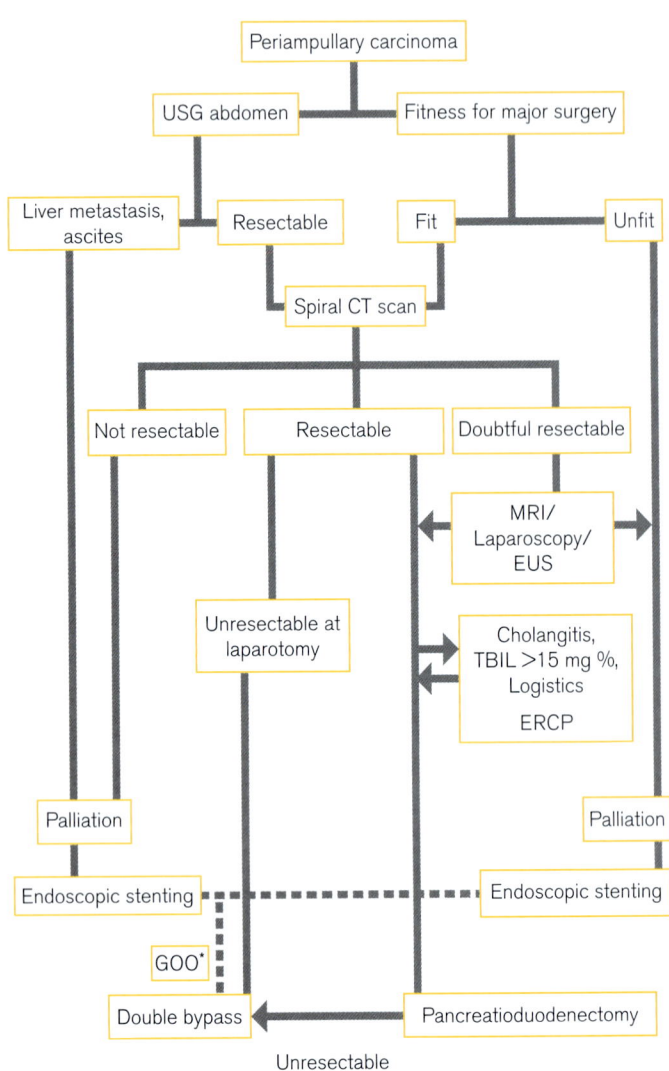

Figure 43.1 Management of periampullary carcinoma

* gastric outlet obstruction

The comparative accuracy of CT and MRI is presented in Table 43.4.

Table 43.4 Accuracy of investigative modalities

	Mass (%)	Vascular invasion (%)	Liver metastasis (%)
CT scan			
Current	96	90	91 for lesions > 1 cm
Historic	80–90	36–64	40–60
MRI	> 90	90	> 90

Other investigations

These include ERCP, endoscopic ultrasound (EUS) and diagnostic laparoscopy (DL). With the availability of state-of-the-art thin section CT scan, DL is not required for routine staging of periampullary carcinoma. Endoscopic ultrasound may be performed for fine needle aspiration cytology (FNAC) when the tumour has doubtful resectability, and for characterisation of rare tumours.

ERCP is required only in selected patients: those in whom there is a dilatation of the biliary and/or pancreatic duct but no mass is seen on CT scan, or when CT scan is suggestive of chronic pancreatitis. ERCP with stenting is indicated in selected patients with cholangitis, when early surgery is not feasible due to logistic or medical problems. Whenever ERCP is being planned, it should always be performed after CT scan of the abdomen as the stent placement and probable post-procedure pancreatitis may obscure the anatomy.

In the appropriate clinical setting and when a periampullary mass lesion is visualised on CT scan, histological confirmation is desirable although not mandatory. For this purpose, side-viewing endoscopy with biopsy is useful. It may provide evidence for ampullary and duodenal carcinomas; endoscopic ultrasound-guided biopsy provides a safe alternative for confirmation of lesions of the head of pancreas. A fine needle aspiration cytology study has a sensitivity of 76 per cent but a false negative test is obtained in 15 per cent of patients. In view of significant complications like bile leak, bleeding, pancreatitis and a 0.05 per cent risk of dying due to the test, FNAC is not recommended. Similarly, routine estimation of tumour markers such as carbohydrate antigen 19-9 (CA 19-9) is no longer recommended.

QUICK FLICK 43

Management

Pancreatoduodenectomy (PD) remains the only available curative treatment for periampullary carcinoma. At specialised centres, the procedure can now be accomplished with a mortality ranging between 1–5 per cent and morbidity of 40–60 per cent. After having excluded distant metastasis, resection can be performed.[1]

Leak from pancreato-enteric anastomosis is the most dangerous complication of the procedure and is associated with increased hospital stay, sepsis, haemorrhage and mortality in 20–40 per cent of patients. The incidence of this complication ranges between 10 and 16 per cent. The important risk factors for this complication include soft gland and a non-dilated pancreatic duct. The management in most patients is expectant and includes nutritional support and control of sepsis. The latter may require CT scan-guided drain placement and/or open surgical drainage. In 5–10 per cent of patients, haemorrhage or continued sepsis may necessitate a completion pancreatectomy.

The other common procedure-related complications of the procedure are listed in Table 43.5.

Table 43.5 Complications of pancreatoduodenectomy

Complication	Incidence (%)
Pancreato-enteric leak	10–16
Delayed gastric emptying	20
Hepato-jejunal leak	5
Sepsis	10–20

Those patients who have unresectable disease are candidates for palliative management. A reasonable approach based on currently available evidence is that patients with biliary obstruction alone may undergo endobiliary stenting, while those with additional gastric outlet obstruction should undergo double bypass surgery. Duodenal stenting provides an alternative to surgical bypass, particularly in patients not fit for surgery.

Prognosis

Only 15–20 per cent of periampullary carcinoma patients are eventually fit for surgical resection due to significant co-morbidities or advanced disease at the time of presentation. Of the latter group, those with peritoneal metastasis and local unresectable disease have a median survival of 6 and 10 months respectively.

The patients who do undergo a surgical margin-negative resection have a median survival of 12 to 20 months; a margin-positive resection confers no survival advantage and has an outcome similar to that of local unresectable disease. A study of the pattern of recurrence revealed that the recurrence was local in 80 per cent of patients, and as liver and peritoneal metastasis in 50 per cent and 25 per cent of patients respectively.

The important factors that determine long-term survival include location of the primary tumour (Table 43.6), lymph node involvement and histological differentiation (patients with well-differentiated tumours do better than those whose tumours are poorly differentiated). Other factors that have been demonstrated to have an impact on survival are the size of the tumour being more than 3 cm, blood transfusion during surgery and the surgeon's experience.

Table 43.6 Post-resection five-year survival of periampullary tumours

Diagnosis	5-year survival (%)
Head of pancreas	15
Ampulla of Vater	40
Distal common bile duct	25
Descending duodenum	60

▷ Proximal biliary tract cancers

These include hilar cholangiocarcinoma (HCCA) and gall bladder cancer (GBC). The investigations, principles of curative resection and palliative management for patients with unresectable tumours are essentially similar; hence, these two entities are considered together in the following section.

Incidence

Hilar cholangiocarcinoma (HCCA) is an uncommon tumour with an annual incidence of 1.2 per 100 000 in the United States, while GBC is one of the commonest cancers in females in North and Central India with a reported annual incidence of 11 per 100 000.

Clinical features

Most patients (> 90%) with proximal biliary tract cancers present with surgical obstructive jaundice (SOJ) characterised by itching, clay-coloured stools and dark urine. In patients with HCCA, typically painless SOJ is accompanied by a firm hepatomegaly and an impalpable gall bladder, whereas patients with GBC experience pain in the right upper quadrant, with a gall bladder mass as the most common presentation.

Investigations

Once a diagnosis of proximal biliary tract carcinoma is suggested by initial ultrasound examination of the abdomen, the next step is to assess medical fitness to undertake major surgery. In patients found fit to undergo surgical intervention, the investigations are planned to delineate the extent of bile duct involvement, encasement of common hepatic artery or main portal vein, and lymph node and distant metastases. For determining the tumour spread along the bile ducts (second-order for HCCA), magnetic resonance cholangiopancreatography (MRCP) is the investigation of choice. The lesion appears as an irregular thickening of the bile duct wall (≥ 5 mm) with upstream asymmetric dilatation of the bile ducts.

The accuracy of MRCP ranges between 78 and 85 per cent for the detection of intraductal extension of the tumour. The vascular involvement that would preclude curative resection is commonly assessed by helical CT scan of the upper abdomen with angiographic reconstruction to provide information regarding the hepatic artery proper and its right and left hepatic branches, and also the main portal vein and its main branches. In addition, the CT scan also provides information pertaining to liver metastases and the extent of lymph node involvement. Recent studies, however, have shown that CT scanning has limitations compared with magnetic resonance imaging (MRI) of the abdomen, particularly in relation to the detection of peritoneal metastases, hepatic artery and lymph node assessment, and segmental biliary pathology. Thus in many centres MRI, together with magnetic resonance angiography (MRA) and MRCP have emerged as the 'one-stop shop' investigations of choice for the assessment of proximal biliary tract cancers.

The addition of Doppler ultrasound has been reported to enhance the accuracy of MRA in the determination of vascular involvement.

Tissue diagnosis in these patients may be obtained by endoscopic exfoliative biliary cytology (low sensitivity, 6–40%), brush cytology (sensitivity 55–70%, specificity 90–100%) and endoscopic ultrasound-guided fine needle aspiration cytology (sensitivity 91%, specificity 89%, accuracy 100%). It is important to remember, however, that 15 to 18 per cent of all hilar lesions that are suspected to be malignant following pre-operative evaluation are finally reported as benign on histopathology of the resected specimen.

Treatment

Malignant hilar blocks (HCCA and GBC) are difficult to treat or palliate, and best managed at tertiary care referral centres only.

Curative surgery

Resection with negative margins is the only treatment option consistent with long-term survival. Therefore, except for patients for whom there are clear indications of unresectability on pre-operative evaluation, all fit patients must be considered for curative surgery, including resection of extrahepatic biliary apparatus, designated lymphadenectomy and liver resection.

For most HCCA patients, liver resection entails major hepatectomy (right or left hepatic lobectomy or, in selected patients, trisegmentectomy) with caudate lobe resection. Innovative strategies to induce hypertrophy of the future remnant liver (FRL)—such as selective biliary drainage (of the FRL) and portal vein embolisation for the hepatic lobe to be removed, four to six weeks prior to surgery—have led not only to an expansion of indications for resection but also to improved perioperative outcome by reducing the incidence of post-resection liver failure. A five-year survival of up to 40 per cent has been reported from high-volume centres following liver resection for HCCA.

For GBC, liver resection usually includes segments IV B and V. Major hepatectomy is indicated only in those patients with involvement of the right hepatic artery, portal vein or duct.

Only 5–20 per cent of patients with proximal biliary tract cancers are candidates for curative resection. The criteria for unresectability are given in Table 43.7.

Table 43.7 Criteria for unresectability of proximal biliary tract tumours

Patient factors	Medically unfit
	Global hepatic cirrhosis
Tumour factors	Tumour extension into secondary biliary radicals bilaterally
	Involvement of common hepatic artery
	Atrophy of one hepatic lobe with contralateral portal vein occlusion or encasement
	Atrophy of one hepatic lobe with contralateral extension of the tumour into secondary biliary radicals
	Unilateral extension to secondary biliary radicals with contralateral portal vein occlusion or encasement
Metastases	Liver, peritoneum, lung
	N2 level lymph nodes

Source: Jarnagin et al.[2]

The symptoms that most often warrant palliative management are intractable pruritus, cholangitis, jaundice and pain. The modalities for palliative management are summarised in Table 43.8.

Table 43.8 Modalities for palliative management of proximal biliary tract cancers

Biliary drainage procedures	Endoscopic stenting
	Percutaneous biliary stenting
	Surgical bypass
Additional therapy	Radiotherapy
	Chemotherapy
	Photodynamic therapy

Source: Singhal et al.[4]

Endoscopic biliary drainage (EBD)

Biliary stenting is the treatment of choice for patients detected to have unresectable tumours on pre-operative evaluation. Either a plastic or a metallic stent can be used. Plastic stents are inexpensive and easy to insert but they have a narrow lumen of 10F which makes them prone to blockage by biliary sludge, thus reducing their average patency period to 126 days. As a result, cholangitis may occur in 20 to 40 per cent of patients palliated with plastic stents.

Self-expanding metallic stents (SEMS) are thus preferred for palliative management of hilar blocks. These stents have a wider lumen of 30F. The incidence of early cholangitis reported with SEMS is 4.9–6 per cent. An additional factor responsible for the low incidence of cholangitis following the insertion of these stents is their open mesh design that allows for the drainage of secondary biliary radicals through the side walls of the stent. The reported median duration of stent patency is 169 days which is similar to median survival of these patients. The main limitation for the use of stents is their higher initial cost; however, this is offset by a low incidence of re-intervention and hospitalisation for complications.

Percutaneous transhepatic biliary drainage (PTBD)

PTBD is a technically simpler procedure than endoscopic biliary drainage. The procedure is performed when endoscopic expertise is not available or has failed, or there are multiple isolated segments with cholangitis. In sick patients with cholangitis or those with unsuccessful endoscopic management, PTBD is done initially with placement of an external drainage catheter (first stage) and subsequently transtumoural stent internalisation is done.

The recently available evidence from high-volume centres appears to favour PTBD over endoscopic stenting for pre-operative drainage as well as palliation. In one study from AMC Amsterdam in resectable HCCA patients, PTBD outperformed EBD, showing fewer infectious complications while using fewer procedures. Similar results have been reported in a recent randomised trial from India on palliative management of unresectable gall bladder cancers. In this study, PTBD with internalised stent had a significantly higher success rate, fewer complications and a lower incidence of cholangitis as compared with EBD.[3]

Surgical cholangiojejunostomy

Segment III cholangiojejunostomy is the preferred operative modality for surgical palliation. In the current scenario its use is mainly restricted to centres that lack expertise in EBD and/or PTBD. The main advantage of segment III bypass is that it provides lasting biliary drainage, but has limitations of associated morbidity (17–51%) and mortality (6–12%).

Summary

The most common benign neoplasms of the gall bladder are polyps. If they are larger than 1.2 cm they may contain malignant cells and should be observed carefully. Carcinomas of the gall bladder and biliary system are divided into:

- carcinomas of the distal bile duct (DBD) and ampulla of Vater
- proximal biliary tract cancers (PBC).

Most tumours in the first category (approximately 75%) are adenocarcinomas. Location of the primary tumour is one of the important prognostic factors for perioperative and long-term outcome.

Periampullary carcinomas are aggressive tumours that are usually at an advanced stage at the time of presentation in most patients, precluding curative resection.

The initial clinical examination should always include an assessment of factors that would preclude resection, such as left supraclavicular lymph node enlargement, ascites and co-morbid conditions. For a patient with suspected periampullary carcinoma based on clinical history and examination, abdominal ultrasonography (USG) should be the initial investigative procedure.

When there are no contraindications for resection on USG abdomen, a triple-phase contrast-enhanced (oral and intravenous) CT scan of the whole abdomen should be done. Pancreatoduodenectomy (PD) is the only available curative treatment for periampullary carcinoma.

In the second category, proximal biliary tract cancers (PBC), GBC is common in some regions, while HCCA is an uncommon tumour. Most patients with PBC present with surgical obstructive jaundice. Investigations include abdominal ultrasound, MRCP, helical CT scan, MRC, MRI with MRA, and endoscopic ultrasound.

Surgical resection with negative margins is the only treatment option consistent with long-term survival.

References

1. Cameron JL, Riall TS, Coleman J, Belcher KA. One thousand consecutive pancreaticoduodenectomies. *Ann Surg*. 2006; 244(1):10–15.

2. Jarnagin WR, Fong Y, DeMatteo RP, Gonen M, Burke EC, Bodniewicz BSJ, Youssef BAM, Klimstra D, Blumgart LH. Staging, resectability, and outcome in 225 patients with hilar cholangiocarcinoma. *Ann Surg*. 2001 Oct; 234(4):507–17; discussion 517–9.

3. Saluja SS, Gulati M, Garg PK, Pal H, Pal S, Sahni P, Chattopadhyay TK. Endoscopic or percutaneous biliary drainage for gallbladder cancer: a randomised trial and quality of life assessment. *Clin Gastroenterol Hepatol*. 2008; 6(8):944–50.

4. Singhal D, van Gulik TM, Gouma DJ. Palliative management of hilar cholangiocarcinoma. *Surg Oncol*. 2005 Aug; 14(2):59–74.

Recommended reading

Blumgart LH, Belghiti J, editors. Surgery of the liver, biliary tract and pancreas. London: WB Saunders; 2006.

Fischer J, Bland KI, editors. Mastery of surgery. Philadelphia: Lippincot Williams & Wilkins; 2007.

Chapter 44: Imaging of biliary tracts

J. Chaganti (Australia)

Key points

- Biliary tract imaging is a multimodality multidisciplinary science.
- Transabdominal ultrasound is the first step in the suspected biliary pathology.
- MDCT and MRI provide excellent cross-sectional imaging. When coupled with cholangiography they are powerful tools for imaging the biliary tract.
- Endoscopic ultrasound is preferred to ERCP in a patient suspected with intermediate probability of having choledocholithiasis.
- MRCP is the investigation of choice in the initial assessment of choledocholithiasis and has equal specificity and sensitivity to ERCP for calculi measuring 3 mm or more.
- MRCP is also the preferred modality in post-operative strictures, sclerosing cholangitis, pancreatic cancers and congenital pancreatic and biliary anomalies.
- Invasive investigative procedures like PTC/ERCP provide excellent spatial resolution but carry risks, and are more often used as therapeutic measures or for obtaining histological samples.
- CT cholangiography is preferred for assessing bile duct anatomy in pre-transplantation work-up.

Introduction

Advances in radiological techniques have greatly enhanced our ability to image the biliary system. The ductal system of the liver has innumerable variations and precise roadmapping of this complex anatomy assumes significance in both pathology and pre-transplantation work-up. The common indications are:

1. Confirmation/ruling out biliary obstruction.
2. Mapping of biliary tract in the pre-operative transplantation work.
3. Evaluation of complications in the post-operative biliary tract.
4. Identification of congenital anomalies.

The established techniques to image the biliary system are percutaneous transhepatic cholangiogram (PTC), endoscopic retrograde cholangiopancreatography (ERCP), intravenous cholangiography, magnetic resonance cholangiopancreatography (MRCP), endoscopic ultrasound (EUS), intraductal ultrasound, helical computed tomography (CT) and helical CT cholangiography (HCTC). These techniques can be broadly classified under two subheadings:

1. Those that are invasive and visualise the anatomy *directly* such as PTC and ERCP.
2. Those that are not invasive and visualise the anatomy *indirectly* with endogenous contrast or exogenously administered contrast.

Although the direct measures have a high spatial resolution and demonstrate extrahepatic and hilar biliary anatomy extremely well, they have the disadvantages of procedure-related morbidity and complications such as cholangitis and pancreatitis. A significant limitation of these invasive methods also lies in their inherent inability to assess the extraluminal causes of obstruction and to evaluate surrounding structures. Modern advances in non-invasive imaging have to a large extent obviated the need to use invasive methods for diagnosis. In most centres, invasive procedures are used primarily for management and their roles are purely therapeutic. Furthermore, their sensitivity in depicting the intrahepatic biliary anatomy is low due to the geographical distribution of the ductal anatomy and the consequent requirement of large volumes of contrast.

Imaging methods

Transabdominal ultrasound (AUS)

Transabdominal sonography is the first step in the evaluation of suspected biliary tract disease and is an extremely versatile imaging modality. AUS is non-invasive and non-ionising, making it ideally suited for the paediatric population as well as for pregnant women, and no harmful effects to the developing foetus have been recorded. Sonography is a portable imaging system and is therefore highly useful in acute care settings for both imaging and guided interventional procedures. The sensitivity and specificity of AUS in evaluating the level and causes of extrahepatic biliary tract obstruction is low due to the limited beam penetration in large patients and in a gaseous abdomen, and its inherent sensitivity for visualising the retroperitoneum is low.[1, 2]

Endoscopic ultrasound (EUS)

EUS combines endoscopy with ultrasound to provide high-resolution images of the pancreatic and biliary systems. Since its development in the 1980s, EUS has dramatically expanded the breadth of gastrointestinal endoscopy.

In the evaluation of suspected biliary obstruction the sensitivity and specificity of EUS are 95 per cent and 88 per cent respectively, which compares favourably with ERCP.[1, 3]

The sensitivity of EUS is roughly equal to that of MRCP; because it is less invasive and has markedly lower complications than ERCP, EUS should be performed before ERCP in evaluating choledocholithiasis.[3]

Intraductal ultrasonography (IDUS)

This is a relatively new technique performed with a highly flexible, thin-calibre non-optic US probe. After performing standard ERCP, the IDUS probe is taken through the standard channel of the duodenoscope to examine the biliary and pancreatic tracts. IDUS provides a better evaluation of the biliary system than EUS and is better able to characterise the cause of obstruction. The chief disadvantage of IDUS is that it is invasive and requires greater technical expertise than EUS.

Percutaneous transhepatic cholangiogram (PTC)

PTC involves puncturing the liver using a very fine needle, usually of 23F, under fluoroscopic guidance and entering a peripheral bile duct. Contrast is injected to visualise the ductal system. Along with ERCP, PTC is considered the 'gold standard' for evaluating the biliary tract. It has high specificity in determining the level of obstruction as well as in characterising the obstruction.

Simultaneous drainage of the obstructed duct system can also be performed. Although a number of complications have been reported, major complications are less than 5 per cent in experienced hands and mortality is less than 0.1 per cent.

Endoscopic retrograde cholangiopancreatography (ERCP)

ERCP is the 'gold standard' for evaluating pancreatic and biliary ductal morphology. Simultaneous therapeutic interventions can be performed, including sphincterotomy, stone extraction, stent insertions and tissue sampling.

Multi-detector CT (MDCT) and CT cholangiogram (CTC)

In a suspected case of biliary obstruction, the MDCT technique involves a dedicated scan of the liver, gall bladder and bile ducts without IV contrast as a base line to identify the lesions independent of contrast, followed by enhanced studies. The use of high attenuating oral contrast should be avoided when using CT for biliary diseases, as contrast density may obscure calculi in the ampulla and may obscure vascular encasement by tumours. Water provides excellent negative enteral contrast and is the agent of choice.

QUICK FLICK 44

MDCT has a reported accuracy of up to 94 per cent in determining the cause and level of obstruction.

CTC involves augmenting the biliary tract with dye either by directly injecting into the biliary tract (post-PTC/ERCP) or alternatively administering intravenous material that is excreted into bile. It has the dual advantage of providing functional information combined with excellent spatial resolution. The current indications for intravenous CTC are to assess the second-order duct anatomy in living transplant donations. In some countries CTC is used routinely to define cystic and bile duct anatomy prior to cholecystectomy. Some studies have shown that CTC has provided clinical diagnosis when ERCP has failed.[4]

Studies performed comparing the CTC with MRCP have shown that CTC may be superior to MRCP in spatial resolution but does not provide superior diagnostic information. CTC has few inherent disadvantages, but noteworthy among them is its dependency on adequate liver function in order to obtain good contrast elimination from the hepatocyte—as is often the case, patients with biliary diseases have compromised liver function and may have suboptimal duct opacification. The other major drawback is risk of adverse reactions to iodinated contrast agents. One meta-analysis study found a mortality rate of 1 in 3000 to 1 in 5000 examinations.[1]

MR cholangiopancreatography (MRCP)

The typical MRCP technique exploits the relatively high signal intensity of static fluids in the biliary tracts with heavily weighted T-2 sequences.[4, 5]

Multiple thin slices are usually obtained using gradient echo technique as 2-D data or 3-D volume; these sequences are often referred to by the acronym HASTE. The acquired 3-D data set can be used to construct an image of the biliary tract using maximum intensity projection algorithms. With present technology, fourth-order biliary ductal anatomy can be readily visualised. Recent meta-analysis of 67 published controlled trials has shown that MRCP has excellent overall sensitivity and specificity of 95 per cent and 97 per cent respectively; however, in choledocholithiasis, the sensitivity for identifying calculi smaller than 3 mm is low compared to ERCP.[1]

The chief disadvantage of MRCP has been its low spatial resolution compared to ERCP, which has led to the introduction of two new techniques: 3-D isotropic MRCP (3DMRCP) and contrast-enhanced MRCP. The 3DMRCP method uses parallel imaging to obtain high resolution images. Its limitation is the formation of ghosting artefacts, usually at the interface of bowel and bile duct.

Contrast-enhanced MRCP

In this novel technique intravenous gadolinium chelates with selective hepatic excretion are used to image the biliary tracts using T-1 weighted sequences: for example, gadobenate dimeglumine (GD-BOPTA) and mangafodipir trisodium (MnDPDP). Contrast-enhanced MRCP has been used to image the biliary tract before anatomical mapping prior to living donor transplantation, and in demonstrating biliary leaks following transplantation. Similar to CTC, it also provides functional information.[4]

The chief disadvantages of this technique are its limited ability to scan patients with ferromagnetic implants and pacemakers or artefacts such as surgical clips. Occasionally a patient with claustrophobia might require sedatives to perform the procedure. Gadolinium chelates have been associated with nephrogenic systemic fibrosis (NSF); therefore using contrast-enhanced MRCP in patients with compromised renal function is not advisable.

◆ Imaging spectrum of biliary tract disease

Obstructive jaundice

Detection

In the evaluation of obstructive jaundice, the role of imaging is to identify the site and cause of obstruction, commonly including impacted calculus, post-inflammatory or post-surgical stricture, and malignant stricture. Uncommon causes such as sclerosing cholangitis and Mirizzi's syndrome should always be considered along with appropriate clinical history.

Imaging signs of obstruction

Non-dilated peripheral intrahepatic ducts (<2 mm) can be visualised by all imaging modalities and appear as scattered tubular structures. If the intrahepatic duct diameters are more than 2 mm the duct visualisation becomes confluent and is a sign of biliary obstruction—referred to as confluent ducts sign. Another notable useful sign of biliary obstruction is parallel tube/duct sign, which reflects dilated biliary ducts forming tubes parallel to the portal channels.

Objective measurements should be made to overcome the pitfalls of making a judgment by sight alone, chief of which is the duct diameter. If the intrahepatic duct diameter exceeds 40 per cent of the diameter of the adjacent intrahepatic portal vein, then the obstruction can be said to be present. The common hepatic duct (CHD) is nearly always visualised by cross-sectional imaging. Although there is some controversy regarding the diameter of CHD/CBD, it is generally accepted by ultrasound criteria that a 6 to 7 mm diameter is the upper limit of normal; in CT the diameter range is greater, with the accepted normal range being 8 to 10 mm.[2]

It is not uncommon to see dilated extrahepatic ducts in elderly or post-cholecystectomy patients. Although the biliary tree dilates beyond the normal range in the presence of an obstruction, there is a time lag before it does so. Awareness of this would avoid potential errors.

Image morphology of obstruction

Knowledge of biliary obstruction would warrant the search for the level and cause. Both MDCT and MRI are eminently suited to do so, as previously outlined.

Regardless of the modality, key to achieving the proper diagnosis with a dilated duct is evaluating the zone of transition. Abrupt termination of the bile duct and irregular, long-segment stricture are cholangiographic signs of malignancy. Smooth, concentric, short-segment tapering more often correlates with benign morphology. Diffuse thickening of the bile ducts is noted both in cholangitis and bile duct cancers. Focal eccentric thickening of the duct proximal to obstruction suggests cholangiocarcinoma.

Biliary stones

The classical imaging finding of a calculus is a filling defect on cholangiography. Transabdominal US has a poor sensitivity (21–63%) in the detection of gallstones. Up to 50 per cent of patients with choledocholithiasis do not exhibit bile duct dilatation, which is an important limitation of US in the diagnosis of duct stones.[1]

Classical radiological findings associated with demonstration of stone disease by CT/MRI are:[2]

- Bile duct stones tend to be in dependent location in the biliary tract and a crescent of bile or gas is commonly seen outlining the anterior portion of the stone.
- Stones are angular in shape and have lamellar appearance on CT.
- Signs of local inflammation commonly coexist with stones, including periductal oedema, wall thickening and mural enhancement; however, caution should be exercised with mural enhancement since it is known to frequently coexist with malignancy and should prompt careful search.

MRCP can demonstrate calculi as small as 3 mm and is comparable to ERCP, with reported sensitivity of 89–100 per cent and specificity of 83–100 per cent. The sensitivity figures drop to 50 per cent when the calculus is smaller than 2 mm.[4]

Other pitfalls in MRCP include pneumobilia, which can be mistaken for stone disease, and a biliary segment filled with calculi with no surrounding bile may be mistaken as normal high density bile.

MDCT sensitivity to stone disease is 72–88 per cent, which falls far short of the desired expectation.

Extrinsic pancreatic disease obstruction

One of the common causes of biliary obstruction is extrinsic disease, of which pancreatic carcinoma is foremost. Abrupt transition of both pancreatic and bile ducts at the ampullary region is highly suggestive of pancreatic cancer and MRCP is the ideal investigation of choice.[5]

Chronic pancreatitis can cause terminal CBD stricture and may mimic pancreatic cancer; however, the changes caused by pancreatitis are gradual rather than abrupt. MRCP also consistently demonstrates biliary ducts above the stricture, whereas ERCP may fail to do so.

Cholangiocarcinoma

Cholangiocarcinoma is the most common tumour of the bile duct. Predominantly an adenocarcinoma at histology, there are three morphological types classically described with this tumour:[5]

- Mass-forming and commonly intrahepatic in location and poorly differentiated.
- Periductal infiltrating (Klatskin tumour), usually located at the hilar region and well differentiated.
- Intraductal and least common of all, and papillary in morphology.

The morphology of tumour stroma, which are composed of fibrous tissue, and mucin-producing glandular tumour have a direct impact on the imaging appearances on both CT and MRI.[2]

MDCT/CTC

Multiphase CT obtained with arterial, portal and delayed studies (3–5 min) is considered an ideal technique for evaluating these bile duct tumours.[6]

The CT appearances of cholangiocarcinoma vary depending upon the location relative to the biliary tree. Intrahepatic tumours are usually hypo- to iso-attenuating relative to normal hepatic parenchyma at unenhanced CT. Post-contrast studies show that most of these tumours remain hypoattenuating during the arterial and portal phases, and show enhancement during the delayed phase. This delayed enhancement may simulate a haemangioma enhancement pattern, but the lack of enhancement in the dynamic arterial pool studies negate the diagnosis of haemangioma.

Volumetric MDCT and CTC with advanced post-processing algorithms allow comprehensive evaluation of cholangiocarcinoma. This multiphase data can provide precise images of the vascular anatomy and the tumour's relationship to it, as well as associated vascular and biliary tract anomalies for precise surgical planning.

MRI/MRCP

Dynamic contrast-enhanced MRA and MRCP are other multifaceted modalities for a comprehensive evaluation of cholangiocarcinoma. Characteristic MR appearances of cholangiocarcinoma show a tumour which is relatively isointense to mildly hypointense on T-1 and variably hyperintense on T-2. These characteristics are based on the amount of mucin and fibrous tissue, as well as haemorrhage and necrosis, that are associated with the tumour. Post-contrast dynamic studies demonstrate minimal enhancement in the periphery on early images and progressive central filling in the late phases, reflecting tumoural cells at the periphery and desmoplastic reaction in the centre. Smaller tumours with less fibrotic reaction may show intense vascular enhancement, mimicking metastasis. MRCP evaluation of ductal tumour is superior to the CTC method. Concurrent arterial reconstruction adds information similar to that obtained from MDCT about vascular encasement/invasion and similar conditions.

PET-CT

The fusion of the benefits of the functional environment of PET with the morphological data obtained by CT appears to be superior to all other known modalities; further confirmatory work is needed.

◯ Pre-transplantation work-up

Both MRCP and CTC are used to evaluate the biliary tract anatomy in the pre-transplantation work-up of donors. CTC appears to be the preferred investigation due to its better spatial resolution and excellent demonstration of second-order biliary ducts.[4]

◯ Post-operative complications

MRI plays a crucial role in the evaluation of the biliary tract following surgical procedures such as cholecystectomy, liver transplantation, hepatic resection and biliary enteric fistulas. MRCP allows analysis of the biliary tract below the level of obstruction developed as a complication following surgery. This essential information cannot be obtained by either ERCP or PTC. MRCP is particularly useful for the evaluation of biliary enteric anastomoses, for which an endoscopic surgery is precluded.[7]

Contrast-enhanced MRCP is very useful to detect biliary fistulas and is the imaging investigation of choice.

◐ Congenital anomalies

Wide spectra of congenital anomalies of the pancreatic and biliary ductal system are encountered during radiological evaluation. Imaging these anomalies is challenging but is also of immense prognostic significance. Foremost of the congenital anomalies of the biliary tract are choledochal cysts. MRCP is ideally suited not only for identifying and characterising the types of cyst, but also for helping to identify associated anomalies and complications.[8]

Summary

Rapidly developments in imaging technology have brought a new challenge to the radiologist, to the point where the boundary between knowledge and technology has become indistinct. Regardless of the modality, optimal imaging of the biliary tract requires specific imaging techniques and collegial multidisciplinary collaboration to obtain the useful diagnostic information.

References

1. Tse F, Barkun JS, Romagnuolo J, Friedman G, Bornstein JD, Barkun AN. Nonoperative imaging techniques in suspected biliary tract obstruction. *HPB (Oxford)*. 2006; 8(6):409–25.

2. Baron RL, Tublin ME, Peterson MS. Imaging the spectrum of biliary tract disease. *Radiol Clin N Am*. 2002; 40:1325–54.

3. Anandasabhapathy S. Endoscopic ultrasound: indications and applications. *Mt Sinai J Med*. 2006; 73(4):702–7.

4. Yeh BM, Liu PS, Soto JA, Corvera CA, Hussain HK. MR Imaging and CT of the biliary tract. *Radiographics*. 2009 Oct; 29(6):1669–88.

5. Razzaq R, Sukumar SA. Imaging of jaundiced adult. *Imaging*. 2004; 16:287–300.

6. Sainani NI, Catalano OA, Holalkere NS, Zhu AX, Hahn PF, Sahani DV. Cholangiocarcinoma: current and novel imaging techniques. *Radiographics*. 2008; 28:1263–87.

7. Hoeffel C, Azizi L, Lewin M, Laurent V, Aubé C, Arrivé L, Tubiana JM. Normal and pathological features of the post operative biliary tract at 3D MR cholangiopancreaticography and MR imaging. *Radiographics*. 2006 Nov–Dec; 26(6): 1603–20.

8. Mortele KJ, Rocha TC, Streeter JL. Multimodality imaging of pancreatic and biliary congenital anomalies. *Radiographics*. 2006; 26:715–31.

Recommended reading

Stroszczynski C, Hunerbein M. Malignant biliary obstruction: value of imaging findings. *Abdom Imaging*. 2005; 30:314–23.

Zandrino F, Curone P, Benzi L, Ferretti ML, Musante F. MR versus multislice CT cholangiography in evaluating patients with obstruction of the biliary tract. *Abdom Imaging*. 2005; 30:77–85.

Section 5

Traditional cultural medicine

Chapter 45: Traditional Chinese medicine

Z. Bian (Hong Kong, China)

Key points

- ▶ Increasing numbers of patients suffering from functional GI disorders seek help from traditional Chinese medicine (TCM), a major form of complementary and alternative medicine.
- ▶ TCM has its unique system of describing human physiology, pathophysiology and treatment. The syndrome is the core of TCM theory, and syndrome diagnosis is based on observation, auscultation and olfaction, interrogation and palpation.
- ▶ The commonly used treatment methods are herbal medicine and acupuncture.
- ▶ Liver and spleen dysfunction are major causes of irritable bowel syndrome (IBS). Tonifying the spleen *qi* and suppressing the liver are the major treatment principles for IBS patients.
- ▶ Dampness is the major pathogenic evil of inflammatory bowel disease (IBD). Treatment is based on tonifying the spleen and eliminating dampness.
- ▶ Dampness in the liver is the major factor of chronic hepatitis B. Treatment of chronic hepatitis B is based on eliminating dampness and regulating the liver and spleen functions.
- ▶ Liver cirrhosis is diagnosed as 'abdominal mass' in Chinese medicine. Treatment focuses on regulating the liver *qi*, eliminating the blood stasis, strengthening the spleen function, and eliminating dampness.

○ Introduction

Complementary and alternative medicine (CAM) has penetrated mainstream medical practice in Western countries such as the USA and Germany.[1, 2]

Its use is related to cultural, ethnic, social, regional, educational and economic factors. Its theories and practices are significantly different from those of conventional medicine in terms of heterogeneity, disease mechanisms, diagnostic approaches, therapeutic methods and efficacy assessment. The major type of CAM involves traditional Chinese medicine (TCM), involving herbal medicine, acupuncture, bone setting, Ayurvedic medicine, homeopathy, massage, holistic medicine and bioelectromagnetic field therapy. Among these, herbal medicine and acupuncture are commonly used in many countries because of their systematic theories and history of clinical practice.

This chapter briefly introduces the use of herbal medicine and acupuncture for common gastrointestinal diseases: irritable bowel syndrome, inflammatory bowel disease, chronic hepatitis B and liver cirrhosis.

�‣ Basic theory of TCM

TCM is the summary of clinical experiences of the Chinese struggle against diseases over thousands of years. It is an important component of Chinese traditional culture and continues to contribute to human health around the world. It differs from Western medicine with its unique system of physiology, pathophysiology and treatment. *Yin–yang* and the five elements are the key to its theories. Treatment is based on differentiation of symptoms.

�‣ *Yin–yang* and the five elements

The unique medical theory of TCM has its roots in two philosophical systems: the theory of *yin* and *yang* and the theory of the five elements. The former, *yin* and *yang*, represents the properties of two opposing forces which are interrelated and interdependent. The relationship between *yin* and *yang* is constantly changing while mutual transformation can happen under certain circumstances. The other theory refers to the five elements (wood, fire, earth, metal and water), which are in a continuing cycle of promoting and controlling each other. For example, wood is promoted by water and promotes fire. In turn, it is controlled by metal and controls earth. These two theories are used to explain the physiological function and pathological changes of the human body as well as formulate treatment principles.[3, 4]

�‣ Aetiology: the cause of disease

TCM holds the body to be an organic integrity and views the relationship between the human being and nature as an integrated one. Normally, health is secured by maintaining the balance between parts of the body and between the body and its environment (equilibrium of *yin* and *yang*). When this balance is threatened, pathology and disease arise. Accordingly, there are three types of pathogenic factors (causes of disease), including exogenous, endogenous and non-exo-endogenous factors.

Exogenous pathogenic factors involve the extreme climatic conditions of wind, cold, summer heat, dampness, dryness and fire.

Endogenous pathogenic factors are the emotional upsets of excessive joy, anger, worry, pensiveness, grief, fear and fright, which disrupt the normal

QUICK FLICK
45

ascending and descending flow of *qi* and disturb the function of *zangfu* organs (internal organs).

Non-exo-endogenous pathogenic factors include intemperate diet, imbalance between work and rest (overwork and too much rest), trauma, injury by insects and animals, and so on.[3]

◗ Diagnostic methods

Based on the concept of integrity, anything inside is bound to manifest outwardly. Therefore, the outward manifestations may reveal the inside condition of the *zangfu* organs and *qi*-blood level. TCM has evolved a systematic diagnostic approach consisting of four classic diagnostic methods: observation, auscultation and olfaction, interrogation and palpation. The data gathered by these methods is then interpreted according to the principles of differentiating syndromes.[3–6]

Observation

TCM practitioners inspect the physique, general expression, the colour of the complexion, head and facial features and tongue, as well as body secretions and excretions. TCM places emphasis on the inspection of the tongue for the reason that the tongue is connected both directly and indirectly with *zangfu* organs via the channels (pathways throughout the body).

Auscultation and olfaction

The sound and odour produced when people speak, breathe, cough, hiccup and belch are important clues for TCM practitioners to determine the state of *qi* flow and the *zangfu* organs' condition.

Interrogation

Interrogation is the key for TCM doctors to make diagnoses. As for Western medical practitioners, inquiry as to the patient's main complaints, development and duration of the illness, past history, lifestyle and diet are necessary.

Palpation

This includes palpation of the body and limbs for inspecting the temperature, swelling, pain, perspiration and, most importantly, pulse-taking. TCM has developed a well-defined theory for taking and interpreting the pulse. In performing pulse palpation, the practitioner places the index, middle and ring fingers on the regions of *cun*, *guan* and *chi* respectively, or the area next to the crease starting from the wrist where the radial artery throbs. Any abnormality in its depth, frequency, rhythm, strength, smoothness or amplitude is a mirror of pathological changes of reflected *zangfu* organs.

Differentiation of syndrome

Differently from conventional medicine, TCM practitioners make diagnoses based not only on the disease but also the syndrome of the patient. 'Syndrome' refers to the pathological generalisation of a group of symptoms and signs at a certain stage in the course of disease development. It represents the aetiology, location, nature and prognosis of a disease. Along with the development of TCM, a variety of differentiation methods has evolved, the most important of which is the 'eight guiding principles': *yin* and *yang*, interior and exterior, cold and heat, deficiency and excess.[4]

CAM treatment principles and basic methods for typical GI diseases

The treatment principles for a disease are normally established based on the syndromes. For example, *qi* stagnation and spleen insufficiency is a common syndrome of irritable bowel syndrome, thus the treatment will focus on regulating *qi* movement and strengthening the spleen function. Generally, there are eight commonly used therapeutic methods: diaphoresis, emesis, purgation, harmonisation, invigoration, heat reduction, elimination and tonification.[5, 6]

Irritable bowel syndrome (IBS)

IBS is always diagnosed as either 'abdominal pain' or 'diarrhoea' in TCM theories.

Liver and spleen dysfunctions are a major cause of IBS, and psychosocial factors, food, cold and dampness, and lack of rest are the key elements affecting the development and recurrence of this disease. A clinical survey has shown that among 211 IBS patients, in 88.2 per cent the disease was related to spleen dysfunction, 33.2 per cent to liver dysfunction, and 6.2 per cent to kidney dysfunction. Tonifying the spleen *qi* and suppressing the liver are the major treatment principles for IBS.[7]

Clinical manifestation

IBS can be majorly categorised into the four following types:

1. Liver *qi* stagnation: Abdominal pain, with diarrhoea or constipation, or alternation of diarrhoea and constipation. The abdominal pain can be precipitated by passions or emotional stress. Other symptoms may involve chronic chest and flank distension, eructation, and reduced or lack of appetite. The tongue is pale and the pulse taut.

2. Spleen insufficiency: Recurrent borborygmus, abdominal pain, loose or watery faeces, sometimes containing undigested food. Other possible manifestations include postprandial epigastric distress, small amounts of greasy foods followed by increased frequency of defecation, sallow complexion and fatigue, a white coating on the tongue, and a threadlike, weak pulse. In this pattern, most patients demonstrate diarrhoea, not constipation. If this pattern continues for a long time, it indicates a spleen *yang* deficiency, with possible symptoms of cold intolerance and cold body and limbs.

3. Liver *qi* stagnation and spleen *qi* deficiency: Recurrent borborygmus, abdominal pain, diarrhoea with pain (which starts with the urge to defecate and subsides after completion), a thin, white tongue coating, and a moderate or wiry, thin pulse. There will also probably be chronic chest and flank distension, eructation and anorexia. Passions or emotional stress can induce recurrence or aggravate the symptoms. The key factors for diagnosis of this syndrome are anorexia, passion or emotional stress-related symptom aggravation. Normally, constipation is not common in this pattern of IBS.

4. Kidney insufficiency: Recurrent borborygmus, abdominal pain, loose or watery faeces, sometimes containing undigested food. In spleen insufficiency syndrome, a possible manifestation is postprandial epigastric distress, and small amounts of greasy foods will be followed by increased frequency of defecation, sallow complexion and fatigue, and a white tongue coating, threadlike and weak pulse. For kidney insufficiency, the symptoms may involve cold body and limbs, cold intolerance, aches in the waist and knees, and faecal incontinence. The tongue is pale, with a white coating. The pulse is deep, weak and threadlike. Most patients with this pattern demonstrate diarrhoea, not constipation.

◊ Treatment for IBS

Liver *qi* stagnation

The therapeutic principle is to suppress the liver and promote the movement of *qi*. The representative herbal formula is a four milled-herb decoction.

Composition

Radix ginseng (*ren shen*) 5–10 g, Semen arecae catechu (*bing lang*) 10–15 g, Lignum aquilariae (*chen xiang*) 3–6 g, Radix linderae strychnifoliae (*wu yao*) 9–12 g.

Acupuncture

The typical acupuncture formula is: *taichong* (LR-3), *zhangmen* (LR-13), *zusanli* (ST-36), *qimen* (LR-14).

Spleen insufficiency

The therapeutic principle is to strengthen the spleen and augment *qi*. The representative herbal formula is *shen ling bai zhu san*.

Composition

Radix ginseng (*ren shen*) 10–15 g, Rhizoma atractylodis macrocephalae (*bai zhu*) 15–20 g, Sclerotium poriae cocos (*fu ling*) 15–30 g, honey-fried Radix glycyrrhizae uralensis (*zhi gan cao*) 5–10 g, Radix dioscoreae oppositae (*shan yao*) 15–20 g, Semen dolichoris lablab (*bai bian dou*) 15–20 g, Semen nelumbinis nuciferae (*lian zi*) 10–15 g, Semen coicis lachryma-jobi (*yi yi ren*) 15–20 g, Fructus amoni (*sha ren*) 5–10 g, Radix platycodi grandiflori (*jie geng*) 5–10 g.

Acupuncture

The commonly used acupoints for this syndrome of IBS are: *zhongwan* (CV-12), *sanyinjiao* (SP-5), *tianshu* (ST-25), *liangmen* (ST-21).

Liver *qi* stagnation and spleen *qi* deficiency

The therapeutic principle is to suppress the liver *qi* and to strengthen the spleen. The representative herbal formula is *tong xie yao fang*.

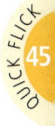

QUICK FLICK 45

Composition

Dry-fried Rhizoma atractylodis macrocephalae (*chao bai zhu*) 10–15 g, dry-fried Radix paeoniae lactiflorae (*chao bai shao*) 10–20 g, dry-fried Pericarpium citri reticulatae (*chao chen pi*) 5–10 g, Radix ledebouriellae divaricatae (*fang feng*) 6–12 g.

Acupuncture

The typical acupuncture formula for this syndrome is: *taichong* (LR-3), *qimen* (LR-14), *zhongwan* (CV-12), *zusanli* (ST-36).

Kidney insufficiency

The therapeutic principle is to warm and strengthen the kidney and stop diarrhoea. *Zhen ren yang zang tang* is a representative herbal formula.

Composition

Radix ginseng (*ren shen*) 10–15 g, Rhizoma atractylodis macrocephalae (*bai zhu*) 15–20 g, Cortex cinnamomi cassiae (*rou gui*) 3–6 g, dry-fried Semen myristicae fragrantis (*wei rou dou kou*) 10–15 g, Fructus terminaliae chebulae (*he zi*) 10–15 g, Radix paeoniae lactiflorae (*bai shao*) 10–15 g, Radix angelicae sinensis (*dang gui*) 10–15 g, Radix aucklandiae lappae (*mu xiang*) 5–10 g, honey-fried Radix glycyrrhizae uralensis (*zhi gan cao*) 5–10 g.

Acupuncture

The typical acupuncture formula could be: *mingmen* (GV-4), *shenshu* (BL-23), *shenque* (CV-8), *qihai* (CV-6), *guanyuan* (CV-4), *sanyinjiao* (SP-6).

◊ Inflammatory bowel disease (IBD)

IBD can be diagnosed as 'dysentery', 'diarrhoea', 'evil in organs' and so on, in terms of TCM. The major related organs of IBD are the spleen and the intestines. Dampness is the main pathogenic evil. A clinical survey has shown that spleen insufficiency with dampness accumulation and heat–dampness accumulation with intestinal damage are the major syndromes of IBD. The major treatment principles for IBD are to tonify the spleen and eliminate dampness.[8]

Clinical manifestation of IBD

The clinical manifestation of IBD may be identified as three main types:

1. Dampness–heat syndrome: Abdominal pain, bloody diarrhoea with mucus, tenesmus, burning in the anus, tightness in the chest and epigastrium. The tongue coating is yellow and greasy, and the pulse slippery and rapid. There is probably a bitter taste in the mouth, yellow urine, and heavy head and limbs.
2. Cold–dampness syndrome: Spastic abdominal pain, diarrhoea with mucus but without blood, tenesmus, anorexia, epigastric discomfort and tightness. The tongue is pale, with white and greasy coating. The pulse is soft and even. There is probably a sweet taste in the mouth, heavy head and limbs, clear urine, and fever without sweating.
3. Spleen–kidney insufficiency: Normally, the patient in the non-active period demonstrates this pattern: the most common symptoms are thin faeces with white gel-like grains, impeded defecation, continual abdominal pain with preference for pressure, warmth and massage; reduced appetite, fatigue and cold aversion. The tongue is pale with a thin coating. The pulse is depletive and threadlike. If the illness worsens, there may be rectal prolapse, aches in the waist and knees, cold intolerance, cold body and limbs, and reduced libido.

◊ Treatment for IBD

Dampness–heat syndrome

The therapeutic principle is to clear the heat, eliminate dampness and stop the bleeding. The representative formula is *huai hua sang* plus *bai tou weng tang*.

Composition of *huai hua sang*
Flos sophorae japonicae (*huai hua*) 10–30 g, Cacumen biotae orientalis (*ce bai ye*) 10–15 g, Herba seu flos schizonepetae tenuifoliae (*jing jie sui*) 10–12 g, Fructus citri seu ponciri (*zhi ke*) 10–12 g.

Composition of *bai tou weng tang*
Radix pulsatillae (*bai tou weng*) 10–15 g, Rhizoma coptidis (*huang lian*) 5–10 g, Cortex phellodendri (*huang bai*) 5–10 g, Cortex fraxini (*qin pi*) 10–12 g.

Acupuncture
For acupuncture treatment: *zhongwan* (CV-12), *tianshu* (ST-25), *shangjuxu* (ST-37), *yinlingquan* (SP-9), *quchi* (LI-11), *neiting* (ST-44).

Cold–dampness syndrome
The therapeutic principle is to warm the *yang* and eliminate dampness. The typical formula is *liu he tang*.

Composition
Radix ginseng (*ren shen*) 5–10 g, Fructus amoni (*sha ren*) 5–10 g, Rhizoma pinelliae ternatae (*ban xia*) 5–10 g, Semen pruni armeniacae (*xing ren*) 5–10 g, Rhizoma atractylodis macrocephalae (*bai zhu*) 5–10 g, Herba agastaches seu pogostemi (*huo xiang*) 10–15 g, Semen dolichoris lablab (*bai bian dou*) 5–10 g, Sclerotium poriae cocos rubrae (*chi fu ling*) 10–15 g, Fructus chaenomelis lagenariae (*mu gau*) 5–10 g, Cortex magnoliae officinalis (*hou po*) 5–10 g, Radix glycyrrhizae uralensis (*gan cao*) 5 g.

Acupuncture
The acupuncture treatment can select: *zusanli* (ST-36), *tianshu* (ST-25), *shangjuxu* (ST-37), *zhongwan* (CV-12), *yinlingquan* (SP-9).

Spleen–kidney insufficiency
The aim of the treatment is to warm the spleen and kidney, and eliminate dampness. The representative formula is *zhen wu tang*.

Composition
Radix lateralis aconiti carmichaeli praeparata (*fu zi*) 10 g, Rhizoma atractylodis macrocephalae (*bai zhu*) 10–15 g, Sclerotium poriae cocos (*fu ling*) 15–30 g, Rhizoma zingiberis officinalis recens (*sheng jiang*) 5–10 g, Radix paeoniae lactiflorae (*bai shao*) 5–10 g.

Acupuncture

Acupuncture treatment can be selected with the following acupoints: *guanyuan* (CV-4), *shenque* (CV-8), *qihai* (CV-6), *zusanli* (ST-36).

▷ Chronic hepatitis B (CHB)

CHB is diagnosed as 'jaundice' (a disease name in TCM, not merely a symptom). The liver, gall bladder, spleen and stomach are the main organs related to CHB, and the major evil is dampness. When dampness attacks the human body it cause dysfunction of these organs—thus the gall bladder is unable to discharge bile normally and jaundice occurs. The treatment of CHB focuses on eliminating dampness and regulating the liver and spleen functions.

Clinical manifestation of CHB

1. Dampness–heat accumulation: Severe to mild jaundice with colour resembling a fresh tangerine, epigastric fullness, anorexia, yellow urine, heaviness and pain in the head and body. The tongue coating is yellowy and greasy, and the pulse is slippery and rapid. For the syndrome of more heat than dampness, possible symptoms are fever, thirst, dysphoria, nausea, vomiting, dark urine and constipation. The tongue may be red, and the pulse is rapid. For the syndrome of more dampness than heat, a possible syndrome is jaundice where the colour is not very fresh, chest and epigastric tightness, stickiness in the mouth without thirst, and the tongue coating is slightly yellow but thick and greasy.
2. Dampness–cold accumulation: Possible jaundice of the whole body and sclera, with the colour of non-fresh yellow, reduced appetite, epigastric fullness, fatigue, cold, and loose or watery faeces. The tongue is pale, with a white thick or thin greasy coating, and the pulse is deep and slow.
3. Liver–spleen dysfunction: Fatigue, a bitter or sweet taste in the mouth, dry mouth and throat, anorexia, loose faeces, abdominal discomfort or distension, with a pale-red tongue and a wiry, deficient pulse.

▷ Treatment for CHB

Dampness–heat accumulation

The therapeutic principle is to clear the heat, eliminate the dampness and reduce the jaundice. The representative recipe is *yin chen hao* decoction.

Composition

Herba artemisiae (*yin chen hao*) 15–20 g, Fructus gardeniae jasminoidis (*zhi zi*) 10–12 g, Radix et rhizoma rhei (*da huang*) 6–10 g.

Acupuncture

The following acupoints can be selected for this syndrome: *ganshu* (BL-18), *danshu* (BL-19), *yanglingquan* (GB-34), *shangjuxu* (ST-37), *yinlingquan* (SP-9).

Dampness–cold accumulation

The therapeutic aim is to warm and strengthen the spleen, eliminate dampness and reduce jaundice. The representative recipe is *yin chen zhu fu tang*.

Composition

Herba artemisiae yinchenhao (*yi chen hao*) 5–10 g, Rhizoma atractylodis macrocephalae (*bai zhu*) 10–12 g, Rhizoma zingiberis officinalis (*gan jiang*) 3–5 g, Radix lateralis aconiti carmichaeli praeparata (*fu zi*) 6–9 g, Cortex cinnamomi cassiae (*rou gui*) 3–5 g, honey-fried Radix glycyrrhizae uralensis (*zhi gan cao*) 3–5 g.

Acupuncture

The acupuncture treatment can be applied selecting the following points: *ganshu* (BL-18), *danshu* (BL-19), *zusanli* (ST-36), *shangjuxu* (ST-37), *zhongwan* (CV-12), *sanyinjiao* (SP-6).

Liver–spleen dysfunction

The therapeutic aim is to spread the liver *qi* and strengthen the spleen. The typical formula for this syndrome is *xiao yao san*.

Composition

Radix bupleuri (*chai hu*) 6–9 g, Radix angelicae sinensis (*dang gui*) 6–9 g, Radix paeoniae lactiflorae (*bai shao*) 6–9 g, Rhizoma atractylodis macrocephalae (*bai zhu*) 15–20 g, Sclerotium poriae cocos (*fu ling*) 15–30 g, honey-fried Radix glycyrrhizae uralensis (*zhi gan cao*) 5 g.

Acupuncture

The typical acupuncture formula for this syndrome is: *ganshu* (BL-18), *diji* (SP-8), *qimen* (LR-14), *zhongwan* (CV-12), *zusanli* (ST-36).

▷ Liver cirrhosis

From a TCM perspective, liver cirrhosis (LC) is diagnosed as 'abdominal mass'. The liver, the spleen and the kidney are the main organs related to LC. The major evils in the early stage are liver *qi* stagnation and blood stasis, while in the late stage the accumulation of dampness is another important factor. The treatment of LC by TCM focuses on regulating the liver *qi*, eliminating the blood stasis, strengthening the spleen function and eliminating dampness.

Clinical manifestation

1. Liver–spleen dysfunction: Anorexia, epigastric discomfort or distension, flank distension, loose faeces, lethargy, fatigue, a pale red tongue and a wiry pulse.
2. *Qi* stagnation and blood stasis: Palpable abdominal mass, with distension and pain which is always located in one part of the abdomen. Also, spider-like blood vessels appear on the skin. The pulse is taut and the tongue is cyanotic or speckled with purpuric spots.
3. Spleen–kidney *yang* insufficiency: Ascites, with symptoms of *yang* deficiency, such as cold aversion, lassitude, either oliguria or polyuria, with pallid or grey complexion. The tongue is pale or with speckled with purpuric spots, or cyanotic, and the pulse is deep, slow and weak.

◐ Treatment for liver cirrhosis

Liver–spleen dysfunction

The therapeutic principle is to regulate the *qi* and strengthen the spleen. The typical recipe is *xiang sha liu yun zi tang*.

Composition

Radix ginseng (*ren shen*) 10–15 g, Rhizoma atractylodis macrocephalae (*bai zhu*) 10–15 g, Sclerotium poriae cocos (*fu ling*) 15–20 g, honey-fried Radix glycyrrhizae uralensis (*zhi gan cao*) 5–10 g, Pericarpium citric reticulatae (*chen pi*) 5–10 g, Rhizoma pinelliae ternatae (*ban xia*) 5–10 g, Fructus amomi (*sha ren*) 5–10 g, Radix aucklandiae lappae (*mu xiang*) 5–10 g.

Acupuncture

The acupoints for the treatment are: *ganshu* (BL-18), *pishu* (BL-20), *qimen* (LR-14), *zhongwan* (CV-12), *zusanli* (ST-36), *fuliu* (KI-7).

Qi stagnation and blood stasis

To regulate the *qi*, mobilise the blood, and remove the blood stasis is the therapeutic aim. *Ge xia zhu yu tang* is a representative recipe.

Composition

Radix angelicae sinensis (*dang gui*) 9–10 g, Radix ligustici chuanxiong (*chuan xiong*) 6–10 g, Semen persicae (*tao ren*) 5–10 g, Cortex moutan radicis (*mu dan pi*) 6–10 g, Radix paeoniao rubrae (*chi shao*) 6–10 g, Radix linderae strychnifoliae (*wu yao*) 6–10 g, Rhizoma corydalis yanhusuo (*yan hu suo*) 5–10 g, Radix glycyrrhizae uralensis (*gan cao*) 5–10 g, Rhizoma cyperi rotundi (*xiang fu*) 3–6 g, Flos cartharmi tinctorii (*hong hua*) 6–9 g, Fructus citri seu ponciri (*zhi ke*) 5–10 g.

Acupuncture

The acupuncture treatment can be applied selecting the following points: *ganshu* (BL-18), *pishu* (BL-20), *weishu* (BL-21), *xingjian* (LR-2), *taichong* (LR-3).

Spleen–kidney *yang* insufficiency

The therapeutic principle is to warm the spleen and the kidney, and invigorate *yang*. *Ji sheng shen qi wan* is a representative recipe.

Composition

Radix rehmanniae glutinosae conquitae (*sheng di huang*) 10–12 g, Fructus corni officinalis (*shan zhu yu*) 5–10 g, Radix dioscoreae oppositae (*shan yao*) 20–25 g, Rhizoma alismatis orientalis (*ze xie*) 5–10 g, Sclerotium poriae cocos (*fu ling*) 20–30 g, Cortex moutan radicis (*mu dan pi*) 5–10 g, Cortex cinnamomi loureiroi (*guan gui*) 3–5 g, Radix lateralis aconiti carmichaeli praeparata (*fu zi*) 5–10 g, Radix cyathulae officinalis (*chuan niu xi*) 5–10 g, Semen plantaginis (*che qian zi*) 10–15 g.

Acupuncture

The typical acupuncture treatment formula is: *guanyuan* (CV-4), *shenque* (CV-8), *qihai* (CV-6), *fuliu* (KI-7), *pishu* (BL-20), *shenshu* (BL-23), *zusanli* (ST-36).

QUICK FLICK 45

Summary

Sufferers of IBS, IBD, CHB and LC are increasingly selecting CAM.[9–14]

The extent of the usefulness of CAM treatments for these patients is far from conclusive from an evidence-based medicine perspective. Systematic reviews have indicated that the results from TCM for these diseases are not satisfactory.[15–22]

The major reason for this is due to the quality of the trials. Most studies have recommended further large-scale trials with rigorous methodology be held. These studies still provide useful evidence, however. For example, *tong xie yao fang* was found to be effective in treating IBS, *xiaochaihu tang* appears to be effective in improving liver function and clearance of serum hepatitis B viral markers, and *fuzheng huayu* capsules are useful for anti-fibrosis of the liver, among other findings. These results suggest that further study of TCM in the treatment of these diseases is warranted.[17, 19, 22]

References

1. Liu Yanchi. The essential book of traditional Chinese medicine. Vol. 1. Theory [Fang Tingyu, Chen Laidi, trans]. New York: Columbia University Press; 1988.

2. Liu Yanchi. The essential book of traditional Chinese medicine. Vol. 2. Clinical practice [Fang Tingyu, Chen Laidi, trans]. New York: Columbia University Press; 1988.

3. Xu Yibing, Xu Wu, Wei Qin, editors. An illustrated guide to Chinese medicine. Beijing: People's Medical Publishing House; 2007.

4. Wu J, Shan SW, Pena AS, Retrospective analysis of 115 cases IBD patients treated and etiopathology by TCM view. *Practical Clin J Integrated Tradit Chin West Med*. 2004; 4(1):4–6.

5. Mullin GE, Pickett-Blakely O, Clarke JO. Integrative medicine in gastrointestinal disease: evaluating the evidence. *Expert Rev Gastroenterol Hepatol*. 2008; 2(2):261–80.

6. Hussain Z, Quigley EM. Systematic review: complementary and alternative medicine in the irritable bowel syndrome. *Aliment Pharmacol Ther*. 2006; 23(4):465–71.

7. Tillisch K. Complementary and alternative medicine for gastrointestinal disorders. *Clin Med*. 2007; 7(3):224–7.

8. Langmead L, Rampton DS. Review article: complementary and alternative therapies for inflammatory bowel disease. *Aliment Pharmacol Ther*. 2006; 23(3):341–9.

9. Seeff LB, Lindsay KL, Bacon BR, Kresina TF, Hoofnagle JH. Complementary and alternative medicine in chronic liver disease. *Hepatology*. 2001; 34(3):595–603.

10. Verma S, Thuluvath PJ. Complementary and alternative medicine in hepatology: review of the evidence of efficacy. *Clin Gastroenterol Hepatol*. 2007; 5(4):408–16.

11. Tillisch K. Complementary and alternative medicine for gastrointestinal disorders. *Clin Med*. 2007; 7(3):224–7.

12. Langmead L, Rampton DS. Review article: complementary and alternative therapies for inflammatory bowel disease. *Aliment Pharmacol Ther*. 2006; 23(3): 341–9.

13. Seeff LB, Lindsay KL, Bacon BR, Kresina TF, Hoofnagle JH. Complementary and alternative medicine in chronic liver disease. *Hepatology*. 2001; 34(3):595–603.

14. Verma S, Thuluvath PJ. Complementary and alternative medicine in hepatology: review of the evidence of efficacy. *Clin Gastroenterol Hepatol*. 2007; 5(4):408–16.

15. Liu JP, Yang M, Liu YX, Wei ML, Grimsgaard S. Herbal medicines for treatment of irritable bowel syndrome. *Cochrane Database Syst Rev*. 2009.

16. Lim B, Manheimer E, Lao LX, Ziea E, Wisniewski J, Liu JP, Berman BM. *Cochrane Database Syst Rev*. 2009.

17. Bian ZX, Wu TX, Liu L, Miao JX, Wong HY, Song L, Sung JJ. Effectiveness of the Chinese herbal formula tong xie yao fang for irritable bowel syndrome: a systematic review. *J Altern Complement Med*. 2006; 12(4):401–7.

18. Hanai H, Sugimoto K. Curcumin has bright prospects for the treatment of inflammatory bowel disease. *Curr Pharm Des*. 2009; 15(18):2087–94.

19. Qin XK, Li P, Han M, Liu JP. Xiaochaihu tang for treatment of chronic hepatitis B: a systematic review of randomised trials. *Zhong Xi Yi Jie He Xue Bao*. 2010; 8(4):312–20.

20. Zhang L, Wang G, Hou W, Li P, Dulin A, Bonkovsky HL. Contemporary clinical research of traditional Chinese medicines for chronic hepatitis B in China: an analytical review. *Hepatology*. 2010; 51(2):690–8.

21. Wang SL, Yao NL, Lu WL. Advances in studies on effect superiorities of traditional Chinese medicine on chronic hepatitis B. *Zhongguo Zhong Yao Za Zhi*. 2007; 32(23):2468–70.

22. Zhao CQ, Wu YQ, Xu LM. Curative effects of Fuzheng Huayu capsules on hepatic fibrosis and the functional mechanisms: a review. *Zhong Xi Yi Jie He Xue Bao*. 2006; 4(5):467–72.

QUICK FLICK 45

Ayurveda has the domains of yoga, spiritual practices and meditation as essential components of a healthy, humane and meaningful life. Yogic practice is not restricted to *asanas* (postures leading to physical benefits) but includes the *yama-niyamas*, which cover mental and moral hygiene as well as adaptive strategies to social and emotional stress; as we know, psychosomatic factors have an impact on gastrointestinal health.

◐ *Maha srotas* and *purishvaha srotas*: the GI tract

The gastrointestinal system in Ayurveda is described as the *maha srota,* extending from the mouth to the ileocaecal junction, together with the *purishavaha srotas*, which comprise the colon and rectum. The *yakrut* and *pleeha*—liver and spleen—are often considered together.

Agni is central to health and longevity. The concept of *agni* is complex and pervasive at all levels of biological organisation, from digestion in the GI tract to cellular metabolism. A lifestyle that protects and enhances *agni* is strongly recommended for daily and seasonal regimens (*dinacharya* and *ritucharya*) which are suitable for the constitution (*prakruti*), age (*vaya*), climate (*ritu*), and exercise (*vyayama*).

The *maha srotas* is considered not merely as a site of digestion, absorption and elimination, but is also central for immunity, cognitive–memory function, endocrine balance in metabolism, and longevity. The quality of *rasa-dhatu* generated in the GI tract is the basis of these benefits, which interestingly are enhanced by substances and regimens called *rasayanas* (systems of rejuvenation). The significant role of the GI tract is evident in the *shodhan kriyas*, the cleansing tehniques that are major interventional procedures in Ayurveda: *Vamana* (emesis), *virechana* (purgation) and *basti* (enema) used for the elimination of vitiated *kapha, pitta* and *vata* respectively. *Panchakarma* (the *shodhana* concerned with the GI tract) constitutes an elaborate process for reinstating lasting harmony and health, especially for chronic diseases.

The liver and spleen are dealt with in a complementary functional mode. Periodic purification of the liver and spleen is advised, and specific drugs and formulations also used. Currently in India, people often prefer Ayurvedic treatment for conditions like hepatitis A, non-alcoholic fatty liver disease and tropical splenomegaly.

◐ Mainstream and complementary role

Ayurveda plays a mainstream role for healthcare in India. However, elsewhere in the world it is considered to be a part of complementary and alternative medicine, as it is not recognised as an official system of medicine. It is often grouped, unfortunately, with herbal medicine. Another reason for this is the inadequate number of qualified and experienced *vaidyas* (TIM practitioners) available outside India. It is therefore imperative that physicians who are using Ayurveda as a complementary mode of therapy be careful to obtain an opinion from an expert *vaidya*. The cautions and precautions, and possibility of drug interactions, must also be observed.

◎ Evidence-based translational research

There are several peer-reviewed journals and recently published books. As modes of evidence (*pramanas*) are different in Ayurveda from those in Western medicine, experiential safety documentation is essential in order to choose safe medications for selected diseases. The publications listed for recommended reading at the end of this chapter provide clinically useful guidance.

◎ Selected diseases

Non-ulcer dyspepsia: *ajeerna*

- Derangement of *Agni*
- Alimentation: rhythm and regulation
- Hingvashtaka Churna, Trikatu, *Carica papaya*

Acid peptic disease: *amlapitta*

- Diet in pathogenesis and reversal
- *Glycyrrhiza glabra, Phyllanthus emblica, Musa sapientum* var. *paradiasiaca, Cocos nucifera,* Shankh Bhasma

Constipation: *malavarodha*

- *Apana vayu* and habits
- *Terminalia chebula*, Triphala, Swadishta Virechana Churna

Diarrhoea: *atisara*

- *Kitanu-vishas* and *apathya*
- Medicated soups (*yushas*) and gruels *(vilepi)*
- *Zingiber officinalis, Berberis aristata, Punica granatum*

Irritable bowel syndrome: *aniyata pakwashaya gati*

- Gut–brain relationships
- Colonic flora and prebiotics
- *Aegle marmelos, Holarrhena anti-dysenterica, Cyperus rotundus, Bacopa monnieri*

Viral hepatitis: *Kamala*

- Types and stages of jaundice
- Nutriments and dietary discretion
- *Picrorhiza kurroa, Tinospora cordifolia,* Trikatu, *Phyllanthes amarus.*

○ Non-ulcer dyspepsia: *ajeerna* (see Table 46.1)

Derangement of *agni*

Agni represents the universe of metabolic and enzymatic sets and subsets involved in energy transduction, synthetic and degradative processes, and the regulation of temperature and appetite. *Agni* is central to the maintenance of health and its derangement is a major contributor to diseases. The branch of Ayurveda named *Kaya Chikitsa,* literally means 'therapeutics modulating *agni*'.

Agni is classified into thirteen types on the basis of sites and functions. *Jatharagni,* the governing *agni,* is located in the *maha strotas* (GI tract) which has a far-reaching effect on tissue and cellular metabolism. Disorders of *jatharagni* cause indigestion (*ajeerna*). These can eventually evolve into GI and systemic diseases. *Agni* is vitiated by improper dietary regimens, choice of nutriments, psychodynamic factors, improper bowel habits, physical inactivity and similar. The derangement leads to residual undigested products collectively (*aama*), inducing channel blockage, inflammation and vitiation of *doshas* and *dhatus.*

The central goal is to reduce and eliminate *aama* by both non-drug and drug modalities. An understanding of this therapeutic approach leads to practical benefits in several GI and systemic diseases.

Alimentation: rhythm and regulation

Quantity of food

The *Charaka Samhita* (c. 300 BCE) says, 'Just as excessive or inadequate fuel can burn out a fire, so is the *Agni* influenced by an excessive indulgence or an inadequate intake of food.' It advises that meals be taken in a quantity such that solid foods fill half of the stomach, fluids fill a quarter while the remaining quarter is left empty. Such pragmatic advice has been quite neglected with the widespread availability of food and indulgence in tasty, fast foods. A balanced calorie-restricted diet assures the protection and enhancement of *agni*. A balanced *agni* not only promotes health and prevents diseases, but is also vital for longevity. The anti-ageing effects of such a diet have been conclusively shown in animal studies.

Rhythm and regulation

The discussion of *aahar vidhi,* or the process of alimentation, contains an elaborate description for health promotion. Among the errors to be avoided are eating too quickly or too slowly, without being attentive and savouring the food. Before eating, thanking God and reciting a Sanskrit prayer is still a living custom in India. The *Sushruta Samhita* (*c.* 800 BCE) mentions that after food, one must sit still for a few minutes, then walk a hundred steps and lie in *vamakukshi* (on the left side). This reduces gastric emptying and enhances acid–peptic digestion.

Food should be taken only when one is truly hungry. Eating before the previous meal is digested (*adhyasahana*) contributes to *ajeerna*. The sequence of foods has been specified according to taste and variations are made depending on *prakruti*, season, and age. *Vishamashana,* or eating too little or too much food, too early or too late, also precipitates *ajeerna*. Eating warm foods that are lubricated, not very heavy, not stale, and with the appropriate use of spices such as ginger, pepper and turmeric ensures that *ajeerna* does not set in.

Interventions

Table 46.1 Interventions for *ajeerna*

Drug/diet	Dose	Actions	Precautions
Trikatu*	0.5–1 g after meals	Digestive, carminative, prokinetic, bio-enhancer	Avoid if concomitant hyperacidity exists
Hingvashtaka Churna†	0.5–1 g with meals	Anti-flatulent, reduces abdominal pain	Avoid if sensitive
Carica papaya (fruit)	After meals	Promotes digestion	Avoid in pregnancy

Notes:
* Trikatu contains equal quantities of dried powders of the rhizome of *Zingiber officinale,* and the fruits of *Piper nigrum* and *Piper longum.*
† Hingvashtaka Churna contains eight parts of the resin of *Ferula asafoetida* and one part each of rock salt, fruits of *Piper nigrum, Piper longum,* rhizome of *Zingiber officinale,* seeds of *Syzygium cumini* and *Apium graveolens.*

▶ Acid–peptic disease: *amlapitta* (see Table 46.2)

Dietary habits in pathogenesis and reversal

Foods with salty, sour and pungent tastes when consumed excessively are pathogenic for hyperacidity. For example, a salt-free diet reduces the gastric acid response to histamine in patients with peptic ulcers. It has recently been shown that increased sodium chloride fosters the expression of virulent genes vacA and cagA in *Helicobacter pylori*. *Ajeerna*, if not properly managed, can also lead to *amlapitta*. Avoidance of acid-inducing foods and withdrawal of salt have a significant complementary role in the reversal of acid–peptic disease.

Interventions

Table 46.2 Interventions for *amlapitta*

Drug/diet	Dose	Actions	Precautions
Glycyrrhiza glabra (root powder)	1–3 g a.c.	Mucosal protection	Avoid if hypertension
Phyllanthus emblica (fruit powder)	2–5 g a.c.	Reduces and neutralises acid	Nil
Musa sapientum var. *paradiasiaca* (banana powder)	5–10 g BD	Improves mucosal defence, prevents ulcers	Nil
Cocos nucifera (candy)	5–10 g BD	Coats mucosa and prevents damage	Nil
Shankh Bhasma (calcined conch shell)	250–500 mg	Used specially for excess *pitta* gastric conditions, anti-dyspeptic, gastric-cytoprotective	Nil

◗ Constipation: *malavarodha* (see Table 46.3)

Apana vayu and habits

Vayu, the *dosha* associated mainly with movement, plays the most significant role in health and disease. Its subset, *apana vayu*, is involved in defecation and micturition reflexes. The interplay of the sympathetic and parasympathetic outflows to the nerve plexuses is supposed to result in an orderly and timely peristaltic movement. *Apana vayu* constitutes the functional control system of the tone, rhythm and frequency of such movements. Any derangement of *apana vayu* leads to GI motility disorders.

Good, early and non-obsessive toilet training, a certain posture and the cultural habit of evacuation every morning are some of the reasons why constipation was not a major problem in the past. With the advent of a sedentary lifestyle, refined foods, diapers hampering early toilet training and social inhibitions of natural urges, constipation has become quite prevalent.

Traditional Asian diets are generally rich in fibre and provide the necessary bulk for stools. Fluid intake is advised when thirsty and when needed. Fats like ghee enhance *snigdhata* (lubrication) and *agni*. This improves digestion and facilitates bowel motility. Traditional Ayurvedic practitioners emphasise lifestyle changes and do not rely heavily on the long-term use of laxatives.

Interventions

Table 46.3 Interventions for constipation

Drug	Dose	Actions	Precautions
Terminalia chebula (dried fruit)	1–2 g at bedtime	Prokinetic *rasayana*	Titrate dose according to stool consistency/frequency
Triphala*	2–3 g at bedtime	*Doshic* balance, *rasayana*	Take with warm water and ghee if excessive *vata*
Swadishta Virechan Churna†	3–5 g	Laxative	Do not take on a long-term basis

* Triphala: fruits of *Terminalia chebula*, *Phyllantus emblica* and *Terminalia bellerica*.
† Swadishta Virechan Churna: contains *Cassia angustifolia*, *Foeniculum vulgare* and *mishri*.

◑ Diarrhoea: (*Atisara*) (see Table 46.4)

Kitanu-vishas and *apathya*

Food and water hygiene were heavily ritualised in Ayurveda. The concept of infections and causative micro-organisms has existed for a long time, with mention of organisms, invisible to the eyes, spreading through impure food, fluids and fomites. There is a description of cholera (*visuchika*) caused by an invisible, curved, needle-like organism hiding in nails, palm folds and dirty clothes. It was also emphasised that diarrhoea often resulted from the ingestion of impure water and foods (*apathya anna*). Susceptibility to diarrhoea is based on the derangement of *agni*.

Medicated soups (*yushas*) and gruels (*vilepi*)

A drastic reduction in the frequency of bowel movement was not advised in mild to moderate cases. Diarrhoea is a response for eliminating the noxious extrinsic and intrinsic factors (*aama*). With premature control before the elimination of *aama*, one may encounter more flatulence, aggravation of fever and systemic toxic effects. Oral supplementation with *pachaka pramathyas* is used—digestive formulations with herbs such as dried fruits of *Piper longum*, and dried rhizome of *Zingiber officinalis*.

Medicated soups with easily digestible lentils like *Vigna radiata* address the calorie, fluid and electrolyte requirements. *Laja mand*, a liquid diet prepared from puffed rice, is particularly given for diarrhoea. As the diarrhoea recedes and *agni* improves, semi-solid gruels can be given incrementally.

Interventions

Table 46.4 Interventions for diarrhoea

Drug	Dose	Actions	Precautions
Zingiber officinalis (dry rhizome powder)	1–2 g TDS/QDS	Astringent, anti-microbial, anti-motility	Gastric sensitivity to ginger. Careful titration
Berberis aristata (dry rhizome powder)	0.5–1 g TDS	Anti-bacterial, anti-cholinergic, anti-secretory	Not to be used in pregnancy
Punica granatum (rind of the fruit)	2–5 g TDS	Astringent, anti-microbial, anti-motility	Nil

◯ Irritable bowel syndrome: *aniyata pakwashaya gati* (see Table 46.5)

Gut–brain relationships

Irritable bowel syndrome (IBS) is a clinically complex conglomeration of symptoms and signs, with varying manifestations of colonic motility influenced by psychosomatic factors. As a consequence, IBS has been correlated closely with *grahani roga* (chronic diarrhoea) by several *vaidyas* and investigators. Reversing somatopsychic mechanisms in *grahani* is an effective therapeutic approach. Current knowledge of the enteric nervous system needs to be explored *vis-à-vis* the Ayurvedic concept of gut health and its influence on the central nervous system.

Colonic flora and prebiotics

The human symbiont of one hundred trillion cells has only ten trillion human eukaryotes. Colonic microflora constitutes a major fraction of the rest of the ninety trillion prokaryotes. It has been calculated that one gram of faeces contains around 10^{14} microbes. In Ayurveda, for health and disease, colonic functions and flora play a central role. Noxious influences on the microflora lead to *vata prakopa* (an imbalance in *vata*) and vitiation of *pitta* and *kapha*. As a consequence, dietary milk and milk products which help to retain healthy colonic flora are encouraged. The prebiotic and probiotic approaches, currently popular in nutraceuticals, can be traced back to this concept.

Medicated retentive and eliminative enemas (*bastis*) are used in IBS. The main ingredients are *takra* (Indian buttermilk), *Bombax malabaricum*, *Cyperus rotundus*, *Holarrhena anti-dysenterica* and *Randia spinosa*. Other ingredients added in small quantities to several types of *bastis* include Trikatu, rock salt, sesame oil and *Foeniculum vulgare*, among others.

Interventions

Table 46.5 Interventions for irritable bowel syndrome

Drug	Dose	Actions	Precautions
Aegle marmelos (immature fruit)	3–5 g BD	Anti-microbial, demulcent	Safe
Holarrhena anti-dysenterica (seed powder)	1–3 g BD	Anti-motility, anti-dysentery, digestive	Neurotoxicity of connesine reported
Cyperus rotundus (dried root)	1–3 g TDS	Anti-microbial, astringent, anti-motility	Local skin irritation
Bacopa monnieri (leaves)	2–3 g BD	Anxiolytic, anti-microbial, astringent	Sedative effect

◖ Viral hepatitis: *kamala*

Types and stages of jaundice

Viral hepatitis has been well studied in modern medicine. In Ayurveda, jaundice has been studied as a syndrome and characterised as several types of *kamala*. In the recent past, several studies have been conducted with Ayurvedic interventions in viral hepatitis and hepatitis B carriers. The therapeutic approach in viral hepatitis is based on the Ayurvedic stage-specific drug and non-drug modalities. In the early stage of hepatitis, when cell necrosis is a dominant feature, cytoprotective and antioxidant plants/formulations are advocated. When cholestatic changes emerge, plants and formulations having hydrocholeretic activity are preferred. During the sub-acute or early chronic stage characterised by fibroblast proliferation and lobular destruction, measures which prevent or regress fibrosis are indicated.

Nutriments and dietary discretion

In hepatitis, diet and specific items/spices are considered, not only for management of the disease, but are also regarded as relevant to the prevention of hepatitis and promotion of healthy liver structure and function. High fat intake is not advocated, but specific formulations in *ghritas* (medicated oils), such as Phalatrikadi, are central in management of the early stages of jaundice. Diets with items which are *guru* (heavy to digest) and *snigdha* (unctuous) are to be limited in quantity. For ready energy, sugar cane juices, black raisins and glucose are used.

Interventions

Table 46.6 Interventions for viral hepatitis

Drug	Dose	Actions	Precautions
Picrorhiza kurroa (rhizome)	0.75–1 g TDS	Hydrocholeretic, anti-inflammatory, prevent fatty infiltration	Care in patients with low cardio-respiratory reserve
Tinospora cordifolia (stem)	1–2 g TDS	Anti-inflammatory, hepato-protective, immunomodulatory, adaptogen	Safe
Trikatu	1–2 g TDS	Anti-cholestatic, appetite enhancer, *rasayana* (rejuvenation)	Gastric sensitivity to spices

◐ Cautions

The remedies and measures described above, though generally safe, need to be used in a complementary consultation with a physician trained in Ayurveda. Self-medication is generally not advisable unless approved by a primary physician.

Summary

Ayurveda, the traditional Indian medicine (TIM) has been practised for more than 5000 years in India. It is based on the principles of *doshas*, *dhatus* and *malas*. Scientific research in Ayurveda has been significantly enhanced in the past three decades. Diseases of the digestive tract that are treated include non-ulcer dyspepsia, acid–peptic disease, constipation, diarrhoea, IBS and viral hepatitis.

Ayurveda has an integrative approach to health and disease which combines diet, lifestyle and interventions.

Information for patients

Who should I see to get involved in Ayurvedic medicine?

Your physician should be informed and involved. It is important that you or your physician consult with a qualified Ayurvedic practitioner.

Is there anything I should be aware of regarding traditional medicines?

Always check the source of safe, effective and quality medicines. Care must be taken regarding dosage frequency and duration of drug use.

Do traditional drugs have side effects?

There can be side effects and interactions between different drugs. Even with good advice, you should leave about 60 minutes between inter-system medicines.

Could I just start a course of treatment on my own?

No. Self-medication is not advisable.

Recommended reading

Dahanukar SA, Thatte UM. Ayurveda revisited. Mumbai: Popular Prakashan; 2000.

Dwarkanath C. Digestion and metabolism in Ayurveda. Calcutta: Baidyanath; 1967.

Gogte VM. Ayurvedic pharmacology and therapeutic uses of medicinal plants (Dravyagunavignyan). Mumbai: Bhavan's SPARC; 2000.

Lele RD. Ayurveda and modern medicine. 2nd ed. Mumbai: Bhartiya Vidya Bhavan; 2002.

Mishra LC, editor. Scientific basis of Ayurvedic therapeutics. Boca Raton, Florida: CRC Press; 2004.

Nagral KS. Ayurveda for modern medical practitioners. Delhi: Chaukhamba; 2008.

Patwardhan B, Mashelkar RA. Traditional medicine-inspired approaches to drug discovery: can Ayurveda show the way forward? *Drug Discov Today*. 2009; 14(15–16):804–11.

Vaidya ADB. Reverse pharmacological correlates of Ayurvedic drug actions. *Ind J Pharmacol*. 2006; 38:311–5.

Valiathan MS. The legacy of Caraka. Chennai: Orient Blackswan; 2003.

QUICK FLICK 46

Index